THERAPEUTIC HYPOTHERMIA

MOLECULAR AND CELLULAR BIOLOGY OF CRITICAL CARE MEDICINE
Robert S. B. Clark and Joseph A. Carcillo, Series Editors

THERAPEUTIC HYPOTHERMIA

edited by

Samuel A. Tisherman, MD
University of Pittsburgh, PA, USA

and

Fritz Sterz, MD
Medical University of Vienna, Vienna, Austria

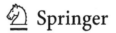 Springer

Samuel A. Tisherman, MD
Department of Critical Care
University of Pittsburgh
Pittsburgh, PA 15213
USA

Fritz Sterz, MD
Emergency Medicine
Medical University of Vienna
1090 Vienna
Austria

Series Editors
Robert S. B. Clark, MD
Pediatric Critical Care Medicine
Children's Hospital of Pittsburgh
Pittsburgh, PA 15213
USA

Joseph A. Carcillo, MD
Pediatric Intensive Unit
Children's Hospital of Pittsburgh
Pittsburgh, PA 15213
USA

Library of Congress Cataloging-in-Publication Data

Therapeutic hypothermia / edited by Samuel A. Tisherman and Fritz Sterz.
　　p. ; cm. – (Molecular and cellular biology of critical care medicine ; 4)
　　Includes bibliographical references and index.
　　ISBN-13: 978-0-387-25402-9 (alk. paper)
　　ISBN-10: 0-387-25402-1 (alk. paper)
　　　1.Cold—Therapeutic use. I. Tisherman, Samuel A. II. Sterz, Fritz. III. Series.
　　　[DNLM: 1. Hypothermia, Induced. 2. Ischemia—therapy. 3. Resuscitation—methods.
　　WO 350 T398 2005]
　　RM863.T48 2005
　　616.9'89—dc22
2005046418

ISBN-10: 0-387-25402-1　　e-ISBN-10: 0-387-25403-X　　Printed on acid-free paper.
ISBN-13: 978-0387-25402-9　　e-ISBN-13: 978-0387-25403-6

Printed in the United States of America.

9 8 7 6 5 4 3 2 1　　　　SPIN 11052159

springeronline.com

Dedication

*This book is dedicated to our
wives and children, who tolerate
our long hours and dedication
to our patients and our
research. We are also indebted
to Peter Safar who inspired so
many of us to care for the
critically ill and to pursue
research in resuscitation.*

Contents

Contributors

Wilhelm Behringer, MD
Associate Professor
Department of Emergency Medicine
Medical University of Vienna
Vienna, Austria

Laura Bennet, PhD
Senior Research Fellow
Department of Physiology
University of Auckland
Auckland, New Zealand

Stephen Bernard, MD
Intensive Care Unit
Dandenong Hospital
Dandenong, Victoria, Australia

Clifford W. Callaway, MD
Associate Professor
Department of Emergency Medicine
Associate Director, Safar Center for
* Resuscitation Research*
University of Pittsburgh
Pittsburgh, PA, USA

Robert S.B. Clark, MD
Associate Professor
Departments of Critical Care Medicine
* and Pediatrics*
Associate Director, Safar Center for
* Resuscitation Research*
University of Pittsburgh
Pittsburgh, PA, USA

W. Dalton Dietrich, III, PhD
Kinetic Concepts Distinguished Chair in
* Neurosurgery*
Professor of Neurological Surgery,
* Neurology, and Cell Biology and*
* Anatomy*
Vice Chair for Research, Neurosurgery
Scientific Director, The Miami Project to
* Cure Paralysis*
University of Miami
Miami, FL, USA

Niels Einer-Jensen, DVM
Institute of Medical Biology, Physiology,
* and Pharmacology*
University of Southern Denmark
Odense, Denmark

Elena Espinosa, MD, PhD
Department of Anesthesiology
Hospital Universitario NS de Candelaria
Santa Cruz de Tenerife, Canary Islands,
* Spain*

Larry M. Gentilello, MD
Professor of Surgery
Chairman, Division of Burns, Trauma
* and Critical Care*
University of Texas Southwestern
* Medical School*
Dallas, TX, USA

James D. Guest, MD, PhD
Assistant Professor
Department of Neurological Surgery
The Miami Project to Cure Paralysis
University of Miami
Miami, FL, USA

Alistair Jan Gunn, MBChB, PhD
Associate Professor
Department of Physiology
University of Auckland
Auckland, New Zealand

Sharon Hale, BS
Senior Scientist

Heart Institute
Good Samaritan Hospital
University of Southern California
Los Angeles, CA, USA

Hyung Soo Han, MD, PhD
Assistant Professor
Department of Physiology
Kyungpook National University School of
  Medicine
Daegu, Korea

Robert W. Hickey, MD
Associate Professor
Department of Pediatrics
Division of Pediatric Emergency
  Medicine
University of Pittsburgh
Pittsburgh, PA, USA

Michael Holzer, MD
Department of Emergency Medicine
Medical University of Vienna
Vienna, Austria

Takeshi Ishii, MD
Clinical Lecturer and Vice-director of
  Surgical High Care Unit
Department of Emergency and Critical
  Care Medicine
University of Tokyo
Tokyo, Japan

Rajiv Jalan, MD
Senior Lecturer in Hepatology
Institute of Hepatology
University College London Medical
  School and Hospital
London, UK

Larry W. Jenkins, PhD
Associate Professor

Departments of Neurological Surgery
  and Neurology
Associate Director, Safar Center for
  Resuscitation Research
University of Pittsburgh
Pittsburgh, PA, USA

Lars Peter Kammersgaard, MD
Staff Physician
Department of Neurology
Gentofte University
Hellerup, Denmark

Shoichi Katada, MD
Clinical Lecturer and Vice-director of
  Emergency Service
Department of Emergency and Critical
  Care Medicine
University of Tokyo
Tokyo, Japan

Robert A. Kloner, MD, PhD
Director of Research
Heart Institute
Good Samaritan Hospital
Professor of Medicine
University of Southern California
Los Angeles, CA, USA

Patrick M. Kochanek, MD
Professor
Departments of Critical Care Medicine
  and Pediatrics
Director, Safar Center for Resuscitation
  Research
University of Pittsburgh
Pittsburgh, PA, USA

Derk W. Krieger, MD, PhD
Staff Physician
Department of Neurology
Section of Stroke and Neurological
  Critical Care

The Cleveland Clinic Foundation
Cleveland, OH, USA

Gernot Kuhnen, PhD
Head, Büro für Thermophysiologie
Pohlheim, Germany

Donald W. Marion, MD, MSc
Senior Research Fellow
The Brain Trauma Foundation
New York, NY, USA

Susumu Nakajima, MD
Associate Professor
Vice-director of Emergency Service
Department of Emergency and Critical
　Care Medicine
University of Tokyo
Tokyo, Japan

Ram Nirula, MD, MPH
Assistant Professor
Department of Surgery
Division of Trauma/Critical Care
Medical College of Wisconsin
Milwaukee, WI, USA

Toshihiko Obayashi, MD
Associate and Vice-director of Intensive
　Care Unit
Department of Emergency and Critical
　Care Medicine
University of Tokyo
Tokyo, Japan

Christopher Rose, PhD
Postdoctoral fellow
Fundacion Valenciana de Investigaciones
　Biomedicas
Valencia, Spain

Stefan Schwab, MD, PhD
Vice Chairman

Neurologische Klinik
University of Heidelberg
Heidelberg, Germany

Fritz Sterz, MD
Professor
Department of Emergency Medicine
Medical University of Vienna
Vienna, Austria

Samuel A. Tisherman, MD
Associate Professor
Departments of Surgery and Critical
　Care Medicine
Associate Director, Safar Center for
　Resuscitation Research
University of Pittsburgh
Pittsburgh, PA, USA

Jesús Villar, MD, PhD
Director, Research Institute
Hospital Universitario NS de Candelaria
Santa Cruz de Tenerife, Canary Islands,
　Spain
Adjunct Scientist
Research Center
St. Michael's Hospital
Toronto, ON, Canada.
Associate Scientist
Centro de Investigaciones Biológicas,
　Consejo Superior de Investigaciones
　Científicas
Madrid, Spain

Naoki Yahagi, MD, MSc
Professor and Chairman
Department of Emergency and Critical
　Care Medicine
University of Tokyo
Tokyo, Japan

Midori A. Yenari, MD
Associate Professor

University of California, San Francisco
San Francisco Veterans Affairs Medical
  Center
San Francisco, CA, USA

PREFACE

Samuel A. Tisherman, MD[1], Fritz Sterz, MD[2]
[1]University of Pittsburgh, Pittsburgh, PA, USA
[2]Medical University of Vienna, Vienna, Austria

The use of hypothermia for a variety of therapeutic purposes has a long and erratic history. Hippocrates recommended the use of topical cooling to stop bleeding. Fay used cooling of the extremities for patients with tumors in the 1930s. It wasn't until the 1950s, when the effects of hypothermia on systemic oxygen metabolism became better defined, that systemic hypothermia became a commonly used modality, particularly for cardiac surgery. Hypothermia was used for *protection* (treatment before the insult) and *preservation* (treatment during the insult) of the heart and entire organism during planned operative ischemia. Shortly thereafter, attempts were made to use hypothermia for *resuscitation* (treatment after the insult) from cardiac arrest and for management of head trauma. At that time, it was felt that moderate hypothermia (28-32°C) was needed. This was difficult to achieve and manage. Multiple complications were noted. Consequently, therapeutic, resuscitative hypothermia lay dormant for many years while mild (32-35°C) to moderate hypothermia became common for many cardiothoracic and neurosurgical procedures.

In the early 1990s, it was found that mild hypothermia, even after cardiac arrest, had benefit for the brain. Similar results were found with head trauma. This lead to a burst of enthusiasm for research into resuscitative hypothermia for a variety of insults, most of which have tissue ischemia as a major component. These laboratory studies demonstrated significant improvement in outcome (survival, neurologic function). In addition, the mechanisms of the beneficial effects of hypothermia were explored in greater detail. It is clear that the effects are not just related to suppression of oxygen demands of tissues. Multiple deleterious chemical cascades are attenuated by hypothermia while beneficial responses are enhanced, or at least decreased to a lesser degree.

These promising laboratory studies have lead to clinical trials for cardiac arrest, head trauma, and stroke. The results for cardiac arrest are extremely encouraging, while those for head trauma are difficult to interpret. Data for stroke are too preliminary. Clinical studies of resuscitative hypothermia for other insults should not be far away.

Peter Safar deserves much of the credit for the use of hypothermia for resuscitation. Even when cardiopulmonary resuscitation was first described as the ABCs (airway, breathing, circulation), Dr. Safar added 'D' for drugs defibrillation, 'E' for EKG (defibrillation), 'F' for fluids, 'G' for gauge (determine and treat the cause of arrest), and *'H' for hypothermia*. With his fellow, Sven Erik Gisvold, he conducted one of the first controlled animal studies utilizing hypothermia as part of a multifaceted therapy after global brain ischemia. He later made the observation that relatively small differences in pre-ischemia brain temperature had significant effects on neurologic outcome. This led to work by Safar's group and others demonstrating that mild hypothermia had beneficial effects after cerebral ischemia. His encouragement led to clinical trials of resuscitative hypothermia, particularly the successful studies of mild hypothermia after cardiac arrest.

This book is designed to review the current state of knowledge regarding therapeutic hypothermia, particularly resuscitative hypothermia, including known mechanisms of action and results from laboratory studies (both mechanistic and outcome) and clinical trials. Cooling methods and potential side effects of hypothermia will be addressed. Unanswered questions and recommendations for future laboratory and clinical research will be presented. This is meant to serve both the researcher interested in therapeutic hypothermia, as well as the clinician interested in the potential use of therapeutic hypothermia in his or her patient population.

Chapter 1

GLOBAL BRAIN ISCHEMIA: ANIMAL STUDIES

Wilhelm Behringer, MD
Medical University of Vienna, Vienna, Austria

INTRODUCTION

This chapter will describe the background of therapeutic hypothermia with regard to animal models with cardiac arrest or vessel occlusion that led to the recent trials of therapeutic hypothermia after cardiac arrest in humans (1-7). In addition, future potentials of intra-ischemic hypothermia (suspended animation) are discussed.

The history of induced hypothermia began in the 1950s with elective moderate hypothermia (28-32°C) of the brain, introduced under anesthesia, for protection-preservation during brain ischemia needed for surgery on the heart or brain (8, 9) *Protective* hypothermia, induced before cardiac arrest, has to be differentiated from *preservative* hypothermia, induced during cardiac arrest, and from *resuscitative* hypothermia, induced during resuscitation after cardiac arrest. The first animal studies of *resuscitative* hypothermia after cardiac arrest were reported in the 1950s (10, 11). Already in the early 1960s, Peter Safar recommended the use of therapeutic resuscitative hypothermia for humans in his cardiopulmonary-cerebral resuscitation algorithm (12). Resuscitative hypothermia research was then given up for 25 years, because experimental and clinical trials had been complicated by the injurious systemic effects of total body cooling, such as shivering, vasospasm, increased plasma viscosity, increased hematocrit, hypocoagulation, arrhythmias (including ventricular fibrillation when temperatures dropped below 30°C), and lowered resistance to infection during prolonged moderate hypothermia (13-16). At that time, it was felt that moderate hypothermia was required for brain protection.

PROTECTIVE-PRESERVATIVE HYPOTHERMIA

It was in the mid-1980s, when therapeutic hypothermia was re-discovered. Hossmann (17) reported the beneficial effect of mild hypothermia (35-36°C), unintentionally induced before the experiment, on electroencephalogram recovery in cats subjected to one hour of global brain ischemia followed by blood recirculation for 3 h or longer. At the same time, Safar analysed the outcome data of several cardiac arrest dog studies and found that dogs that were mildly hypothermic at the beginning of the experiment had better neurologic outcome than dogs that were normothermic at the beginning of the experiment (18). These observations were followed by controlled, randomized animal studies in various laboratories. In dogs (19), ventricular fibrillation cardiac arrest of 12.5-min no-flow was accompanied by head immersion in iced water (which reduced brain temperature by only 1°C during no flow) and followed by reperfusion cooling with brief cardiopulmonary bypass to 34°C for one hour. Functional and morphologic brain outcome variables were significantly improved in the hypothermic groups four days after the insult. Busto, et al (20), found in a 20-min four-vessel occlusion rat model that small increments of intra-ischemic brain temperature (33, 34, 36, or 39°C) markedly accentuated histopathological changes following 3-day survival, despite severe depletion of brain energy metabolites during ischemia at all temperatures. Siesjö, et al (21, 22), confirmed the beneficial effects of intraischemic hypothermia in a two-vessel occlusion rat model with various durations of ischemia. Intentional lowering of brain temperature from 37 to 35°C markedly reduced, and to 33°C virtually prevented, neuronal necrosis.

Importantly, the benefit of intra-ischemic mild to moderate hypothermia on neuronal death is regarded as long lasting. Green, et al (23), found in a 12.5-min four-vessel occlusion rat model that intra-ischemic hypothermia to 30°C provided protection from behavioural deficits as well as neuronal injury up to 2 months. This long lasting effect of intra-ischemic hypothermia was confirmed by the same group in a 10-min two-vessel occlusion rat model (24), and by Corbett, et al (25), in a 5-min global ischemia gerbil model with brain temperature of 32°C.

The critical finding in these studies was that mild hypothermia (33-35°C), which is safe, could have a significant impact on the brain. Cooling to moderate hypothermia levels, which is difficult to achieve and maintain, and is associated with many extracerebral complications, may not be needed.

RESUSCITATIVE HYPOTHERMIA

The re-discovery of protective-preservative mild to moderate hypothermia in brain ischemia led to widespread research of *resuscitative* mild to moderate hypothermia in several animal models in the 1990s. Safar and colleagues conducted a systematic series of major outcome studies in dogs of prolonged normothermic cardiac arrest followed by *mild resuscitative* cerebral hypothermia (34°C), induced immediately after reperfusion and maintained for 2-3 h (26-28) or 12 h (29). In these studies, controlled ventilation was maintained for 24 h, and intensive care was provided for three to four days, with final evaluation of neurologic outcome and histologic damage in various brain regions. In one study (26), ventricular fibrillation cardiac arrest of 10 min no-flow was reversed by standard external cardiopulmonary resuscitation. Cooling to 34°C for 2 hours was with a combination of head-neck-trunk surface cooling, plus cold fluid loads administered intravenously, intragastrically, and nasopharyngeally; in one group induced at the beginning of resuscitation, in another group induced after restoration of spontaneous circulation. In both hypothermia groups, neurologic recovery in terms of functional outcome and histologic damage was improved compared to normothermic control animals. In the next study (27), ventricular fibrillation cardiac arrest of 12.5 min no-flow was reversed with brief cardiopulmonary bypass. Immediate post-arrest mild (34°C) or moderate (30°C) hypothermia improved functional and morphologic brain outcome, but deep post-arrest hypothermia (15°C) did not improve function and worsened brain histology. In the same model (28), delaying cooling (to 34°C for one hour) until 15 mins after normothermic reperfusion did not improve functional outcome, but did improve histologic damage, compared to normothermia. In the last study of this series (29), after ventricular fibrillation cardiac arrest of 11 min, reversed by brief cardiopulmonary bypass, a combination treatment of mild hypothermia induced by head-neck-surface cooling plus peritoneal instillation of cold Ringer's solution to keep brain temperature 34°C from reperfusion until 12 h, plus cerebral blood flow promotion by induced moderate hypertension until 4 h and colloid induced hemodilution until 12 h, led to the best functional outcome with least histologic damage ever achieved in dogs. Mild cooling in all dog studies caused no cardiovascular or other side effects.

At the same time, resuscitative hypothermia was studied in rodent ischemia models as well. First, Busto, et al (30), reduced hippocampal CA1 injury with 3 h of immediate, but not 30-min delayed, post-ischemic hypothermia to 30°C in a two-vessel occlusion rat model with 10 min of ischemia and survival to 3 days. Buchan, et al (31), reduced hippocampal CA1 injury with 8 h of immediate hypothermia to 34.5°C in gerbils after 5 min of ischemia and survival to 5 days. Coimbra, et al (32), reduced hippocampal CA1 injury after 5 h of immediate hypothermia to 29°C in gerbils with 5 min of ischemia and survival to 7 days. Chopp, et al (33), reduced hippocampal CA1 injury with 2 h of immediate hypothermia to 34°C in a in a two-vessel occlusion rat model after 8 min of ischemia, but not 12 min of ischemia, and survival to 7 days. Carroll, et al (34), progressively reduced hippocampal CA1 injury with immediate hypothermia to 28-32°C for 1/2, 1, 2, 4, and 6 hours in gerbils after 5 min of ischemia, and survival to 4 days; 6 h of hypothermia delayed for 1 hour after reperfusion resulted in protection as well, delayed for 3 h was not effective. In another study by Coimbra, et al (35), hippocampal CA1 injury was reduced with 5 h of hypothermia to 33°C, delayed for 2 h after reperfusion, in a two-vessel occlusion rat model after 10 min of ischemia and survival to 7 days. The same group (36) reduced hippocampal CA1 injury with 5 h of hypothermia to 33°C, delayed for 2, 6, and 12 h, but not for 24 and 36 h, after reperfusion in a two-vessel occlusion rat model after 10 min of ischemia and survival to 7 days; 3.5 h of hypothermia delayed for 2 h after reperfusion was less effective, and 30 min of hypothermia delayed for 2 h after reperfusion was ineffective in the same model.

While the benefit of intra-ischemic hypothermia on preventing neuronal death seems to be long lasting (23, 25), long lasting effects of post-ischemic hypothermia have been more controversial. Dietrich, et al (24), found hippocampal CA1 protection in a in a two-vessel occlusion rat model with 10 min of ischemia and post-arrest immediate hypothermia to 30°C for 4 h, when histologic evaluation was at 3 days after the insult. This protection significantly declined by 7 days and was completely absent by 60 days after the insult.

Colbourne, et al (37-39), conducted a series of studies in gerbils to systematically explore factors affecting neuro-protection of hypothermia. In the first study (37), two experiments were performed. In experiment 1, after 3 min of ischemia, 12 h of hypothermia (32°C), delayed for 1 h after reperfusion, attenuated the early (<10 days) ischemia-induced open-field habituation impairments and substantially reduced hippocampal CA1 necrosis when assessed at 10 and 30 days. Hypothermia was only partially effective after 5 min ischemia. In experiment 2, prolonged hypothermia (32°C) for 24 h, delayed for 1 h after reperfusion, resulted in near total preservation of CA1 neurons at 30 days even after 5 min of ischemia. In the second study, with ischemia of 5 min (38), the observation period was extended to 6 months. Hypothermia (32°C) for 24 h delayed for 1 h after reperfusion, provided substantial CA1 protection at 6 months, although there was less protection than at 1 month. Delaying hypothermia (32°C, 24 h) to 4 h after reperfusion also provided significant protection at 6 months survival, but significantly less than that found with delaying hypothermia for only 1 h. In the third study, with ischemia of 5 min (39), increasing the duration of hypothermia to 48 h resulted in long lasting protection of neurons at 1 month, even when hypothermia was delayed to 6 h after reperfusion. The long lasting effect of delayed (6 h), prolonged (48 h) hypothermia (32-34°C) on functional and histologic outcome at 1 month was confirmed in rats after 10 min of severe four-vessel occlusion ischemia (40).

The studies described above suggest that minimal delay and longer durations of hypothermia are of critical importance to extend the therapeutic window and to provide permanent protection.

SUSPENDED ANIMATION

About one half of out-of-hospital resuscitation attempts for sudden cardiac death fail to restore heartbeat. Resuscitation of these patients is often given up in the field (41). It is suspected that many of these deaths occur in patients with potential for complete cardiac and cerebral recovery if oxygen delivery could be rapidly restored. For example, initiation of cardiopulmonary bypass before loss of cerebral viability could support the heart until it recovers from stunning or it can be repaired or replaced (42, 43). Cardiopulmonary bypass is not currently available in the field. Therefore preservation of the organism is needed until cardiopulmonary bypass can be initiated in the emergency department. In 1984, Colonel Ronald Bellamy and Professor Peter Safar introduced the concept of "suspended animation for delayed resuscitation", starting with a focus on rapidly exsanguinating trauma patients. Suspended animation is hypothermic and pharmacologic "preservation of the organism during transport and surgical hemostasis, under prolonged controlled clinical death, followed by delayed resuscitation to survival without brain damage" (44).

Preservative hypothermia, induced and reversed with cardiopulmonary bypass before cardiac arrest, has been shown to preserve the organism for up to 15 min by mild hypothermia (33°-36°C) (18), for up to 20 min by moderate hypothermia (28°-32°C) (8), for up to 30 min by deep hypothermia (11°-27°C) (45, 46), and for up to 60 min by profound hypothermia (6°-10°C) (47). To rapidly preserve the brain with mild to moderate hypothermia until more prolonged preservation with profound hypothermic circulatory arrest could be induced and reversed by cardiopulmonary bypass (43, 47, 48), the use of an aortic cold saline flush, via a balloon catheter, was introduced (49-52). In a clinically realistic exsanguination cardiac arrest dog outcome model, the induction of suspended animation by use of cold (4°C) saline aortic flush within the first 5 min of CA, has shown to preserve brain viability for a cardiac arrest time of 15 min (49), 20 min (50), 30 min (51), 90 min, and, perhaps, 120 min (52).

This approach of preserving the organism with rapidly induced mild to moderate cerebral hypothermia to buy time for transport to the hospital needs to also be explored for normovolemic cardiac arrest patients who are temporarily resistant to conventional resuscitation attempts (42, 44). The clinical scenario might be (modified after [42]): After cardiac arrest, a bystander will initiate basic life support and already induce cooling by exposure; ambulance personnel arrives at the scene and begins advanced life support with hypothermic intravenous infusion with a vasoconstrictor and defibrillation attempts; if restoration of spontaneous circulation can not be achieved within 10 min, the emergency physician will further attempt cooling to achieve systemic temperatures as low as possible to preserve the brain and heart, leaving the patient in cardiac arrest for transport to the emergency department, where cardiopulmonary bypass will be initiated. This suspended animation hypothermic no-flow scenario during transport should be compared with hypothermic low-flow, i.e. continued external cardiac massage after cold aortic flush, and with normothermic low-flow, i.e. conventional external cardiac massage, in a large animal outcome study.

REFERENCES

1. Yanagawa Y, Ishihara S, Norio H, et al. Preliminary clinical outcome study of mild resuscitative hypothermia after out-of-hospital cardiopulmonary arrest. *Resuscitation* 1998; 39:61-66.
2. Zeiner A, Holzer M, Sterz F, et al. Mild resuscitative hypothermia to improve neurological outcome after cardiac arrest. A clinical feasibility trial. Hypothermia After Cardiac Arrest (HACA) Study Group. *Stroke* 2000; 31:86-94.
3. Hachimi-Idrissi S, Corne L, Ebinger G, et al. Mild hypothermia induced by a helmet device: a clinical feasibility study. *Resuscitation* 2001; 51:275-281.
4. Bernard SA, Jones BM, Horne MK. Clinical trial of induced hypothermia in comatose survivors of out-of-hospital cardiac arrest. Ann Emerg Med 1997; 30:146-153.
5. Bernard SA, Gray TW, Buist MD, et al. Treatment of comatose survivors of out-of-hospital cardiac arrest with induced hypothermia. *N Engl J Med* 2002; 346:557-563.
6. The Hypothermia after Cardiac Arrest (HACA) Study Group. Mild therapeutic hypothermia to improve the neurologic outcome after cardiac arrest. *N Engl J Med* 2002; 346:549-556.
7. Nolan JP, Morley PT, Hoek TL, Hickey RW. Therapeutic hypothermia after cardiac arrest. An advisory statement by the Advancement Life support Task Force of the International Liaison committee on Resuscitation. *Resuscitation* 2003; 57:231-235.
8. Bigelow WG, Linsay WK, Greenwood WF. Hypothermia: Its possible role in cardiac surgery. *Ann Surg* 1950; 132:849-866.
9. Rosomoff HL, Holaday A. Cerebral blood flow and cerebral oxygen consumtion during hypothermia. *Am J Physiol* 1954; 179:85-88.
10. Zimmermann JM, Spencer FC. The influence of hypothermia on cerebral injury resulting from circulatory occlusion. *Surg Forum* 1959; 9:216.
11. Wolfe KB. Effect of hypothermia on cerebral damage resulting from cardiac arrest. *Am J Cardiol* 1960; 6:809-812.
12. Safar P. Community-wide cardiopulmonary resuscitation. (The CPCR system). *J Iowa Med Soc* 1964; 54:629-635.
13. Friedman EW, Davidoff D, Fine J. Effect of hypothermia on tolerance to hemorrhagic shock. In: Dripps RD, editor. The physiology of induced hypothermia. Washington, DC: *National Academy of Science Publication*, 1956: 369-380.
14. Reuler JB. Hypothermia: pathophysiology, clinical settings, and management. *Ann Intern Med* 1978; 89:519-527.
15. Steen PA, Soule EH, Michenfelder JD. Detrimental effect of prolonged hypothermia in cats and monkeys with and without regional cerebral ischemia. *Stroke* 1979; 10:522-529.
16. Steen PA, Milde JH, Michenfelder JD. The detrimental effects of prolonged hypothermia and rewarming in the dog. Anesthesiology 1980; 52:224-230.
17. Hossmann KA. Resuscitation potentials after prolonged global cerebral ischemia in cats. *Crit Care Med* 1988; 16:964-971.
18. Safar P. Resuscitation from clinical death: pathophysiologic limits and therapeutic potentials. *Crit Care Med* 1988; 16:923-941.
19. Leonov Y, Sterz F, Safar P, et al. Mild cerebral hypothermia during and after cardiac arrest improves neurologic outcome in dogs. *J Cereb Blood Flow Metab* 1990; 10:57-70.
20. Busto R, Dietrich WD, Globus MY, et al. Small differences in intraischemic brain temperature critically determine the extent of ischemic neuronal injury. *J Cereb Blood Flow Metab* 1987; 7:729-738.

21. Minamisawa H, Smith ML, Siesjo BK. The effect of mild hyperthermia and hypothermia on brain damage following 5, 10, and 15 minutes of forebrain ischemia. *Ann Neurol* 1990; 28:26-33.

22. Minamisawa H, Nordstrom CH, Smith ML, Siesjo BK. The influence of mild body and brain hypothermia on ischemic brain damage. *J Cereb Blood Flow Metab* 1990; 10:365-374.

23. Green EJ, Dietrich WD, van Dijk F, et al. Protective effects of brain hypothermia on behavior and histopathology following global cerebral ischemia in rats. *Brain Res* 1992; 580:197-204.

24. Dietrich WD, Busto R, Alonso O, Globus MY, et al. Intraischemic but not postischemic brain hypothermia protects chronically following global forebrain ischemia in rats. *J Cereb Blood Flow Metab* 1993; 13:541-549.

25. Corbett D, Nurse S, Colbourne F. Hypothermic neuroprotection. A global ischemia study using 18- to 20-month-old gerbils. Stroke 1997; 28:2238-2242.

26. Sterz F, Safar P, Tisherman S, et al. Mild hypothermic cardiopulmonary resuscitation improves outcome after prolonged cardiac arrest in dogs. *Crit Care Med* 1991; 19:379-389.

27. Weinrauch V, Safar P, Tisherman S, et al. Beneficial effect of mild hypothermia and detrimental effect of deep hypothermia after cardiac arrest in dogs. *Stroke* 1992; 23:1454-1462.

28. Kuboyama K, Safar P, Radovsky A, et al. Delay in cooling negates the beneficial effect of mild resuscitative cerebral hypothermia after cardiac arrest in dogs: a prospective, randomized study. *Crit Care Med* 1993; 21:1348-1358.

29. Safar P, Xiao F, Radovsky A, et al. Improved cerebral resuscitation from cardiac arrest in dogs with mild hypothermia plus blood flow promotion. *Stroke* 1996; 27:105-113.

30. Busto R, Dietrich WD, Globus MY, Ginsberg MD. Postischemic moderate hypothermia inhibits CA1 hippocampal ischemic neuronal injury. Neuroscie Let 1989; 101:299-304.

31. Buchan A, Pulsinelli WA. Hypothermia but not the N-methyl-D-aspartate antagonist, MK-801, attenuates neuronal damage in gerbils subjected to transient global ischemia. *J Neurosci* 1990; 10:311-316.

32. Coimbra CG, Cavalheiro EA. Protective effect of short-term post-ischemic hypothermia on the gerbil brain. *Braz J Med Biol Res* 1990; 23:605-611.

33. Chopp M, Chen H, Dereski MO, Garcia JH. Mild hypothermic intervention after graded ischemic stress in rats. *Stroke* 1991; 22:37-43.

34. Carroll M, Beek O. Protection against hippocampal CA1 cell loss by post-ischemic hypothermia is dependent on delay of initiation and duration. *Metab Brain Dis* 1992;7:45-50.

35. Coimbra C, Wieloch T. Hypothermia ameliorates neuronal survival when induced 2 hours after ischaemia in the rat. *Acta Physiol Scan* 1992; 146:543-544.

36. Coimbra C, Wieloch T. Moderate hypothermia mitigates neuronal damage in the rat brain when initiated several hours following transient cerebral ischemia. *Acta Neuropathologica* 1994; 87:325-331.

37. Colbourne F, Corbett D. Delayed and prolonged post-ischemic hypothermia is neuroprotective in the gerbil. *Brain Res* 1994; 654:265-272.

38. Colbourne F, Corbett D. Delayed postischemic hypothermia: a six month survival study using behavioral and histological assessments of neuroprotection. *J Neurosci* 1995; 15:7250-7260.

39. Colbourne F, Auer RN, Sutherland GR. Behavioral testing does not exacerbate ischemic CA1 damage in gerbils. *Stroke* 1998; 29:1967-1970.

40. Colbourne F, Li H, Buchan AM. Indefatigable CA1 sector neuroprotection with mild hypothermia induced 6 hours after severe forebrain ischemia in rats. *J Cereb Blood Flow Metab*; 19:742-749.

41. Eisenberg MS, Horwood BT, Cummins RO, et al. Cardiac arrest and resuscitation: a tale of 29 cities. *Ann Emerg Med* 1990; 19:179-186.

42. Safar P, Tisherman SA, Behringer W, et al. Suspended animation for delayed resuscitation from prolonged cardiac arrest that is unresuscitable by standard cardiopulmonary-cerebral resuscitation. *Crit Care Med* 2000; 28 (11 Suppl):N214-N218.

43. Safar P, Abramson NS, Angelos M, et al. Emergency cardiopulmonary bypass for resuscitation from prolonged cardiac arrest. *Am J Emerg Med* 1990; 8:55-67.

44. Bellamy R, Safar P, Tisherman SA, et al. Suspended animation for delayed resuscitation. *Crit Care Med* 1996; 24(2 Suppl):S24-S47.

45. Hickey PR. Deep hypothermic circulatory arrest: current status and future directions. *Mt Sinai J Med* 1985; 52:541-547.

46. Livesay JJ, Cooley DA, Reul GJ, et al. Resection of aortic arch aneurysms: a comparison of hypothermic techniques in 60 patients. *Ann Thorac Surg* 1983; 36:19-28.

47. Capone A, Safar P, Radovsky A, et al. Complete recovery after normothermic hemorrhagic shock and profound hypothermic circulatory arrest of 60 minutes in dogs. *J Trauma* 1996; 40:388-395.

48. Tisherman SA, Safar P, Radovsky A, et al. Profound hypothermia (less than 10 degrees C) compared with deep hypothermia (15 degrees C) improves neurologic outcome in dogs after two hours' circulatory arrest induced to enable resuscitative surgery. *J Trauma* 1991; 31:1051-1061.

49. Woods RJ, Prueckner S, Safar P, et al. Hypothermic aortic arch flush for preservation during exsanguination cardiac arrest of 15 minutes in dogs. *J Trauma* 1999; 47:1028-1036.

50. Behringer W, Prueckner S, Safar P, et al. Rapid Induction of Mild Cerebral Hypothermia by Cold Aortic Flush Achieves Normal Recovery in a Dog Outcome Model with 20-minute Exsanguination Cardiac Arrest. *Acad Emerg Med* 2000; 7:1341-1348.

51. Behringer W, Prueckner S, Kentner R, et al. Rapid hypothermic aortic flush can achieve survival without brain damage after 30 minutes cardiac arrest in dogs. *Anesthesiology* 2000; 93:1491-1499.

52. Behringer W, Safar P, Wu X, et al. Survival without brain damage after clinical death of 60-120 mins in dogs using suspended animation by profound hypothermia. *Crit Care Med* 2003; 31:1523-1531.

Chapter 2

GLOBAL CEREBRAL ISCHEMIA: CLINICAL STUDIES

Michael Holzer, MD[1], Stephen A. Bernard, MD[2], Fritz Sterz, MD[1]
[1]*Medical University of Vienna, Vienna, Austria*
[2]*Dandenong Hospital, Dandenong, Victoria, Australia*

INTRODUCTION

The single most important clinically relevant cause of global cerebral ischemia is cardiac arrest. Other causes like hanging will not be covered in this chapter. The estimated rate of sudden cardiac arrest lies between 40 to 130 cases per 100,000 people per year in industrialized countries (1,2). Unfortunately full cerebral recovery is still a rare event. Almost 80% of patients who initially are resuscitated from cardiac arrest remain comatose for more than one hour. One year after cardiac arrest only 10-30% of these patients survive with good neurological outcome (3). Current therapy after cardiac arrest has concentrated on resuscitation efforts (4) but until recently no specific therapy for brain resuscitation was available.

The ability to survive anoxic no-flow states is dramatically increased with protective (before the insult) and preservative (during the insult) hypothermia (5). Intraischemic hypothermia for brain protection has been used for several years in combination with particular surgical procedures and circulatory arrest states. Experimental results showed a marked neuroprotective effect of hypothermia also if started after ischemic situations (resuscitation) (6).

NON-RANDOMIZED TRIALS

The first experiences with therapeutic hypothermia after cardiac arrest were gained by Williams and Spencer (7) in 1958; they presented a case series of two children and two middle-aged adults after cardiac arrest (Tables 2-1, 2-2). The cardiac arrests were due to respiratory failure and traumatic injury of the heart. They cooled their patients with a water-cooled mattress to a temperature of 30 to 34°C until the patients regained consciousness (24 to 72 hours). Only one individual had a residual moderate neurological defect (visual impairment). One year later Benson and coworkers (8) compared hypothermia treatment in 12 patients to 7 normothermic controls after in-hospital cardiac arrest in the operating room. All patients had moderate to severe neurological dysfunction prior to cooling. A blanket containing circulating coolant was used to reduce the temperature to 30-32°C until improvement of neurological function was observed. Patients treated with hypothermia had a favorable neurological recovery in 50% compared to 14% in the control group.

Although the target temperature was lower and the method and duration of cooling also differed compared to recent studies, the results of these pioneering studies were similar. However, the once common use of prolonged hypothermia as a therapeutic tool in cardiac arrest patients was largely abandoned until the 1990s. A review of the literature did not give a satisfactory explanation for this change in practice, but inconclusive findings and the rate of cardiovascular problems with temperatures below 30°C might have been important factors (9). Moderate hypothermia (28-32°C) can cause coagulopathy and risk of infection if prolonged. Furthermore, reports on the detrimental effect of hypothermia in experimental stroke might have also intensified this change in practice (10).

Studies in the late 1980s found that mild hypothermia (32-34°C), which should have fewer side effects than moderate hypothermia, provided significant benefit during and after global cerebral ischemia. This led to renewed interest in the efficacy of therapeutic hypothermia after localized and global ischemia in the 1990s and to the first modern clinical studies of mild (32-34°C) therapeutic hypothermia after cardiac arrest.

Bernard and colleagues (11) studied 22 consecutive patients who were comatose after an out-of-hospital cardiac arrest, excluding trauma, drug overdose or stroke. In contrast to the studies of the 1950s all patients were intubated, mechanically ventilated, sedated and relaxed. They cooled the patients by surface cooling with ice packs to 33°C core temperature for 12 hours and compared the results to a group of historical controls fulfilling the same inclusion and exclusion criteria. The target temperature in the hypothermia group was reached within 74 min. Hypothermia caused reduction of pulse during cooling and an increase in cardiac index and decrease in systemic vascular resistance during rewarming. Compared to historical controls, patients who were cooled for 12 hours had better functional neurological recovery as measured with the Glasgow Outcome Coma Scale (normal/moderate disability: 11 of 22 vs. 3 of 22).

Table 2-1. Non Randomized trials of hypothermia after cardiac arrest - Inclusion

Study	Year	N	Cause of cardiac arrest	VF(%)	ROSC(min)
Williams (7)	1958	4	respiratory and trauma	0	5-14
Benson (8)	1959	12	respiratory		
Bernard (11)	1997	22	all	77	17
Yanagawa (12)	1998	13	all	54	31
Zeiner (13)	2000	27	cardiac	100	21
Nagao (14)	2000	23	all	91	58
Felberg (15)	2001	9	all	78	24
Holzer (16)	2002	19	all	63	21
Bernard (17)	2003	22	Cardiac	63	26

VF, rate of ventricular fibrillation; ROSC, time to return of spontaneous circulation

Table 2-2. Non Randomized trials of hypothermia after cardiac arrest - Cooling

Study	Year	Method	T_{targ}(°C)	t_{targ}(min)	t_{cool}(h)
Williams (7)	1958	Blanket	30-34	n.a.	24-72
Benson (8)	1959	Blanket	31-32	n.a.	3-192
Bernard (11)	1997	ice-pack	33	74	12
Yanagawa (12)	1998	Blanket	33-34	414	48
Zeiner (13)	2000	cold-air	32-34	276	24
Nagao (14)	2000	blood cooling by hemodialysis coil	34	360	72
Felberg (15)	2001	Blanket	32-34	378	24
Holzer (16)	2002	cooling catheter	32-34	95	24
Bernard (17)	2003	ice cold saline; ice	33	~ 30	12

T_{targ}, target temperature, t_{targ}, time until target temperature was reached; t_{cool}, duration of cooling

A combination of water filled cooling blankets and topical alcohol was used by Yanagawa and co-workers (12) to cool cardiac arrest survivors to a core temperature between 33 and 34°C over 48 hours. The patients had to be hemodynamically stable on admission. Cardiac arrest due to trauma or central nervous disease was excluded. One of 15 patients in the historical control group survived without severe disabilities (Glasgow outcome scale 1 and 2) as compared to 3 of 13 patients in the hypothermia group. Among the patients who survived, the duration of no cerebral perfusion was longer in the cooled patients.

Table 2-3. Blood Chemical Values, Hematologic and Coagulation Values, and Arterial Blood Gas Values Uncorrected for Temperature in the 27 patients cooled in the pilot study of Zeiner et al. (13)

	Admission	24 hours	36 hours	P
Potassium, mmol/l	3.8 (3.5 – 3.9)	3.7 (3.6 – 4.0)	4.2 (3.9 – 4.8)	NS
Sodium, mmol/l	139 (138 – 139)	139 (138 – 142)	139 (135 – 142)	NS
Creatinine, μmol/L	122 (113 – 116)	73 (60 – 97)	83 (73 – 88)	<0.05
Urea nitrogen, mmol/L	7.0 (5.8 – 7.9)	5.7 (4.5 – 8.2)	4.8 (3.3 – 6.0)	NS
Total bilirubin, μmol/L	10 (7 – 14)	16 (11 – 34)	15 (7 – 18)	NS
Asparate aminotransferase, U/l	53 (30 – 88)	72 (32 – 98)	55 (24 – 126)	NS
Alanine aminotransferase, U/l	53 (35 – 73)	38 (35 – 58)	37 (26 – 102)	NS
Amylase, U/l	87 (80 – 118)	190 (45 – 397)	187 (48 – 362)	NS
Lipase, U/l	82 (66 – 124)	35 (10 – 234)	33 (10 – 109)	<0.05
Glucose, mmol/L	14.9 (11.8 – 17.8)	6.9 (6.6 – 10.3)	7.1 (6.6 – 10.1)	<0.05
C-reactive protein, mg/dl	0.05 (0.05 – 0.05)	4.59 (3.22 – 5.40)	9.28 (7.54 – 11.80)	<0.05
Lactate, mmol/l	8.6 (6.5 – 11.0)	1.8 (1.0 – 4.7)	1.6 (0.8 – 3.0)	<0.05
White-cell count, G/l	13.4 (11.9 – 14.9)	8.0 (6.4 – 11.4)	7.2 (6.2 – 1.32)	NS
Platelet count, G/l	227 (211 – 300)	157 (118 – 100)	157 (125 – 178)	<0.05
Hemoglobin, g/L	144 (138 – 148)	129 (114 – 133)	120 (114 – 135)	<0.05
Fibrinogen, g/L	3.1 (2.6 – 3.6)	3.5 (3.0 – 3.6)	4.0 (2.4 – 4.4)	NS
Prothrombin Time, s	0.79 (0.51 – 0.99)	0.57 (0.16 – 0.77)	0.54 (0.07 – 0.66)	NS
PH	7.28 (7.19 – 7.35)	7.38 (7.34 – 7.44)	7.40 (7.36 – 7.44)	<0.05
PaO_2, mmHg	335 (212 – 461)	89 (83 – 95)	90 (80 – 102)	<0.05
$PaCO_2$, mmHg	38.5 (33.0 – 45.0)	34.0 (32.0 – 39.0)	38.9 (35.0 – 41.0)	NS
PaO_2/FiO_2	396 (230 – 470)	243 (175 – 275)	225 (175 – 287)	NS
Base excess, mmol/l	-8.30 (-13.40 - -4.70)	-1.55 (-2.70 - -1.00)	0.00 (-2.70 – 1.40)	<0.05

Values are median (95% CI). n=27
Adapted with kind permission from the American Heart Association, Stroke 2000; 31:86-94.

Zeiner and colleagues (13) included 27 comatose patients with ventricular fibrillation (VF) cardiac arrest in a pilot trial (Table 2-3). A water filled blanket and cold air were used to surface cool the patients within 62±33 minutes after cardiac arrest. After 287±145 minutes the target temperature of 33±1°C was reached, which was maintained for an additional 24 hours. The patients were passively rewarmed within 7±4 hours to a temperature above 35°C. The laboratory results did show a decrease in platelet counts, but this was within the physiologic range. All other values changed as expected after a cardiac arrest of this severity.

After six months good neurological recovery (cerebral performance category score 1 and 2), was achieved by 14 (52%) patients; 2 (7%) had poor neurological recovery and 11 (41%) died before discharge. Compared to historical controls this was a two-fold improvement of outcome.

In a small feasibility study of therapeutic hypothermia after cardiac arrest Felberg (15) and associates cooled 9 patients with water filled cooling blankets, ice bags and cold gastric lavage to 33°C. This temperature was maintained for 24 hours and neurologic function on discharge was recorded. Three of the included patients (33%) had a favorable neurological outcome.

A different approach was used by Nagao and co-workers (14). A combined cardiac and cerebral resuscitation strategy with emergency cardiopulmonary bypass and the intra-aortic balloon pump for patients in cardiac arrest on arrival to the emergency department (40% of included patients) was used in this study. Comatose survivors after successful resuscitation were subjected to hypothermia therapy, which was performed by direct blood cooling (34°C) via a coil over a minimum of 48 (71±49) hours. Thirteen of 23 (57%) patients treated with hypothermia had a favorable neurological recovery. Factors for good neurological outcome were higher cardiac index and oxygen delivery during cooling.

In a recent study, the feasibility of using a central venous cooling catheter was evaluated (16). In these cooling system cold fluid is pumped through a balloon at the tip of the catheter (Icy®, Alsius Corp., Irvine, USA) when inserted in the superior or inferior vena cava. Nineteen comatose patients after witnessed cardiac arrest were included, 16 were of cardiac origin, and in 12 patients the first recorded rhythm was VF. The 'no-flow-time' was 5 (1-11) minutes. Time to return of spontaneous circulation was 21 (15-28) minutes. Within 95 (70-134) minutes after start of cooling the patients were cooled to a temperature below 34°C, which led to a cooling rate of 1.4 (1.0-1.9)°C/h. In patients with VF, favorable neurological recovery at 1 month occurred in 67% of patients; 1 of 3 patients with pulseless electrical activity and 1 of 4 with a primary rhythm of asystole also achieved good neurological recovery.

A very simple and cost effective way of induction of hypothermia was used by Bernard (17) and colleagues. In this study the effectiveness and safety of rapid infusion of large volume, ice-cold intravenous fluid for induction of hypothermia was investigated. With an infusion of 30 ml/kg of ice-cold (4°C) lactated Ringer's solution over 30 minutes, 22 comatose survivors of out-of-hospital cardiac arrest were cooled. This infusion resulted in a rapid decrease in median core temperature from 35.5 to 33.8°C (cooling rate 3.4°C/h). This reduction in temperature was accompanied by significant improvements in mean arterial blood pressure, renal function and acid/base status. No patient developed pulmonary edema. This is an inexpensive and effective technique of inducing mild hypothermia.

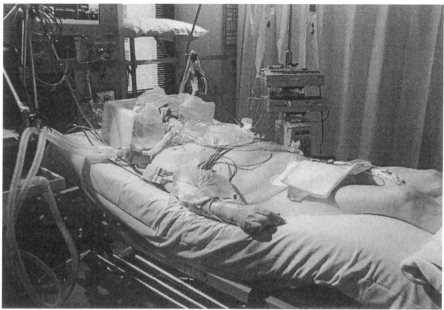

Figure 2-1. Cooling with ice packs in the Australian study (19).

RANDOMIZED CLINICAL TRIALS

Three randomized studies on hypothermia after cardiac arrest have been published so far (Tables 2-4, 2-5, 2-6).

Hachimi-Idrissi and colleagues (18) studied 30 comatose survivors after cardiac arrest of presumed cardiac origin with primary rhythms of asystole or pulseless electrical activity. This patients were randomized either to cooling with a cooling helmet or to standard treatment. The cooling helmet was changed every hour to yield the maximum cooling capability. The patients were cooled with this device to a target temperature of 34°C for a maximum of 4 hours and then rewarmed spontaneously over the next 8 hours. Favorable neurological recovery occurred in 2 of 16 patients in the hypothermia group and in none of the patients in the normothermia group.

In the Australian study by Bernard and associates (19), 77 patients with return of spontaneous circulation after cardiac arrest of cardiac origin and primary rhythm of VF were randomly assigned to treatment with hypothermia or normothermia (Table 2-5). The patients in the hypothermia group were cooled to 33°C core temperature over 12 hours with ice packs

(Figure 2-1). In the hypothermia group 59% required an infusion of epinephrine as compared to 49% in the normothermia group. The blood pressure was higher and the cardiac index was lower after induction of cooling in the hypothermia group, but were consistent with the values in the normothermia group later on. The pulse rate was lower and the systemic vascular resistance was higher during the whole cooling process.

Nine of the 34 patients treated with normothermia (26%) survived and had a good outcome as compared to 21 of the 43 patients treated with hypothermia (49 %, P=0.046). After adjustment for base-line differences, the odds ratio for a good outcome with hypothermia as compared with normothermia was 5.25 (95 percent confidence interval, 1.47 to 18.76; P=0.011).

Table 2-4. Randomized trials of hypothermia after cardiac arrest - Eligibility and General Management

	Hachimi-Idrissi (18)	Bernard (20)	HACA (19)
N	30	77	275
Comatose	●	●	●
Hemodynamically stable	●	●	●
Not pregnant	●	●	●
T_{tymp} (°C)	> 30		> 30
No known coagulopathy	●		●
Collapse to First-EMS-CPR-Attempts 5 - 15 min			●
Collapse to ROSC interval < 60 min			●
Age (years)	>18	>18 (>50 female)	18-75
Cause	cardiac	All	Cardiac
Rhythm	Asystole/PEA	VF	VF/VT
Sedation	Midazolam 0.13 mg/kg/h	Midazolam 2-5 mg	Midazolam 0.13 mg/kg/h
Analgesia	Fentanyl 2µg/kg/h		Fentanyl 2µg/kg/h
Relaxation	Pancuronium 0.1 mg/kg every 2 h	Vecuronium 8-12 mg	Pancuronium 0.1 mg/kg every 2 h

T_{tymp}, tympanic temperature; EMS, emergency medical service; ROSC, return of spontaneous circulation; PEA, pulseless electrical activity; VF, ventricular fibrillation; VT, ventricular tachycardia

In the European multicenter trial, Hypothermia After Cardiac Arrest (HACA) (20), patients who had been resuscitated after cardiac arrest due to VF or pulseless ventricular tachycardia (VT) were randomly assigned to therapeutic hypothermia (32-34°C bladder temperature, cooled with cold air) over a period of 24 hours or to standard treatment with normothermia (Figure 2-2). According to a detailed protocol all patients received standard intensive care, including the use of sedation (midazolam, initially 0.125 mg/kg/h, and fentanyl, initially 0.002 mg/kg/h), and pancuronium (initially 0.1 mg/kg every 2 h, then as needed to prevent shivering) for 32 hours, with mandatory mechanical ventilation.

Table 2-5. Physiological and hemodynamic values in the study of Bernard et al. (20)*

VARIABLE	GROUP	ADM. TO ED	6 h	12 h	24 h
Number of patients	Hypoth.	43	39	39	38
	Normoth.	34	32	32	31
Temperature (°C)	Hypoth.	35.0±1.18	32.7±1.19†	33.1±0.89†	37.4±0.85†
	Normoth.	35.5±0.90	37.1±0.75	37.4±0.58†	37.3±0.59†
	P value‡	0.02	<0.001	<0.001	0.60
Mean arterial pressure	Hypoth.	90.4±18.89	97.0±14.92	89.5±13.16	89.1±12.9
(mm Hg)	Normoth.	87.2±21.46	92.2±13.00	90.8±14.16	92.1±11.76
	P value‡	0.51	0.16	0.82§	0.24
Pulse (per minute)	Hypoth.	97±22.5	72±17.1§	70±17.6	89±17.9†
	Normoth.	105±30.4	100±21.9	94±17.9	99±15.5
	P value‡	0.18	<0.001	<0.001	0.02
Cardiac index (l/min/m²)¶	Hypoth.		2.1 (0.9–4.2)	2.4 (0.8–4.9)	3.4 (1.6–6.8)§
	Normoth.		2.7 (1.4–6.1)	3.2 (1.2–6.1)	3.0 (1.8–5.7)
P value‡			0.16	0.10	0.54
SVR (dyn·sec·cm-5)¶	Hypoth.		1808 (836–4531)	1564 (439–4280)	987 (551–2500)§
	Normoth.		1278.5 (346–2841)	1056 (340–3163)	1072 (591–1998)
P value‡			<0.001	0.002	0.50

*Plus–minus values are means ±SD. Medians and ranges (in parentheses) are given for the cardiac index and systemic vascular resistance, which were log-transformed before analysis of variance was performed, because of nonparametric distribution. One patient in the hypothermia group and two in the normothermia group died during the first 24 hours. ED denotes emergency department.

†P<0.05 for the comparison with the value on admission to the emergency department.

‡P values are for the differences between the hypothermia and the normothermia groups.

§P<0.01 for the comparison with the value on admission to the emergency department.

¶Cardiac index and systemic vascular resistance values are given for the 32 patients treated with hypothermia and the 22 patients treated with normothermia who had a pulmonary-artery catheter.

Adapted with kind permission from the Massachusetts Medical Society, *N Engl J Med* 2002; 346:557-563.

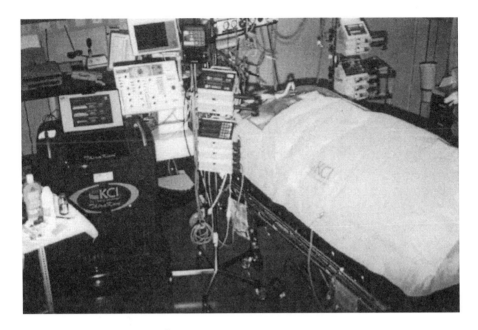

Figure 2-2. Cooling device from the HACA study (20) - Cooling with cold air (TheraKool, Kinetic Concepts, Wareham, United Kingdom)

Favorable neurological outcome within six months after cardiac arrest was the primary end point. Secondary end points were mortality within six months and the rate of complications within seven days. In the hypothermia group 75 of the 136 patients (55%) had a favorable neurological recovery (cerebral performance category 1 or 2), as compared with 54 of 137 (39%) in the normothermia group (risk ratio, 1.40; 95% confidence interval 1.08 to 1.81). At six months 56 of 137 (41%) patients had died in the hypothermia group, as compared with 76 of 138 patients in the normothermia group (55%; risk ratio, 0.74; 95% confidence interval 0.58 to 0.95) (Figure 2-3). Only 8% of the patients assessed for eligibility could be included in this trial, as there were very strict inclusion and exclusion criteria. Whether or not these results can be extrapolated to patients with other causes of brain damage or to those with cardiac arrest due to rhythms other than VF needs to be evaluated in further studies.

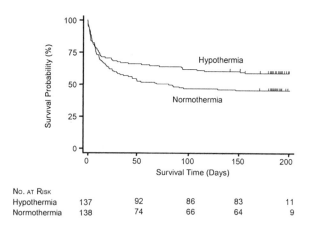

Figure 2-3. Cumulative Survival in the Normothermia and Hypothermia Groups. Censored data are indicated by tick marks. Data of the HACA trial. (20) Reprinted with kind permission from the Massachusetts Medical Society, *N Engl J Med* 2002; 346:549-556.

Table 2-6. Randomized trials of hypothermia after cardiac arrest – Cooling process

Study	Method	T_{targ} (°C)	t_{targ} (min)	Cooling Rate (°C/h)	t_{cool} (h)	t_{rw} (h)
Hachimi-Idrissi (18)	cooling helmet	30-34	180	0.7	Max 4	8
Bernard (20)	ice-pack	33	120	1.5	12 (18)	6
HACA (19)	cold air	32-34	480	0.3	24	8

ROSC, time to return of spontaneous circulation; T_{targ}, target temperature, t_{targ}, time until target temperature was reached; t_{cool}, duration of cooling; t_{rw}, duration of rewarming

COMPLICATIONS OF THERAPEUTIC HYPOTHERMIA

From previous experiences with moderate (26-32°C) hypothermia in the beginning of the therapeutic hypothermia era it was feared that the beneficial effect of hypothermia would be nullified by the arising complications. The fact is that the advantageous effect of therapeutic hypothermia after cardiac arrest outweighs the complications by far, particularly with mild hypothermia (32-34°C). Nevertheless there are complications that have to be considered if patients are treated with therapeutic hypothermia.

Table 2-7. Complications of therapeutic hypothermia

Study	Arrhythmia	Hemodyn. Instability	Bleeding	Pneumonia	Sepsis	Seizures
Bernard 1997 (11)	O		-		-	①
Yanagawa 1998 (12)	-		-	●		
Zeiner 2000 (13)	O	O	-	-	-	
Nagao 2000 (14)		O	O		O	
Felberg 2001 (15)	O	-	O	O	-	O
Holzer 2002 (16)	-	-	O	-	-	
Bernard 2003 (17)	-	-	-	-	-	-
Idrissi 2001 (18)	-		-	-	-	
Bernard 2002 (20)	-	①	-	-	-	
HACA 2002 (19)	①	-	①	①	①	-

●   significantly higher complication rate in hypothermia group
①   higher complication rate in hypothermia group (NS)
O   complication mentioned without comparison to control group
-    no complications
blank, no data on specific complication presented

Significantly higher rates of pneumonia were only reported in one study, (12) but pulmonary infection was not a direct cause of death in these patients (Table 2-7). Higher, but not statistically significant, rates were found for arrythmias, hemodynamic instability, bleeding events, thrombocytopenia, pneumonia, sepsis and seizures. The total complication rate was not significantly higher in the hypothermia groups in any of the reported studies, but the number of studied patients is still low. If patients are treated with hypothermia, extra care should be taken to document and possibly avoid these complications.

SUMMARY

After resuscitation from out-of-hospital cardiac arrest, induced therapeutic mild hypothermia (32-34°C) can improve neurological outcome and reduce mortality in comatose survivors. Until now no specific therapy existed to improve outcome after cardiac arrest. One could expect that broad implementation of this therapy could save thousands of lives worldwide. If possible complications are prevented by strict protocols, this therapy is recommended for all patients who are admitted comatose to the hospital after a VF cardiac arrest.

Although therapeutic induced mild hypothermia was effective, the optimal temperature range and duration still remains the subject of investigation. Existing evidence, however, suggests that cooling should be started as soon as possible to yield maximum benefit. Additional advancement would be the design of new techniques or cooling devices, which can be already used in the ambulance or even during cardiopulmonary resuscitation. To facilitate the widespread use of therapeutic hypothermia in these clinical settings, these techniques should be easy to use and inexpensive. Whether this therapy is also beneficial to patients at lower risk for brain damage or to those with cardiac arrest due to causes other than VF needs further evaluation.

The best current treatment regimen in our opinion consists of rapid induction of cooling with an ice-cold intravenous saline bolus and maintenance with an intravascular cooling device, which has the advantage of precise and easy control of body temperature over the whole cooling period.

Recently the International Liaison Committee on Resuscitation has formulated an advisory statement for therapeutic hypothermia after cardiac arrest. It was recommended that "unconscious adult patients with spontaneous circulation after out-of-hospital cardiac arrest should be cooled to 32 to 34°C for 12 to 24 hours when the initial rhythm was VF. Such cooling may also be beneficial for other rhythms or in-hospital cardiac arrest" (21).

REFERENCES

1. Becker LB, Smith DW, Rhodes KV. Incidence of cardiac arrest: a neglected factor in evaluating survival rates. *Ann Emerg Med* 1993; 22:86-91.
2. Vreede-Swagemakers JJ, Gorgels AP, Dubois-Arbouw WI, et al. Out-of-hospital cardiac arrest in the 1990's: a population-based study in the Maastricht area on incidence, characteristics and survival. *J Am Coll Cardiol* 1997; 30:1500-1505.
3. Paradis N, Halperin H, Novak R. Cardiac Arrest. The Science and Practice of Resuscitation Medicine. Baltimore: Williams & Wilkins; 1996:
4. International Guidelines 2000 for CPR and ECC : A Consensus on ScienceCirculation 2000; 102:I-1-I-384
5. Ginsberg MD, Sternau LL, Globus MY, et al. Therapeutic modulation of brain temperature: relevance to ischemic brain injury. *Cerebrovasc Brain Metab Rev* 1992; 4:189-225.
6. Marion DW, Leonov Y, Ginsberg M, et al. Resuscitative hypothermia. *Crit Care Med* 1996; 24:S81-S89.
7. Williams GR, Spencer FC. Clinical use of hypothermia after cardiac arrest. *Ann Surg* 1958; 148:462-468.
8. Benson DW, Williams GR, Spencer FC. The use of hypothermia after cardiac arrest. *Anesth Analg* 1959; 38:423-428.
9. Steen PA, Soule EH, Michenfelder JD. Detrimental effect of prolonged hypothermia in cats and monkeys with and without regional cerebral ischemia. *Stroke* 1979; 10:522-529.
10. Michenfelder JD, Milde JH. Failure of prolonged hypocapnia, hypothermia, or hypertension to favorably alter acute stroke in primates. *Stroke* 1977; 8:87-91.
11. Bernard SA, Jones BM, Horne MK. Clinical trial of induced hypothermia in comatose survivors of out-of-hospital cardiac arrest. *Ann Emerg Med* 1997; 30:146-153.
12. Yanagawa Y, Ishihara S, Norio H, et al. Preliminary clinical outcome study of mild resuscitative hypothermia after out-of-hospital cardiopulmonary arrest. *Resuscitation* 1998; 39:61-66.
13. Zeiner A, Holzer M, Sterz F, et al. Mild resuscitative hypothermia to improve neurological outcome after cardiac arrest. A clinical feasibility trial. Hypothermia After Cardiac Arrest (HACA) Study Group. *Stroke* 2000; 31:86-94.
14. Nagao K, Hayashi N, Kanmatsuse K, et al. Cardiopulmonary cerebral resuscitation using emergency cardiopulmonary bypass, coronary reperfusion therapy and mild hypothermia in patients with cardiac arrest outside the hospital . *J Am Coll Cardiol* 2000; 36:776-783.
15. Felberg RA, Krieger DW, Chuang R, et al. Hypothermia after cardiac arrest: feasibility and safety of an external cooling protocol. *Circulation* 2001; 104:1799-1804.
16. Holzer M, Kliegel A, Schreiber W, et al. Effectiveness and feasibility of rapid endovascular cooling for resuscitative hypothermia. *Circulation* 2002; 106 (Suppl):II-404.
17. Bernard S, Buist M, Monteiro O, Smith K. Induced hypothermia using large volume, ice-cold intravenous fluid in comatose survivors of out-of-hospital cardiac arrest: a preliminary report. *Resuscitation* 2003; 56:9-13.
18. Hachimi-Idrissi S, Corne L, Ebinger G, et al. Mild hypothermia induced by a helmet device: a clinical feasibility study. *Resuscitation* 2001; 51:275-281.
19. Bernard SA, Gray TW, Buist MD, et al. Treatment of comatose survivors of out-of-hospital cardiac arrest with induced hypothermia. *N Engl J Med* 2002; 346:557-563.
20. The Hypothermia After Cardiac Arrest (HACA) study group. Mild therapeutic hypothermia to improve the neurologic outcome after cardiac arrest. *N Engl J Med* 2002; 346:549-556.

21. Nolan JP, Morley PT, Vanden Hoek TL, et al. Therapeutic hypothermia after cardiac arrest. An advisory statement by the Advanced Life Support Task Force of the International Liaison Committee on Resuscitation. *Resuscitation* 2003; 57:231-235.

Chapter 3

FOCAL CEREBRAL ISCHEMIA: MECHANISMS

Hyung Soo Han, MD, PhD[1], Midori A. Yenari, MD[2]

[1]*Kyungpook National University School of Medicine, Daegu, South Korea*
[2]*University of California, San Francisco, San Francisco, CA, USA*

INTRODUCTION

Hypothermia can be neuroprotective when applied during or after focal cerebral ischemia. Its neuroprotective effect is especially robust in the laboratory where it has been shown to ameliorate many of the damaging effects of cerebral ischemia. Most laboratory research on therapeutic cooling in stroke models has been conducted in rodent models of temporary and permanent middle cerebral artery occlusion. Intra-ischemic cooling vastly reduces infarct size in most occlusion models. Although hypothermia has effects on excitotoxicity, apoptosis, inflammation, and the breakdown of the blood–brain barrier, any of which may lead to protection, the exact pathophysiologic mechanisms of protection by hypothermia during and after ischemia remain a matter of debate. This chapter will summarize potential mechanisms underlying the protective effect of hypothermia in focal cerebral ischemia.

ENERGY METABOLISM

Hypothermia's protective effect has long been thought to be due to preservation of metabolic stores, as cooling the brain leads to approximately 5% reduction in oxygen and glucose consumption per degree centigrade (1-4). In addition to simple reduction of metabolism, cooling of the brain couples both energy metabolism and blood flow to a lower rate for the entire tissue (5).   Cerebral metabolism can be divided generally into two compartments: (i) cellular integrity and structure, as maintained by the basal compartment; and (ii) cellular function, such as neuronal firing, related to the functional compartment. Protein synthesis and ion-balancing adenosine triphosphatases (ATPases) are the dominant energy-consuming processes in mammalian metabolism. Thus, decreased ATP demand, as a consequence of decreased pump activity and lowered membrane permeability, down-regulates energy turnover in metabolically depressed states (6).

Disturbances in cerebral tissue ATP during acute ischemia can lead to brain tissue damage. In sedated and paralyzed mammals, acute hypothermia for 0.5 to 3 h decreases global cerebral metabolic rate for glucose (CMRglc) and oxygen (CMRO$_2$) but maintains a slightly better energy level, which indicates that ATP breakdown is reduced more than its synthesis. Intracellular alkalinization stimulates glycolysis and independently enhances energy generation. Decreased temperature during hypoxia$^-$ ischemia slows the rate of glucose, phosphocreatine, and ATP breakdown. Hypothermia also decreases lactate and inorganic phosphate formation and improves recovery of energetic parameters during reperfusion. Mild hypothermia of 12 to 24-h duration after normothermic hypoxic$^-$ ischemic insults seems to prevent or ameliorate secondary failures in energy parameters. Thus it can be concluded that lowered brain temperatures help to protect and maintain normal central nervous system (CNS) function by preserving brain ATP supplies and levels (7).

In contrast, studies in complete or near complete ischemia models have failed to show an effect of hypothermia on preservation of brain ATP. Despite the profound effects of hypothermia on lowering the rate of cerebral oxygen consumption, a complete lack of substrate will inevitably result in the depletion of energy stores.

Using autoradiography, Tohyama, et al (8), measured local glucose utilization in rats subjected to focal cerebral ischemia. Although ischemia suppressed glycolysis in the ischemic core regardless of brain temperature, glycolysis was increased within regions that extended to the infarct periphery. Interestingly, in rats cooled to 30°C, such increases were not observed, suggesting that moderate hypothermia mainly influences glucose metabolism in the lesion periphery or "penumbra." However, Dietrich, et al (9), showed that while cooling applied during both the ischemic period and shortly into the reperfusion period produces long-lasting neuroprotection, neuroprotection from cooling initiated only during reperfusion is transient. Furthermore, the extent of metabolite recovery (10-20%) was not proportionate to the extent of neuroprotection (35-45%) by cooling. Therefore, the mechanisms of hypothermic protection may involve factors other than hypothermia's influence on brain metabolism.

Whether protection by mild hypothermia against cerebral ischemic insults is necessarily due to the preservation of metabolic stores is far from clear. Barbiturates suppress cerebral metabolism to a similar or even greater degree than hypothermia (10), yet there is little conclusive evidence that barbiturates are truly neuroprotective (11). Hypothermia is also known to reduce the extent of focal cerebral ischemic injury in some models of permanent cerebral artery occlusion (12-14). This observation that hypothermia protects even in settings where ATP is depleted suggest that lower temperatures may exert a protective effect by interfering with other pathologic processes.

EXCITOTOXICITY

The amino-acid glutamate acts as a neurotransmitter. Ischemia severe enough to damage the brain causes flooding of excitatory synapses with glutamate due to failure of energy dependent reuptake pumps that normally remove glutamate from the synapse into glia (15, 16). The high levels of glutamate, in turn, lead to strong activation of glutamate receptors, especially the N-methyl-D-aspartate (NMDA)-type glutamate receptor. Energy failure also leads to depolarization and voltage-dependent loss of magnesium, which normally blocks this receptor (17). Elevated synaptic levels of glutamate lead to large amounts of calcium entering cells (Figure 3-1).

Mild hypothermia alters neurotransmitter release (18). During focal cerebral ischemia, neurotransmitter release increases within 10-20 min of ischemia onset, peaks within 60 minutes, decreases by 50-90 min and then returns to baseline or decreases substantially by 90–120 min (18-21). Intra-ischemic mild hypothermia appears to blunt this peak and, in some instances, delays it by 20 minutes (20, 21). A few studies have shown that mild postischemic hypothermia is still effective even when applied after glutamate peaks (21, 22). Hypothermia between 30 and 33°C completely inhibits glutamate release (18). Greater protection was observed at 30°C than at 33°C (23), even though both levels reduced excitotoxic transmitter efflux equally (18). These data suggest that hypothermic effects on ischemic transmitter release per se cannot completely explain its neuroprotective effects.

By reducing of the glutamate surge, with subsequent reduction of calcium mobilization and ATP expenditure, mild hypothermia is likely to ameliorate cytotoxic edema (24). Even though reduction of presynaptic glutamate release is an important mediator of hypothermic neuroprotection, few reports are available regarding the mechanisms for attenuation of ischemia-induced effluxes of neurotransmitters by hypothermia. As it is generally accepted that biosynthesis and uptake of neurotransmitters are

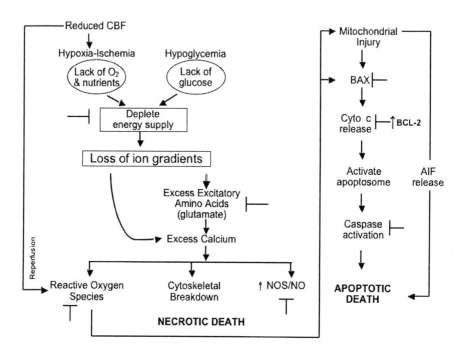

Figure 3-1. The ischemic cascade and apoptosis: influence of hypothermia. Following cessation of blood flow, loss of metabolic stores leads to reversal of ATP-dependent ion pumps and flow of Na+, K+ and Ca++ down their concentration gradients leading to voltage-dependent Ca++ channel opening and accumulation of extracellular glutamate. Glutamate can then stimulate its N-methyl-D-aspartate (NMDA) receptors leading to further intracellular calcium influx, which then activates various damaging signaling pathways ultimately leading to typically necrotic cell death. Among the pathways activated, NMDA stimulation leads to upregulation of nitric oxide synthase (NOS) in neurons, which leads to generation of nitric oxide (NO). In some instances such as during reperfusion, injury can also lead to the generation of reactive oxygen species, which can either directly damage mitochondria or activate the pro-apoptotic protein, Bax. This leads to the creation of a mitochondrial transition pore and subsequent release of cytochrome c (Cyto c) into the cytosol. Cytosolic cytochrome c can activate the apoptosome (pro-caspase-9 and Apaf-1) followed by caspase activation and apoptotic cell death. Apoptosis can also occur independent of caspase activation by mitochondrial release of apoptosis inducing factor (AIF) which translocates directly to the nucleus causing chromatin condensation and DNA fragmentation. The anti-apoptotic protein Bcl-2 can prevent mitochondrial loss of cytochrome c and possibly AIF, thereby conferring protection. Hypothermia can ameliorate this process at multiple levels, such as preventing loss of energy stores, glutamate and NO accumulation, Bax upregulation, cytochrome c release, and caspase activation. Some studies have even shown that hypothermia can upregulate Bcl-2 expression.

temperature-dependent, the degree of glutamate surge is largely depressed and the onset of calcium mobilization is significantly delayed by hypothermia. The hypothermia-induced effects on ion exchangers and co-transporters involved in cell regulation are still poorly understood. One study suggests that protein kinase C (PKC) is involved in the hypothermia-dependent reduction of extracellular glutamate levels in the striatum during ischemia (25). Another study using a focal ischemia model demonstrated that intra-ischemic hypothermia attenuates the activation of PKC (26). These observations support the hypothesis that hypothermia prevents delayed brain injury through inhibition of glutamate receptor-mediated activation of PKC.

Cortical spreading depressions (CSDs) have been thought to contribute to the growth of the ischemic area due to increased calcium influx (27). Following focal cerebral ischemia, CSDs are increased in number, and their onset is delayed by cooling (28-30). The reasons for these observations are not clear, but lower temperatures are known to alter membrane fluidity and ion channels (31). Other reports describe slowing and reduced frequency of propagated waves by hypothermia. These results are consistent with the observation that hypothermia attenuates spreading depression (6). The reduced incidence of spreading depression during ischemia could be an important component of the neuroprotective effect of hypothermia, since spreading depression is believed to increase the size of necrotic regions during focal ischemia (27). However, in a recent study, hypothermia did not affect the number extracellular potassium ion peaks, another measure of spreading depression during acute focal ischemia (32).

APOPTOSIS

Suppression of apoptotic death is another possible mechanism of the protective effect of hypothermia (Figure 3-1). The intrinsic apoptotic pathway, the best characterized pathway in ischemic pathophysiology, proposes that Bax, a pro-apoptotic protein, translocates during ischemia-reperfusion to the mitochondria and forms a pore within the inner membrane (33, 34). Once a mitochondrial pore is formed, cytochrome c is released into the cytosol and activates complexes of procaspase-9 and Apaf-1 (35). This activation leads to cleavage of caspase-9, which in turn activates caspase-3. However, the release of cytochrome c can be inhibited by the anti-apoptotic protein, Bcl-2 (36, 37), which may explain the protective effect of Bcl-2. Caspase-3 and other effector caspases then act in a final common pathway leading to deoxyribonucleic acid (DNA) cleavage and, ultimately, cell death.

The limited literature addressing the effect of temperature on apoptotic cell death is conflicting, and the effects may depend on the nature and severity of the insult as well as whether apoptosis is even observed in some models. Some reports demonstrated that hypothermia decreased the number of apoptotic cells (22, 38-41). Other studies showed reduced expression of Bax (38), caspase 3 (40), and cytosolic cytochrome c (42), but increased Bcl-2 (41, 43). These data support the anti-apoptotic effect of hypothermia. However, another study showed that in the absence of caspase activation, mild hypothermia significantly decreased the amount of cytosolic cytochrome c release 5 hours after the onset of ischemia, but mitochondrial translocation of Bax was not observed until 24 hours and Bcl-2 levels were unchanged (42). These data suggest that, although mild hypothermia inhibits cytochrome c release, its protective effect does not appear to be due to alterations in classic apoptosis-related proteins. Others have recently shown that Bax and other factors can induce mitochondrial damage and cause apoptosis even in the absence of caspase activity (44, 45). In this scenario, apoptosis-inducing factor (AIF) is released from the mitochondria and translocates to the nucleus, resulting in chromatin condensation and DNA fragmentation (46). Furthermore, using an *in vitro* model of neuronal death largely due to apoptosis, Xu, et al (47), showed that incubator temperatures of 33°C inhibited the intrinsic pathway compared to neurons subjected to apoptosis at 37°C. Together, these data indicate that hypothermia likely decreases apoptosis following focal cerebral ischemia.

INFLAMMATION

It is known that inflammation contributes to cerebral ischemic injury, and recent work indicates that mild hypothermia also has anti-inflammatory effects (Figure 3-2). Neutrophils appear within hours of focal cerebral ischemia, peaking 1-2 days later in the rodent, and are then replaced by monocytes/macrophages at 3-7 days (48). Leukocytes enter injured tissue and contribute to secondary injury by releasing reactive oxygen species (ROS), generating lipid mediators, activating thrombosis, damaging the blood brain barrier (BBB), increasing cerebral edema, and plugging the cerebral microvasculature. Many reports have shown that inhibition of neutrophil infiltration into the brain decreases ischemic injury (49, 50), and mild hypothermia is associated with decreased tissue neutrophils (51-55).

Following focal cerebral ischemia, adhesion molecules are needed to attract leukocytes to microvessels (56). Inflammatory cell migration requires interactions between adhesion molecules on the surfaces of the endothelial cells and leukocytes (48). The selectins, designated E- (endothelium), P-(platelet) and L- (leukocyte) selectin, are involved in leukocyte rolling. E and P selectin have been identified on endothelial cells, whereas L-selectin is expressed on leukocytes. Leukocyte rolling stops when leukocytes encounter activated endothelium and bind to the endothelial adhesion molecule, ICAM

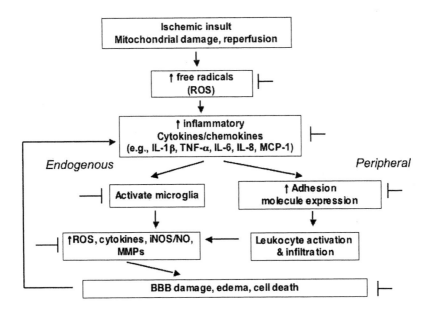

Figure 3-2. Inflammation and stroke. Following ischemic insults, inflammatory responses arise from the peripheral circulation as well as within the brain itself. Such responses are triggered by reactive oxygen species generated in the brain from hypoxic mitochondria and other pathways. These reactive species can then upregulate inflammatory cytokines which stimulate endothelial cells to produce adhesion molecules and peripheral leukocytes to upregulate integrins. Integrin-adhesion molecule interactions permit leukocyte binding to vessels in ischemic brain followed by transmigration into the parenchyma. At the same time, reactive species and endogenously produced cytokines can activate the brain's resident inflammatory cell, the microglia. Once in the brain, activated inflammatory cells can generate a variety of potentially toxic substances such as more reactive species, cytokines, and MMPs. This leads to BBB damage, edema, and more cell death as well as further activation of immune molecules. Hypothermia can interfere with inflammation by preventing inflammatory cell activation and migration as well as suppressing their ability to generate damaging substances.

-1 through its CD11/CD18 leukointegrin. L-selectin is shed from the leukocyte's surface, and transendothelial migration occurs. Blocking CD11/CD18 (50), ICAM-1 (49) or E- and P-selectin (57, 58) decrease neutrophil infiltration and reduces injury from experimental stroke. Furthermore, mice lacking ICAM-1 are protected against transient focal cerebral ischemia (59). Hypothermia has been shown to reduce leukocyte migration (60) and infiltration (52, 53, 55) into ischemic brain by downregulating adhesion molecule expression (51, 53-55).

In addition to peripheral leukocytes, the brain's endogenous inflammatory cells are also influenced by hypothermia. Microglia are often viewed as resident monocytes, which when activated assume a morphology that is indistinguishable from macrophages. After a stroke occurs, microglial activation follows, with noticeable morphologic changes at the infarct periphery by 3 h, within the infarct core by 4-12 h, and increases 3 to 7 days later (61). Activated microglia have been observed even as late as 4 weeks. Inhibitors of microglial activation (62) have recently been shown to be neuroprotective. In fact, mild hypothermia appears to inhibit microglial activation following focal cerebral ischemia (51, 52, 55, 63).

In addition to preventing inflammatory cell activation and infiltration, hypothermia also appears to suppress leukocyte generation of potential toxic mediators. Leukocytes and microglia produce significant quantities of superoxide and nitric oxide (NO). Superoxide and other ROS are well known to potentiate ischemic injury (64), and NO, generated from L-arginine by nitric oxide synthase (NOS), is similarly damaging. It is now known that there are several isoforms of NOS, which have varying roles in mediating ischemic injury, some being protective and others being damaging (65). Of particular relevance to the study of inflammation, the inducible form (iNOS) is now thought to be present mostly in microglia and macrophages, and studies indicate that it is most certainly involved in potentiating ischemic damage (66, 67). Another ROS, peroxynitrite, is generated from superoxide and nitric oxide, and is a potent oxidant and nitrating agent. Several studies have shown that hypothermia reduces the generation of all of these reactive species (63, 68-72). Furthermore, hypothermia attenuates NO and superoxide release in cultured microglia in response to activating stimuli (73). Hypothermia also appears to reduce NO generation by suppressing NOS (63, 69). The mechanism for suppressing superoxide is less straightforward as brain cooling does not alter superoxide dismutase (SOD) levels (72), but does prevent consumption of other endogenous antioxidants (74).

Once activated, microglia and other inflammatory cells also generate cytokines, including IL-1beta and tumor necrosis factor-alpha (TNF-alpha), that induce adhesion molecule expression, initiate thrombosis, and further activate other inflammatory cells (75). IL-1beta expression appears to be localized to microglia and endothelial cells (76, 77), though there are conflicting reports as to whether there is expression in astrocytes (77). TNF-alpha has been observed in neurons, microglia (78) and some astrocytes (79). Very little work has been conducted in the area of inflammatory cytokine generation and mild hypothermia following cerebral insults, and the few reports are conflicting. Hypothermia decreased IL-1beta levels in animal models of brain hypoxia (80) and traumatic brain injury (81), but did not appear to affect levels after focal cerebral ischemia (82). Some reports indicate that hypothermia reduces the levels of TNF-alpha (83), IL-6 (80) and the chemokine, monocyte chemoattractant protein-1 (MCP-1) (82) after brain ischemia. Sutcliffe and colleagues demonstrated that hypothermia inhibits leukocyte rolling and adhesion possibly by inhibiting transcription of inflammatory genes such as IL-8 and IL-1 beta (84). However, another study showed that while cultured human monocytes exposed to most activating factors appear to generate less TNF-alpha at 30°C compared to 37°C, the opposite effect was observed in the presence of lipopolysaccharide (LPS) (85). Hypothermia was also reported to reduce levels of the anti-inflammatory cytokine, IL-10 in cultured human monocytes activated by phytohemagglutinin, but did not change levels of TNF-alpha, IL-6 and IL-8 (86). Reasons for these contradictory results are unclear, but they may represent the complexity and redundancy of the immune system, and perhaps differences depending on the model used.

BLOOD BRAIN BARRIER

Ischemic brain edema appears to involve two distinct processes, the relative contribution and time course of which depend on the duration and severity of ischemia and the presence of reperfusion. The first process involves an increase in tissue Na+ and water content accompanying increased pinocytosis and Na+, K+ ATPase activity across the endothelium. This is apparent during the early phase of infarction and before any structural damage is evident. This phenomenon is augmented by reperfusion. A second process results from a more indiscriminate and delayed blood brain barrier (BBB) breakdown that is associated with infarction of both the parenchyma and the vasculature itself. Although tissue Na+ level still seems to be the major osmotic force for edema formation at this second stage, the extravasation of serum proteases is an additional potentially deleterious factor. Degradation of the extracellular matrix conceivably leads to further BBB disruption and softening of the tissue, setting the stage for the most pronounced forms of brain swelling. A number of factors mediate or modulate ischemic edema formation, with recent studies implicating proteases such as matrix metalloproteinases (MMPs) and plasminogen activators (PAs) (87, 88).

Hypothermia was shown to prevent BBB disruption and edema formation following experimental cerebral ischemia (89, 90). Leukotriene B4, an arachidonic acid metabolite, produced by ischemic degradation of membrane lipid, has been reportedly linked to the development of ischemia-induced vasogenic edema. The postischemic production of leukotriene B4 was decreased by mild hypothermia (91). Recent studies have also correlated reduced MMPs and PAs with reduction in edema and hemorrhage by hypothermia (92, 93). There is also evidence that oxygen free radicals may play a significant role in the development of microvascular brain damage and subsequent breakdown of the BBB. By reducing the $CMRO_2$ and depressing the rates of all enzymatic reactions, hypothermia may blunt the generation of free radicals and protect the BBB (94). Since stimulated leukocytes also release oxygen free radicals and damaging proteases, the hypothermia-induced protection of BBB integrity may be partly mediated by attenuation of leukocyte accumulation. The direct relationship between reduced brain edema formation and preservation of the BBB by hypothermia suggests that one part of the neuroprotective effect of hypothermia is mediated by its restoration (6).

GENE REGULATION

Four pathophysiologic mechanisms have been suggested by which hypothermia produce changes in gene expression: (i) generalized cold-induced inhibition of transcription and translation; (ii) inhibition of ribonucleic acid (RNA) degradation; (iii) increased transcription, mediated by a cold response element in the promoter region of cold-inducible RNA-binding protein (CIRP); and (iv) an enhanced efficiency of translation at lower temperatures that is mediated by specialized regions within the mRNA 5'-leader sequences (internal ribosome entry sites of RBM3, a cold shock protein) (24).

It is now well recognized that following ischemia, dramatic changes in gene expression occur. A growing body of evidence indicates that many different kinds of transcription factors encoded by the immediate early genes such as the Fos and Jun families are induced in cerebral tissues after ischemic insults, with hypothermia altering their expression (28, 95). There are limited reports in focal cerebral ischemia, but one report showed that mild hypothermia inhibits nuclear translocation of the inflammatory transcription factor nuclear factor-kappa B (NF-κB) by suppressing the activation of its inhibitor, I-κB (83). Yet another report demonstrated that hypothermia increased c-Fos expression and AP-1 DNA binding activity in peri-infarct cortex (95). It remains to be established whether such responses are a cause or consequence of cell survival, but these results clearly establish that altered transcription is a key feature of tissue sparing following hypothermic focal ischemia.

CONCLUSIONS

In sum, hypothermia is a robust neuroprotectant. Although the precise mechanism of protection is unknown, it is associated with a host of changes ranging from alterations in metabolism to genetic reprogramming. Likely, hypothermia targets multiple facets of ischemic injury leading to the marked and consistent neuroprotection observed by several laboratories. As such, it could be argued that hypothermia represents the ultimate "cocktail" approach to treating stroke and other brain injuries.

REFERENCES

1. Frietsch T, Krafft P, Piepgras A, et al. Relationship between local cerebral blood flow and metabolism during mild and moderate hypothermia in rats. *Anesthesiology* 2000; 92:754-763.
2. Hagerdal M, Harp J, Nilsson L,Siesjo BK. The effect of induced hypothermia upon oxygen consumption in the rat brain. *J Neurochem* 1975; 24:311-316.
3. Krafft P, Frietsch T, Lenz C, et al. Mild and moderate hypothermia (alpha-stat) do not impair the coupling between local cerebral blood flow and metabolism in rats. *Stroke* 2000; 31:1393-1400.
4. Palmer C, Vannucci RC, Christensen MA,Brucklacher RM. Regional cerebral blood flow and glucose utilization during hypothermia in newborn dogs. *Anesthesiology* 1989; 71:730-737.
5. Sakoh M, Gjedde A. Neuroprotection in hypothermia linked to redistribution of oxygen in brain. *Am J Physiol Heart Circ Physiol* 2003; 285:H17-25.
6. Schaller B, Graf R. Hypothermia and stroke: the pathophysiological background. *Pathophysiology* 2003; 10:7-35.
7. Erecinska M, Thoresen M, Silver IA. Effects of hypothermia on energy metabolism in Mammalian central nervous system. *J Cereb Blood Flow Metab* 2003; 23:513-530.
8. Tohyama Y, Sako K, Yonemasu Y. Hypothermia attenuates hyperglycolysis in the periphery of ischemic core in rat brain. *Exp Brain Res* 1998; 122:333-338.
9. Dietrich WD, Busto R. Alonso O, et al. Intraischemic but not postischemic brain hypothermia protects chronically following global forebrain ischemia in rats. *J Cereb Blood Flow Metab* 1993; 13:541-549.
10. Nemoto EM, Klementavicius R, Melick JA,Yonas H. Suppression of cerebral metabolic rate for oxygen (CMRO2) by mild hypothermia compared with thiopental, *J Neurosurg Anesthesiol* 1996; 8:52-59.
11. Yenari MA, Steinberg GK. Pharmacological advances in cerebrovascular protection. In I. Awad (Ed.), *Cerebrovascular Neurosurgery.* Current Medicine, Philadelphia, 1998, pp. 98-116.
12. Baker CJ, Onesti ST, Barth KN, et al. Hypothermic protection following middle cerebral artery occlusion in the rat. *Surg Neurol* 1991; 36:175-180.
13. Kader A, Brisman MH, Maraire N, et al. The effect of mild hypothermia on permanent focal ischemia in the rat. *Neurosurgery* 1992; 31:1056-60; discussion 1060-1061.
14. Yanamoto H, Nagata I, Niitsu Y, et al. Prolonged mild hypothermia therapy protects the brain against permanent focal ischemia. *Stroke* 2001; 32:232-239.
15. Andine P, Sandberg M, Bagenholm R, et al. Intra- and extracellular changes of amino acids in the cerebral cortex of the neonatal rat during hypoxic-ischemia. *Brain Res Dev Brain Res* 1991; 64:115-120.
16. Martin LJ, Brambrink AM, Lehmann C, et al. Hypoxia-ischemia causes abnormalities in glutamate transporters and death of astroglia and neurons in newborn striatum. *Ann Neurol* 1997; 42:335-348.
17. Pang Z, Geddes JW. Mechanisms of cell death induced by the mitochondrial toxin 3-nitropropionic acid: acute excitotoxic necrosis and delayed apoptosis. *J Neurosci* 1997; 17:3064-3073.
18. Busto R, Globus MY, Dietrich WD, et al. Effect of mild hypothermia on ischemia-induced release of neurotransmitters and free fatty acids in rat brain. *Stroke* 1989; 20:904-10.19. Baker CJ, Fiore AJ, Frazzini VI, et al. Intraischemic hypothermia decreases the release of glutamate in the cores of permanent focal cerebral infarcts. *Neurosurgery* 1995; 36:994-1001.

20. Graham SH, Shiraishi K, Panter SS, et al: Changes in extracellular amino acid neurotransmitters produced by focal cerebral ischemia. *Neurosci Lett* 1990; 110:124-130.
21. Huang FP, Zhou LF, Yang GY. Effects of mild hypothermia on the release of regional glutamate and glycine during extended transient focal cerebral ischemia in rats. *Neurochem Res* 1998; 23:991-996.
22. Van Hemelrijck A, Vermijlen D, Hachimi-Idrissi S, et al. Effect of resuscitative mild hypothermia on glutamate and dopamine release, apoptosis and ischaemic brain damage in the endothelin-1 rat model for focal cerebral ischaemia. *J Neurochem* 2003; 87:66-75.
23. Busto R, Dietrich WD, Globus MY, et al. Small differences in intraischemic brain temperature critically determine the extent of ischemic neuronal injury. *J Cereb Blood Flow Metab* 1987; 7:729-738.
24. Kataoka K, Yanase H. Mild hypothermia--a revived countermeasure against ischemic neuronal damages. *Neurosci Res* 1998; 32:103-117.
25. Boris-Moller F,Wieloch T. The effect of 4 beta-phorbol-12,13-dibutyrate and staurosporine on the extracellular glutamate levels during ischemia in the rat striatum. *Mol Chem Neuropathol* 1998; 35:133-147.
26. Tohyama Y, Sako K, Yonemasu Y. Hypothermia attenuates the activation of protein kinase C in focal ischemic rat brain: dual autoradiographic study of [3H]phorbol 12,13-dibutyrate and iodo[14C]antipyrine. *Brain Res* 1998; 782:348-351.
27. Busch E, Gyngell ML, Eis M, et al. Potassium-induced cortical spreading depressions during focal cerebral ischemia in rats: contribution to lesion growth assessed by diffusion-weighted NMR and biochemical imaging. J Cereb Blood Flow Metab 1996; 16:1090-1099.
28. Mancuso A, Derugin N, Hara K, et al. Mild hypothermia decreases the incidence of transient ADC reduction detected with diffusion MRI and expression of c-fos and hsp70 mRNA during acute focal ischemia in rats. *Brain Res* 2000; 887:34-45.
29. Ueda M, Watanabe, N, Ushikubo Y, et al. The effect of hypothermia on CSD propagation in rats]. *No Shinkei Geka* 1997; 25:523-528.
30. Yenari MA, Onley D, Hedehus M, et al. Diffusion- and perfusion-weighted magnetic resonance imaging of focal cerebral ischemia and cortical spreading depression under conditions of mild hypothermia. *Brain Res* 2000; 885;208-219.
31. Almeida MT, Ramalho-Santos J, Oliveira CR, de Lima MC. Parameters affecting fusion between liposomes and synaptosomes. Role of proteins, lipid peroxidation, pH and temperature. *J Membr Biol* 1994; 142:217-222.
32. Sick TJ, Tang R, Perez-Pinzon MA. Cerebral blood flow does not mediate the effect of brain temperature on recovery of extracellular potassium ion activity after transient focal ischemia in the rat. *Brain Res* 1999; 821:400-406.
33. Green DR, Reed JC. Mitochondria and apoptosis. *Science* 1998; 281:1309-1312.
34. Murphy KM, Ranganathan V, Farnsworth ML, Kavallaris M, Lock RB. Bcl-2 inhibits Bax translocation from cytosol to mitochondria during drug-induced apoptosis of human tumor cells. *Cell Death Differ* 2000; 7:102-111.
35. Liu X, Kim CN, Yang J, Jemmerson R, Wang X. Induction of apoptotic program in cell-free extracts: requirement for dATP and cytochrome c. *Cell* 1996; 86:147-157.
36. Rosse T, Olivier R, Monney L, et al. Bcl-2 prolongs cell survival after Bax-induced release of cytochrome c, *Nature* 1998; 391:496-499.
37. Zhao H, Yenari MA, Cheng D, Sapolsky RM, Steinberg GK. Bcl-2 overexpression protects against neuron loss within the ischemic margin following experimental stroke and inhibits cytochrome c translocation and caspase-3 activity. *J Neurochem* 2003; 85:1026-1036.

38. Inamasu J, Suga S, Sato S, et al. Postischemic hypothermia attenuates apoptotic cell death in transient focal ischemia in rats. *Acta Neurochir Suppl* 2000; 76:525-527.

39. Maier CM, Ahern K, Cheng ML, et al. Optimal depth and duration of mild hypothermia in a focal model of transient cerebral ischemia: effects on neurologic outcome, infarct size, apoptosis, and inflammation. *Stroke* 1998; 29:2171-2180.

40. Phanithi PB, Yoshida Y, Santana A, et al: Mild hypothermia mitigates post-ischemic neuronal death following focal cerebral ischemia in rat brain: immunohistochemical study of Fas, caspase-3 and TUNEL. *Neuropathology* 2000; 20:273-282.

41. Zhang Z, Sobel RA, Cheng D, Steinberg GK, Yenari MA. Mild hypothermia increases Bcl-2 protein expression following global cerebral ischemia. *Brain Res Mol Brain Res* 2001; 95:75-85.

42. Yenari MA, Iwayama S, Cheng D, et al. Mild hypothermia attenuates cytochrome c release but does not alter Bcl- 2 expression or caspase activation after experimental stroke *J Cereb Blood Flow Metab* 2002; 22:29-38.

43. Prakasa Babu P, Yoshida Y, Su M, et al: Immunohistochemical expression of Bcl-2, Bax and cytochrome c following focal cerebral ischemia and effect of hypothermia in rat. *Neurosci Lett* 2000; 291:196-200.

44. Hansen RS, Braithwaite AW. The growth-inhibitory function of p53 is separable from transactivation, apoptosis and suppression of transformation by E1a and Ras. *Oncogene* 1996; 13:995-1007.

45. Susin SA, Lorenzo HK, Zamzami N, et al. Molecular characterization of mitochondrial apoptosis-inducing factor. *Nature* 1999; 397:441-446.

46. Loeffler M, Daugas E, Susin SA, et al. Dominant cell death induction by extramitochondrially targeted apoptosis-inducing factor *Faseb J* 2001; 15:758-767.

47. Xu L, Yenari MA, Steinberg GK, Giffard RG. Mild hypothermia reduces apoptosis of mouse neurons in vitro early in the cascade. *J Cereb Blood Flow Metab* 2002; 22:21-28.

48. Hallenbeck JM. Significance of the inflammatory response in brain ischemia. *Acta Neurochir Suppl (Wien)* 1996; 66:27-31.

49. Chopp M, Li Y, Jiang N, Zhang RL, Prostak J. Antibodies against adhesion molecules reduce apoptosis after transient middle cerebral artery occlusion in rat brain. *J Cereb Blood Flow Metab* 1996; 16:578-584.

50. Yenari MA, Kunis D, Sun GH, et al. Hu23F2G, an antibody recognizing the leukocyte CD11/CD18 integrin, reduces injury in a rabbit model of transient focal cerebral ischemia. *Exp Neurol* 1998; 153:223-33.

51. Deng H, Han HS, Cheng D, Sun GH, Yenari MA. Mild hypothermia inhibits inflammation after experimental stroke and brain inflammation. *Stroke* 2003; 34:2495-2501.

52. Inamasu J, Suga S, Sato S, et al. Post-ischemic hypothermia delayed neutrophil accumulation and microglial activation following transient focal ischemia in rats. *J Neuroimmunol* 2000; 109:66-74.

53. Inamasu J, Suga S, Sato S, et al. Intra-ischemic hypothermia attenuates intercellular adhesion molecule-1 (ICAM-1) and migration of neutrophil. *Neurol Res* 2001; 23:105-111.

54. Kawai N, Okauchi M, Morisaki K, Nagao S. Effects of delayed intraischemic and postischemic hypothermia on a focal model of transient cerebral ischemia in rats. *Stroke* 2000; 31:1982-1989.

55. Wang GJ, Deng HY, Maier CM, Sun GH, Yenari MA. Mild hypothermia reduces ICAM-1 expression, neutrophil infiltration and microglia/monocyte accumulation following experimental stroke. *Neuroscience* 2002; 114:1081-1090.

56. Zhang R, Chopp M, Zhang Z, Jiang N, Powers C. The expression of P- and E-selectins in three models of middle cerebral artery occlusion. *Brain Res* 1998; 785:207-214.

57. Huang J, Kim LJ, Mealey R, et al. Neuronal protection in stroke by an sLex-glycosylated complement inhibitory protein. *Science* 1999; 285:595-599.

58. Zhang RL, Chopp M, Zhang ZG, et al. E-selectin in focal cerebral ischemia and reperfusion in the rat. *J Cereb Blood Flow Metab* 1996; 16:1126-1136.

59. Kitagawa K, Matsumoto M, Mabuchi T, et al. Deficiency of intercellular adhesion molecule 1 attenuates microcirculatory disturbance and infarction size in focal cerebral ischemia. *J Cereb Blood Flow Metab* 1998; 18:1336-1345.

60. Ishikawa M, Sekizuka E, Sato S, et al. Effects of moderate hypothermia on leukocyte-endothelium interaction in the rat pial microvasculature after transient middle cerebral artery occlusion. *Stroke* 1999; 30:1679-1686.

61. Davies CA, Loddick SA, Stroemer RP, Hunt J, Rothwell NJ. An integrated analysis of the progression of cell responses induced by permanent focal middle cerebral artery occlusion in the rat. *Exp Neurol* 1998; 154:199-212.

62. Yrjanheikki J, Keinanen R, Pellikka M, Hokfelt T, Koistinaho J. Tetracyclines inhibit microglial activation and are neuroprotective in global brain ischemia. *Proc Natl Acad Sci U S A* 1998; 95:15769-15774.

63. Han HS, Qiao Y, Karabiyikoglu M, Giffard RG, Yenari MA. Influence of mild hypothermia on inducible nitric oxide synthase expression and reactive nitrogen production in experimental stroke and inflammation. *J Neurosci* 2002; 22:3921-3928.

64. Chan PH. Role of oxidants in ischemic brain damage. *Stroke* 1996; 27:1124-1129.

65. Iadecola C. Bright and dark sides of nitric oxide in ischemic brain injury. *Trends Neurosci* 1997; 20:132-139.

66. Iadecola C, Zhang F, Casey R, Nagayama M, Ross ME. Delayed reduction of ischemic brain injury and neurological deficits in mice lacking the inducible nitric oxide synthase gene. *J Neurosci* 1997; 17:9157-164.

67. Love S. Oxidative stress in brain ischemia. *Brain Pathol* 1999; 9:119-131.

68. Kader A, Frazzini VI, Baker CJ, Solomon RA, Trifiletti RR. Effect of mild hypothermia on nitric oxide synthesis during focal cerebral ischemia. *Neurosurgery* 1994; 35:272-277.

69. Karabiyikoglu M, Han HS, Yenari MA, Steinberg GK. Attenuation of nitric oxide synthase isoform expression by mild hypothermia after focal cerebral ischemia: variations depending on timing of cooling. *J Neurosurg* 2003; 98:1271-1276.

70. Kil HY, Zhang J, Piantadosi CA. Brain temperature alters hydroxyl radical production during cerebral ischemia/reperfusion in rat. *J Cereb Blood Flow Metab* 1996; 16:100-106.

71. Kumura E, Yoshimine T, Takaoka M, et al. Hypothermia suppresses nitric oxide elevation during reperfusion after focal cerebral ischemia in rats. *Neurosci Lett* 1996; 220:45-48.

72. Maier CM, Sun GH, Cheng D, et al. Effects of mild hypothermia on superoxide anion production, superoxide dismutase expression, and activity following transient focal cerebral ischemia. *Neurobiol Dis* 2002; 11:28-42.

73. Si QS, Nakamura Y, Kataoka K. Hypothermic suppression of microglial activation in culture: inhibition of cell proliferation and production of nitric oxide and superoxide, *Neuroscience* 1997; 81:223-229.

75. Kim JS. Cytokines and adhesion molecules in stroke and related diseases. *J Neurol Sci* 1996; 137:69-78.

74. Karibe H, Chen SF, Zarow GJ, et al. Mild intraischemic hypothermia suppresses consumption of endogenous antioxidants after temporary focal ischemia in rats. *Brain Res* 1994; 649:12-18.

76. Buttini M, Sauter A, Boddeke HW. Induction of interleukin-1 beta mRNA after focal cerebral ischaemia in the rat. *Brain Res Mol Brain Res* 1994; 23:126-134.

77. Zhang Z, Chopp M, Goussev A, Powers C. Cerebral vessels express interleukin 1beta after focal cerebral ischemia. *Brain Res* 1998; 784:210-217.

78. Liu T, Clark RK, McDonnell PC, et al. Tumor necrosis factor-alpha expression in ischemic neurons. *Stroke* 1994; 25:1481-1488.

79. Uno H, Matsuyama T, Akita H, Nishimura H, Sugita M. Induction of tumor necrosis factor-alpha in the mouse hippocampus following transient forebrain ischemia. *J Cereb Blood Flow Metab* 1997; 17:491-499.

80. Yanagawa Y, Kawakami M, Okada Y. Moderate hypothermia alters interleukin-6 and interleukin-1alpha reactions in ischemic brain in mice. *Resuscitation* 2002; 53:93-99.

81. Goss .R, Styren SD, Miller PD, et al. Hypothermia attenuates the normal increase in interleukin 1 beta RNA and nerve growth factor following traumatic brain injury in the rat. *J Neurotrauma* 1995; 12:159-167.

82. Li LX, Jiang T, Liu EZ, et al. Effect of intraischemic mild hypothermia on interleukin-1beta and monocyte chemoattractant protein-1 contents in ischemic core of rat cortex after transient focal cerebral ischemia. *Zhonghua Yi Xue Za Zhi* 2003; 83:541-543.

83. Han HS, Karabiyikoglu M, Kelly S, Sobel RA, Yenari MA. Mild hypothermia inhibits nuclear factor-kappaB translocation in experimental stroke. *J Cereb Blood Flow Metab* 2003; 23:589-598.

84. Sutcliffe IT, Smith HA, Stanimirovic D, Hutchison JS. Effects of moderate hypothermia on IL-1 beta-induced leukocyte rolling and adhesion in pial microcirculation of mice and on proinflammatory gene expression in human cerebral endothelial cells. *J Cereb Blood Flow Metab* 2001; 21:1310-1319.

85. Luhm J, Schromm AB, Seydel U, et al. Hypothermia enhances the biological activity of lipopolysaccharide by altering its fluidity state. *Eur J Biochem* 1998; 256:325-333.

86. Matsui T, Ishikawa T, Takeuchi H, Tsukahara M, Maekawa T. Mild hypothermia inhibits IL-10 production in peripheral blood mononuclear cells. *Acta Anaesthesiol Scand* 2004; 48:205-210.

87. Fukuda S, Fini CA, Mabuchi T, et al. Focal cerebral ischemia induces active proteases that degrade microvascular matrix. *Stroke* 2004; 35:998-1004.

88. Lo EH, Wang X, Cuzner ML. Extracellular proteolysis in brain injury and inflammation: role for plasminogen activators and matrix metalloproteinases. *J Neurosci Res* 2002; 69:1-9.

89. Dietrich WD, Busto R, Halley M, Valdes I. The importance of brain temperature in alterations of the blood-brain barrier following cerebral ischemia. *J Neuropathol Exp Neurol* 1990; 49:486-497.

90. Karibe H, Zarow GJ, Graham SH, Weinstein PR. Mild intraischemic hypothermia reduces postischemic hyperperfusion, delayed postischemic hypoperfusion, blood-brain barrier disruption, brain edema, and neuronal damage volume after temporary focal cerebral ischemia in rats. *J Cereb Blood Flow Metab* 1994; 14:620-627.

91. Dempsey RJ, Combs DJ, Maley ME, et al. Moderate hypothermia reduces postischemic edema development and leukotriene production. *Neurosurgery* 1987; 21:177-181.

92. Hamann GF, Burggraf D, Martens HK, et al. Mild to moderate hypothermia prevents microvascular basal lamina antigen loss in experimental focal cerebral ischemia. *Stroke* 2004; 35:764-769.

93. Wagner S, Nagel S, Kluge B, et al. Topographically graded postischemic presence of metalloproteinases is inhibited by hypothermia. *Brain Res* 2003; 984:63-75.
94. Gordon CJ. The therapeutic potential of regulated hypothermia. *Emerg Med J* 2001; 18:81-89.
95. Akaji K, Suga S, Fujino T, et al. Effect of intra-ischemic hypothermia on the expression of c-Fos and c-Jun, and DNA binding activity of AP-1 after focal cerebral ischemia in rat brain. *Brain Res* 2003; 975:149-157.

Chapter 4

FOCAL CEREBRAL ISCHEMIA: CLINICAL STUDIES

Derk W. Krieger, MD, PhD[1], Stefan Schwab, MD[2], Lars P. Kammersgard, MD[3]

[1]*The Cleveland Clinic Foundation, Cleveland, OH, USA*
[2]*University of Heidelberg, Heidelberg, Germany*
[3]*Gentofte University, Hellerup, Denmark*

INTRODUCTION

Acute ischemic stroke is a major leading cause of death and disability throughout the developed world. Although early vascular reperfusion improves the clinical outcome, fewer than 5% of patients with acute ischemic stroke actually receive thrombolytic therapy. The challenge of thrombolytic therapy is that, with time, the ability to recover brain tissue decreases rapidly while vulnerability to reperfusion injury increases. The result of this quandary, a narrow time-window, proved to be the stumbling block in wider dissemination of this treatment. Conceivably, co-administration of a "tissue protectant" could enhance the effectiveness of thrombolysis while expanding the time window and reducing the risks of reperfusion. A promising candidate to serve this purpose is hypothermia. A wealth of animal experiments have demonstrated that hypothermia or simply fever prevention diminishes ischemic damage with transient occlusion followed by reperfusion. In models of permanent occlusion, reduction of infarct size was less impressive (1, 2). In transient ischemia models, hypothermia was most effective when administered during the period of vascular occlusion (intra-ischemic) or immediately after vascular reperfusion (post-ischemic) (3-5). According to these models, hypothermia is efficacious in concert with reperfusion in only a narrow time window. Some investigations suggest that more prolonged periods of hypothermia enhance the benefit of early post-ischemic induction and even may have benefit after permanent occlusion. Consequently, in patients with acute stroke, therapeutic hypothermia will more likely confer benefit in conjunction with early vascular reperfusion and when applied over prolonged periods of time. The use of antipyretic agents has not been shown to effectively reduce core temperature after stroke, although, post-stroke fever can be inhibited. Therapeutic mild (33-36°C) to moderate (28-32°C) hypothermia can be achieved by surface cooling (external cooling) or by using intravenous counter-current heat exchange (endovascular cooling). External cooling is almost invariably associated with imprecise timing and continuation of the hypothermic effect. With endovascular cooling heat is directly removed from, or added to, the thermal core, thus bypassing the heat sink and insulating effects of peripheral tissues. Several early open and controlled studies have shown that endovascular cooling is safe and can effectively manage core temperatures in the mild to moderate hypothermic range. This review of clinical studies will address the advances in the understanding of mechanisms by which hypothermia enhances stroke outcomes and how these insights may help to translate benefits of hypothermia from bench to bedside.

PATHOPHYSIOLOGY OF ISCHEMIC STROKE

Acute ischemic stroke results from the abrupt interruption of focal cerebral blood flow (6, 7). Angiographically visible embolic or thrombotic occlusions have been identified as the cause of stroke in up to 80 percent of patients with symptoms severe enough to warrant early arteriography (8-11). Other causes of decreased cerebral blood flow include abrupt occlusion of small penetrating arteries and arterioles, single or multiple high-grade arterial stenoses with poor blood flow through collateral vessels, arteritis, arterial dissection, venous occlusion, and profound anemia or hyperviscosity (12, 13). The molecular events set off by acute focal ischemia can be simplified as a time-dependent cascade, characterized by decreased energy production, overstimulation of neuronal glutamate receptors (excitotoxicity), excessive intraneuronal accumulation of sodium, chloride, and calcium ions, mitochondrial injury, and eventual cell death (6, 14-16). The fundamental goals of intervention are to restore normal cerebral blood flow as soon as possible and to protect neurons by interrupting or slowing the ischemic cascade (6, 14, 15). Studies using magnetic resonance imaging (MRI) and positron-emission tomography suggest that critical ischemia rapidly produces a core of infarcted brain tissue surrounded by hypoxic but potentially salvageable tissue. (7, 17, 18).

Reperfusion in Ischemic Stroke

Clinical recovery after cerebral ischemia can be hampered by irreversible tissue damage at the time of reperfusion or by ongoing damage as a result of reperfusion, a condition termed "reperfusion injury". Ischemic neuronal damage progresses after stroke onset and becomes irreversible within three hours after onset in non-human primates (19). Reperfusion injury has been demonstrated to peak with reperfusion occurring between three and six hours after onset of ischemia (20, 21). On a cellular level, reperfusion injury appears to be mediated by the accelerated formation of several reactive oxidants including superoxide, hydroxyl, and nitric oxide (NO) radicals. One particularly damaging consequence of reactive oxygen species formation may be single-strand deoxyribonucleic acid (DNA) breakage, leading to activation of the repair enzyme poly (adenosine diphosphate ribose) polymerase (PARP) and PARP-mediated depletion of cellular NAD+ and energy stores (22). Nitric oxide (NO) generated by inducible NO synthase (iNOS or type II NOS), expressed in macrophages, neutrophils, and microglia following immunologic challenge, may also contribute to late tissue injury. In experimental stroke models, post-ischemic reperfusion results in marked endothelial cell dysfunction. Endothelium-dependent vasodilatation is impaired, whereas the responses to endothelium-dependent vasoconstrictors are exaggerated. Increased production of potent vasoconstrictors, such as endothelin-1 and oxygen free radicals, increases vasospasm and reduces blood flow. Furthermore, endothelial dysfunction facilitates a prothrombotic state characterized by platelet and neutrophil activation. Post-ischemic reperfusion induces an inflammatory response further exacerbating tissue injury. Elevation of messenger ribonucleic acid (mRNA) levels of the cytokines tumor necrosis factor (TNF-α) and interleukin (IL)-1β are seen as early as 1 hour after the induction of ischemia. Adhesion molecules on the endothelial cell surface (e.g., intercellular adhesion molecule 1 [ICAM-1], P-selectins, and E-selectins) are also induced, enhancing neutrophil adhesion and passage through the vessel wall into the brain parenchyma. There are several other possible mechanisms by which post-ischemic inflammation can disrupt the blood brain barrier (BBB). Inter-endothelial cell tight junctions, the basal lamina, and perivascular astrocytes comprise the blood brain barrier. Following disruption of the endothelium in focal cerebral ischemia, only the basal lamina prevents extravasation of cellular blood elements into the brain parenchyma. Loss of basal lamina integrity results in interstitial edema and microvascular hemorrhage (23, 24). The main components of the basal lamina include type IV collagen, laminins, fibronectin as well as entactin, nidogen and heparan sulfates (25). These components are degraded at similar rates in non-human primate middle cerebral artery occlusion and reperfusion models (23). Mechanisms of basal lamina degradation are not entirely understood but seem to involve non-cellular proteolytic systems, such as matrix metalloproteinases (MMPs) and the endogenous plasminogen-plasmin system, hydrolyzing components of the basal lamina (26-28). These findings suggest that the ultimate brain injury after cerebral artery occlusion is a result of ischemic damage worsened by reperfusion injury.

THERAPEUTIC HYPOTHERMIA IN ISCHEMIC STROKE

As outlined above, brain injury in cerebral ischemia emerges from the intricate interaction of molecular events set in motion by ischemia and incidents complicating the restoration of cerebral blood flow. Progression of ischemia and reperfusion are time-sensitive suggesting that therapeutic interventions are time-critical and phase specific. The time dependency of thrombolytic therapy is an example of such a time critical intervention. As early as minutes after complete cessation of flow, or up to three hours with ample collateral blood flow, irreversible injury occurs and reperfusion triggers further injury independent of the index ischemic event. Multiple, synergistic effects of hypothermia, affecting ischemia and reperfusion have great potential to be successful in clinical stroke. By nature, hypothermia does not correct the underlying vascular occlusion. Thus, co-administration of hypothermia and thrombolytics must consider time sensitivity and possible interactions between the two. In acute stroke, a correlation between body temperature, initial stroke severity, infarct volume, and clinical outcome has been recognized (29). Several preliminary studies indicate benefit of mild to moderate hypothermia in addition to thrombolytic therapy (30-32). Deep hypothermia (10-20°C) is routinely applied during operative repair of complex intracranial aneurysms or the aortic arch because it can preserve brain tissue from profound ischemia associated with these procedures. Mild to moderate hypothermia can reduce ischemic brain edema in the setting of massive ischemic strokes (33, 34). The hypothermic protection is not simply proportional to a reduction in cerebral metabolic rate, and the traditional view that "colder is better", is being questioned (35).

Time Course of Temperature in Ischemic Stroke

Several studies have claimed that temperature on admission is of prognostic significance in acute stroke (36). Experimental studies showing that *hyper*thermia increases infarct size have lent credibility to this assumption (37). The Copenhagen Stroke Study revealed that admission body temperature is an important determinant even for outcome after stroke. Low body temperature on admission was shown to be an independent predictor of good short and long-term outcome (29, 38). To the contrary, others have suggested that initially low temperature and a later increase in temperature are proportional to stroke severity (39). Similar results were recently reported by the Osaka group. When analyzing the neuroimaging data in their study, the admission temperature was significantly higher in patients with large strokes as opposed to small strokes on computed tomography (CT) imaging over the first four days after stroke onset (40). The hypothalamus presumably plays a pivotal role in body temperature regulation. This region senses changes in local brain temperature, integrates information of temperature from other parts of the body, and sends efferent signals to various regions. Heat-sensitive neurons in the optic area send excitatory signals to vasodilatory neurons in the caudal part of the lateral hypothalamus, ventrolateral periaqueductal gray matter, and the reticular formation, and send inhibitory signals to vasoconstrictive neurons in the rostral part of the ventral tegmental area (41). Experimentally, using a variation of the intraluminal suture middle cerebral artery (MCA) occlusion model, ischemia can be limited to the medial hypothalamus. In these experiments hypothalamic infarcts are unequivocally accompanied by *hyper*thermia, suggesting that damage to the medial hypothalamus is responsible for the rise of body temperature (42). Although these results support the notion that large infarcts disturb temperature regulation they do not exclude the possibility that a sustained rise in temperature during the first days after stroke may have a detrimental effect, further aggravating the neurological deficit.

More importantly, the effects of these uncontrolled temperature fluctuations do not allow conclusions regarding the potential benefits of controlled, therapeutic hypothermia.

Prevention of Fever and Modest Hypothermia

Minimal alterations in temperature have prominent effects on ischemic cell injury and stroke outcome. Antipyretics may reduce body temperature in patients with acute stroke. Three studies have evaluated the efficacy of

acetaminophen and loxoprofen-Na to reduce body temperature in patients
with acute stroke (Table 4-1).

Table 4-1. Studies on prevention of fever and modest hypothermia.

Category	Dippel 2001		Kasner 2002	Naritomi 2002	Kammersgaard 2000
N	25	26	20	17	17
Design	Randomized		Randomized	Case control	Case control
Age	74±14	69±13	70±13	72±8	69±16
Severity (NIHSS)	9±6	10±8	14	18±4	n/a
Severity (SSS)	n/a	n/a	n/a	n/a	26±12
Drug Dose	Acet 3g/d x 5 d	Acet 6g/d x 5 d	Acet 4.5g/d x 24 h	Loxo 180 mg/d x 5 d	"Forced air" x 6 h
Time to Presentation (hrs)	<24	<24	<24	6-12	0-12
Temperature Initial (°C)	37.2	36.9	37.13	36.5	36.8
Temperature Reduction (°C)	- 0.2	0.1	0.22	0.5	1.3
Mortality (%)	1/25 (4%)	4/26 (15%)	1/20 (5%)	2/17 (12%)	1/17 (6%)
Good Outcome [mRS 0-3] (%)	12/25 (48%)	9/26 (35%)	15/20 (80%)	7/17 (41%)	n/a
Poor Outcome [mRS 4-6] (%)	13/25 (52%)	17/26 (65%)	5/20 (20%)	11/17 (59%)	n/a

Acet = acetaminophen, Loxo = loxoprofen-Na, NIHSS = National Institutes of Health Stroke
Scale, SSS = Scandinavian Stroke Scale, mRS = modified Rankin Scale.

The first study (43) randomized seventy-five patients with acute ischemic
stroke confined to the anterior circulation to treatment with either 500 mg
(low dose) or 1000 mg (high dose) acetaminophen compared to placebo,
administered as suppositories 6 times daily during the first 5 days after
stroke onset. The primary outcome measure was rectal temperature at 24
hours after the start of treatment. High-dose acetaminophen resulted in 0.4°C
lower body temperatures than placebo treatment at 24 hours. The mean
reduction from baseline temperature with high-dose acetaminophen was
0.3°C. Low-dose acetaminophen did not lower body temperatures. After 5
days of treatment, no differences in temperature were detectable between the
placebo and the high- or low-dose acetaminophen groups.

The second study (44) randomized 39 patients within 24 hours of onset of
symptoms of stroke to receive 650 mg acetaminophen or placebo every 4
hours for 24 hours. The primary outcome measure was mean core

temperature during the 24-hour study period. The secondary outcome measure was the change in stroke severity. Baseline core temperature was the same: 36.96°C for acetaminophen versus 36.95°C for placebo. During the study period, core temperatures tended to be lower in the acetaminophen group (37.13°C vs 37.35°C). Patients given acetaminophen tended to be more often hypothermic <36.5°C and less often hyperthermic >37.5°C. The change in stroke severity from baseline to 48 hours did not differ between the groups.

The third case control study (40) tested 60 mg of loxoprofen-Na given three times daily for 5 days in 17 patients with acute stroke admitted within six to 12 hours after stroke onset. Control patients consisted of 50 age-matched patients with acute strokes admitted >12 hours after onset. Admission temperatures were identical between the two groups. Axillary temperatures were significantly lower between day two and five in test patients (36.5°C versus >37°C). Stroke severity was similar at admission (National Institutes of Health Stroke Scale [NIHSS] 18±4 in test patients versus 18.7±4.8 in matched controls). The treatment group had less frequent hemorrhagic transformation (3 of 17, 17.5% versus 19 of 50, 38%) and better functional outcome as determined by Barthel Index >75 (7 of 17, 41% versus 6 of 50, 12%).

Feasibility and safety of inducing modest hypothermia by surface cooling in awake patients with acute stroke was evaluated in another case-control study (45). Seventeen patients with acute stroke within 12 hours prior to admission treated with "modest" hypothermia were compared to 56 historic controls admitted within the same time. Directly upon admission the patients received hypothermic therapy for 6 hours using the "forced air" method (Bair Hugger, Augustine Medical, Eden Prairie, Minnesota), which draws room air through a filter, cools the air to a specified temperature (in this study 10°C.), and delivers the air via a hose to a blanket covering the patient. Hence, the surface of the body is cooled through the principle of convection. Compensatory shivering was treated with intravenous administration of meperidine in doses of 25 to 50 mg, given when the patient reported shivering or the investigators observed shivering. All patients developed shivering at some point during the application of forced air cooling. A significant decrease in mean body temperature was achieved after 1 hour of hypothermic therapy (36.4°C vs 36.8°C), the lowest mean body temperature was achieved after 6 hours (35.5°C vs 36.8°C). The hypothermic effect was present until 4 hours after cessation of hypothermic therapy (mean 36.8°C versus 36.5°C). The total mean dose of meperidine given per patient throughout the 6 hour period was 241 mg. Hematocrit, hemoglobin, and albumin increased significantly during hypothermia, suggesting loss of plasma via capillary leak or a cold diuresis. Potassium concentration stayed within normal limits, but increased from a mean of 3.6 mmol/L to 4.1 mmol/L of plasma. There were no significant changes in mean diastolic blood pressure. Mean systolic blood pressure and heart rate, however, decreased significantly from 178 mm Hg to 169 mm Hg and 72 to 68 beats/min, respectively. None of the patients showed signs of significant cardiac arrhythmias or cardiac ischemia on consecutive electrocardiography performed during hypothermic therapy. The frequency of infectious complications was 18% in the patients who underwent hypothermic therapy compared with 13% in the control group. Mortality at 3 months after stroke was 6% in cases vs. 11% in controls, at 6 months, 12% in cases vs. 23% in controls as 6 months (Table 4-1). Final neurological impairment (Scandinavian Stroke Scale score at 6 months) was mean 42.4 points in cases versus 47.9 in controls (lower numbers indicate more severe deficits).

Early administration of antipyretics or modest hypothermia to afebrile patients with acute stroke may result in a small reduction in core temperature that may be beneficial. "Modest" hypothermia can be achieved in wakeful patients with acute stroke by surface cooling with the "forced air" method, using meperidine to treat shivering. Further studies should determine whether this benefit is reproducible and clinically meaningful.

THERAPEUTIC HYPOTHERMIA AND STROKE

Rescue Hypothermia For Massive Stroke

Massive hemispheric strokes typically present with hemiplegia, forced eye and head deviation, and progressive deterioration of consciousness. Almost invariably accompanied by major early infarct signs on computed tomography (CT) this syndrome is caused by terminus internal carotid artery (ICA) and/or proximal middle cerebral artery (MCA) (possibly, anterior cerebral artery) occlusion (46). Even with thrombolysis, the prognosis remains poor and the mortality reportedly high. Transtentorial herniation frequently occurs within 24-96 hours after stroke onset. Medical treatment to counteract intracranial hypertension consists of hyperventilation, osmotherapy, and barbiturate administration and is only rarely effective. Hyperventilation is discouraged because of the concern that hypocarbia may reduce cerebral blood flow and further exacerbate cerebral ischemia. Osmotherapeutics may increase tissue fluid shifts, aggravating brain edema by intracerebral entrapment after passage through the damaged blood brain barrier (47). Barbiturate therapy has also failed to provide benefit in the treatment of postischemic brain edema (48). Decompressive surgery for management of intractable intracranial hypertension as a result of massive stroke and ischemic edema improves cerebral perfusion and mechanical compression of the brain against various intracranial anchors including falx, tentorium, and sphenoid ridge (49). However, there remains controversy as to timing and implementation of hemicraniectomy (50). Ineffectiveness of medical therapy and uncertainties surrounding decompressive surgery necessitate alternative concepts, such as induced hypothermia.

The first clinical investigation, published by the Heidelberg group (33) included data from 25 patients with particularly severe hemispheric infarctions (Table 4-2). Hypothermia was mainly used to curtail intracranial hypertension in the late clinical stages of massive hemispheric strokes. The mean time from onset of symptoms to induction of hypothermia was 14 hours, after which 3.5-6.2 hours were required to achieve a target of 32-33°C. In this study, a cooling blanket with cool ventilator air fanning (Bair Hugger, Augustine Medical, Eden Prairie, Minnesota) was used. Fifty-six percent of patients survived; herniation related to cerebral edema during rewarming was the most concerning complication, being responsible for all mortalities. Among the survivors, the median Scandinavian Stroke Scale was 29 after 4 weeks, and 38 after 4 months; the median Barthel Index was 70 and the mean Rankin scale was 2.6. The same group reported in 2001 on a larger cohort of 50 patients with cerebral infarction involving at least the complete middle cerebral artery territory treated with mild to moderate hypothermia (34) (Table 4-2). Hypothermia was induced within 22±9 hours after stroke onset and maintained for 24 to 72 hours. Subsequently, patients were passively rewarmed over a mean duration of 17 hours. Time required for cooling to <33°C varied from 3.5 to 11 hours. The most frequent complications of hypothermic therapy were thrombocytopenia (70%), bradycardia (62%), and pneumonia (48%). Four patients (8%) died during hypothermia as a result of severe coagulopathy, cardiac failure, or uncontrollable intracranial hypertension. An additional 15 patients (30%) died during or after rewarming because of rebound intracranial hypertension and fatal herniation. Rapid (<16 hours) rewarming, in particular, was associated with this life-threatening complication. At 3 months, the mean Barthel Index was 65 (range, 10 to 85), and the mean Rankin Scale score was 2.9 points (range, 2 to 5). These results suggest that mild to moderate hypothermia decreases elevated intracranial hypertension in massive strokes. Although critical rebound intracranial hypertension upon rewarming and adverse clinical events are frequently encountered, favorable outcomes can be achieved in some patients.

Table 4-2. Studies on rescue-hypothermia for massive hemispheric stroke.

Category	Schwab 1998	Schwab 2001
N	25	50
Age	49±14	57±8
Severity [NIHSS] (range)	n/a	25 (15-32)
Severity [SSS] (range)	24 (18-28)	n/a
Time to Hypothermia (hrs)	14 (4-24)	23 (4-75)
Mortality (%)	11/25 (44%)	19/50 (38%)
Mean mRS (range)	2.6 (2-4)	2.9 (2-5)
Mean Barthel Index (range)	70 (60-85)	65 (10-80)

NIHSS = National Institutes of Health Stroke Scale, SSS = Scandinavian Stroke Scale.

Adjunctive Hypothermia in Acute Ischemic Stroke

The brain is particularly vulnerable to ischemia. In part, the vulnerability of brain tissue to ischemic damage reflects its high metabolic rate. In addition, central neurons have a near exclusive dependence on glucose as an energy substrate; and brain stores of glucose or glycogen are limited. Nevertheless, recent evidence indicates that energetics considerations and energy substrate limitations are not solely responsible for the brain's heightened vulnerability to ischemia. Rather, it appears that the brain's intrinsic cell-cell and intracellular signaling mechanisms, normally responsible for information processing, become harmful under ischemic conditions, hastening energy failure and enhancing the final pathways underlying ischemic cell death in all tissues. Furthermore, reperfusion events, including free radical production, activation of catabolic enzymes, membrane failure, apoptosis, and inflammation contribute to cell death and organ dysfunction independent of the ischemic event.

Hypothermia is known to affect platelet function and coagulation (51, 52). Thrombolytic therapy based on protein interactions may also be affected by hypothermia. *In vitro*, the tissue-type plasminogen activator (t-PA) effect on clot lysis is temperature dependent. Cooling to 30-33°C caused a 2-4% decrease in t-PA activity in a clot lysis assay (53). *In vitro* data from the manufacturer indicate that t-PA activity falls by 50% when the clot temperature decreases to 30°C (Genentech, South San Francisco, CA data unpublished of file). Others have confirmed this finding (54). Data from *in vitro* studies must be interpreted with caution, however, because hypothermia affects all aspects of the clotting cascade and fibrinolytic pathways, including inhibitors. There are two models that have evaluated the interaction of t-PA and hypothermia *in vivo*. In a rat embolic stroke model, intra-ischemic mild hypothermia (32°C) enhanced angiographic reperfusion as effectively as t-PA. Sixteen rats were externally cooled followed by middle cerebral artery embolization. Hypothermia was induced at onset ischemia and maintained for three hours, following which body temperature was allowed to passively rewarm to 37°C. The animals were killed for infarct size determination between 48 and 72 hours. Twenty-six rats were treated with human recombinant t-PA (20 mg/kg i.v. during 45 min), started two hours after embolization. In addition, 14 rats were pre-treated with hypothermia for three hours followed by t-PA infusion starting at the second hour. Thrombolytic therapy reduced median infarct volume by 76% (p = 0.006) compared to controls. Three hours of hypothermia reduced infarct volume by 92% (p = 0.0007). Combinatory hypothermia and thrombolysis had neither additive nor reduced effects on final infarct size (55). In a rabbit carotid thrombosis model t-PA (9mg/kg) was administered intravenously to normothermic and hypothermic animals using a frontloaded protocol over 90 minutes. Time to reperfusion, incidence of re-occlusion, and incisional blood loss were measured. Carotid temperature in the hypothermic animals was 30.4 ± 1.3^0C vs. 38 ± 0.3^0C in the normothermic animals (p<.01). There was no significant difference in median time to reperfusion in hypothermic versus normothermic animals (107 min vs. 106 min, p=ns). The incidence of re-occlusion tended to be higher in the normothermic group than the hypothermic group (5 of 7 vs. 2 of 7), while incisional blood loss was greater in the normothermic animals (41±27 g vs. 14±10 g, p<.05) (56). In view of this data, there is no obvious contraindication to the combination of thrombolysis and mild hypothermia although the effect of thrombolytic activity may be marginally decreased.

The first study published to address the feasibility and safety of thrombolysis and adjunctive hypothermia was the Cooling for Acute Ischemic Brain Damage (COOL AID) open pilot study (33), followed by a comprehensive study published by the Osaka group (40). In both studies hypothermia was only considered in patients with severe strokes when reperfusion was not feasible or ineffectual (Table 4-3).

In COOL AID, hypothermia was induced in 10 patients with massive stroke using surface cooling methods. Although not randomized, this study utilized concurrent patients with severe strokes that underwent thrombolysis but not hypothermia as a control group. Hypothermia was successfully initiated in all 10 patients at a mean of 6.2±1.3 hours after stroke onset. Time to reach core target temperature of 32°C averaged 3.5±1.5 hours (range 2 to 6.5 hours). Hypothermia at 32±1°C was maintained for a mean of 22.8±8 hours (range 11 to 41 hours). For 9 of the 10 patients, the target temperature was overshot (the lowest temperature reached was 28.4°C.). Rewarming of patients to 37°C required 22.6±15.6 hours (range 6.5 to 49.8 hours) as a result of the slow rewarming process at a mean of 0.21°C/h. The total duration of hypothermia (body temperature <36°C.) averaged 47.4±20.4

hours (range 23.5 to 96 hours). Except for sinus bradycardia, there were no significant differences in minor or critical event rates. Bradycardia was temporary and asymptomatic in most cases; one patient required a prophylactic transvenous pacemaker for a heart rate of <40 bpm associated with hypotension. All other events associated with hypothermia therapy did not result in any significant complications. Of all laboratory measures, only pH, PCO_2, and potassium concentrations were significantly altered by hypothermia, and all quickly corrected without sequela on return to normothermia. There were 3 deaths in the hypothermia group. In the non-hypothermia patients there were 2 deaths and 3 patients remained in a vegetative state at three months. Three-month neurologic outcomes using the modified Rankin scale were better in the hypothermia group, although these numbers did not reach statistical significance.

Table 4-3. Pooled data from COOL AID I & II and Osaka patients.

CATEGORY	CONTROLS[1]	REPERFUSION[1]	EXTERNAL COOLING[2]	ENDOVASCULAR COOLING[3]
N	35	23	22	17
Age	66±10	69±12	64±12	61±8
Severity (NIHSS)	20±7	17±3	21±7	15±4
Time to Presentation (hrs)	0-12	0-6	0-6	0-12
Time to Hypothermia (hrs)	n/a	n/a	7.5	9
Mortality (%)	9/36 (26%)	5/23 (22%)	5/22 (23%)	5/17 (29%)
Good Outcome [mRS 0-3] (%)	6/35 (17%)	6/23 (26%)	12/22 (55%)	7/17 (41%)
Poor Outcome [mRS 4-6] (%)	29/35 (83%)	17/23 (74%)	10/22 (45%)	10/17 (59%)
Mean mRS (range)	n/a	2.9 (0-4)	2.4 (0-4)	2.8 (0-5)

[1]COOL AID I non-hypothermic patients, COOL AID II controls, and Osaka matched control patients

[2]COOL AID I hypothermic patients and Osaka hypothermic patients excluding patient 9 (basilar occlusion)

[3]COOL AID II hypothermic patients

NIHSS = National Institutes of Health Stroke Scale, mRS = modified Rankin Scale.

The Osaka study included twelve patients with massive hemispheric strokes induced with surface cooling methodology to 33°C core temperature followed with serial CT imaging (40). Entry criteria included age below 75 years, admission within 4 hours after stroke, hemiplegia and clouded consciousness, major anterior circulation occlusion, and no improvement with thrombolytic therapy. Mild hypothermia was induced in the stroke unit using surface cooling methodology under general anesthesia. There were seven patients with acute internal carotid artery and five with middle cerebral artery occlusions. Eight patients received thrombolytic therapy (7 intravenously and 1 intra-arterially) prior to induction of hypothermia and 4 were cooled without prior thrombolytic therapy. Brain temperature was monitored in the internal jugular bulb and core temperature in the bladder. The initial stroke severity was NIHSS 21.8±9.8, i.e., unaffected by thrombolytic therapy within 4 hours, and cooling was initiated at 3.6±0.8 hours after stroke onset. Target temperature was achieved 1.6±0.7 hours after initiation. The hypothermia was continued for 3-6 days depending on size of stroke and mass effect on serial CT scans. Rewarming was deliberately slow, approximately 1-2°C/day. Five patients developed pneumonia and 3 developed moderate congestive heart failure during induced hypothermia all of which responded to medical therapy. Two patients died of recurrent stroke or massive cerebral hemorrhage during induced hypothermia. One additional patient required evacuation of a large hemorrhagic transformation during hypothermia. Altogether ten patients survived with good functional recovery at three months. In the survivors, subsequent CT revealed no intracranial mass shifts and no or only little parenchymal enhancement on serial contrast CT scans. There was gradual expansion of the ischemic lesion only in patients with carotid occlusions that did not reperfuse. Ischemic lesions were distinctly discriminated from surrounding brain tissue as early as 48 hours after onset.

Delay in heat transfer from the periphery to the core makes precise control of the temperature with surface cooling challenging. Wide fluctuations in temperature require frequent adjustments of the cooling apparatus to prevent overshoot and undershoot. Endovascular cooling using a counter-current heat exchange catheter directly removes heat from the core resulting in rapid induction of hypothermia and precise temperature control (57, 58).

Intubation, sedation, and neuromuscular blockade (all frequently used with therapeutic hypothermia to induce poikilothermia and prevent shivering) preclude clinical assessment in patients with stroke. A method to counteract shivering in awake patients is needed in order for hypothermia to be safely and broadly applicable in patients with ischemic strokes. Recently, the combination of meperidine and buspirone (a 5-HT$_{1A}$ partial agonist) was found to synergistically reduce the shivering threshold in humans without causing significant sedation or respiratory depression (59). COOL AID II was a randomized pilot clinical trial testing whether endovascular cooling with a heat exchange catheter combined with meperidine and buspirone to minimize shivering could achieve hypothermia rapidly without intubation in awake patients with acute ischemic stroke (60) (Table 4-3). Endovascular cooling was found to be feasible and generally safe in patients with moderate to severe anterior circulation territory ischemic infarct. The heat-exchange catheter could be inserted quickly and easily in the critical care unit, emergency department or angiography suite. Reduction in core temperature was rapid with a mean time to target temperature of 77 ± 44 minutes. In contrast to surface cooling, in which 90% of patients overshot the target temperature (the lowest temperature being 28.4°C) (32), no overshoot was observed with endovascular cooling (the lowest temperature was 32.8°C). In a few patients, most commonly due to catheter misplacement, the target temperature of 33°C was not achieved. This issue was readily addressed and reflects a learning curve with the technology. Only one patient, a woman with a massive stroke, was intubated during active cooling. All other 17 hypothermia patients remained awake and responsive throughout the period of hypothermia. Although evidence of clinical efficacy requires a larger trial, there was a trend towards reduced infarct volumes in those treated with hypothermia. Despite having larger, more severe strokes at baseline, the mean infarct volume increase in the hypothermia group was less than that of the control group. This was especially apparent in the subset of patients who cooled well. As anticipated, given the small sample size of this pilot trial, there was no difference in clinical outcomes at 3 months in NIH Stroke Scale scores and Modified Rankin Scale scores.

SUMMARY

Hypothermia attains salutary effects in animal models of focal cerebral ischemia. Experimental work and preliminary clinical studies suggest detrimental effect of early hyperthermia. There is a suggestion of some benefit of temperature management (i.e., prevention of *hyper*thermia) in patients with acute ischemic stroke. In contrast, mild to moderate hypothermia is clearly effective in transient occlusion/reperfusion models. Similar to thrombolysis, favorable results accrue within a three hour time window with reperfusion obtained in two hours and hypothermia induced within the next hour. Prolonged cooling with gradually rewarming may be superior to brief cooling. Imprecise timing and continuation of the hypothermic effect by surface cooling methods can be effectively overcome by use of intravenous heat exchangers. Preliminary studies established reasonable safety and feasibility in wakeful patients with acute ischemic stroke undergoing thrombolysis. Not unexpectedly, adverse events increase with age and stroke severity as well as duration of hypothermia. Larger studies are needed to determine the benefit of adjunctive hypothermia in acute ischemic stroke.

REFERENCES

1. Morikawa E, Ginsberg MD, Dietrich WD et al. The significance of brain temperature in focal cerebral ischemia: Histopathological consequences of middle cerebral artery occlusion in the rat. *J Cereb Blood Flow Metab* 1992; 12:380-389.
2. Ridenour TR, Warner DS, Todd MM, McAllister AC. Mild hypothermia reduces infarct size resulting from temporary but not permanent focal ischemia in rats. *Stroke* 1992; 23:733-738.
3. Maier CM, Ahern K, Cheng ML, et al. Optimal depth and duration of mild hypothermia in a focal model of transient cerebral ischemia. Effects on neurologic outcome, infarct size, apoptosis, and inflammation. *Stroke* 1998; 29:2171–2180.
4. Yanamoto H, Nagata I, Nakahara I et al. Combination of intraischemic and postischemic hypothermia provides potent and persistent neuroprotection against temporary focal ischemia in rats. *Stroke* 1999; 30:2720-2726.
5. Maier CM, Sun G, Kunis D, et al. Delayed induction and long-term effects of mild hypothermia in a focal model of transient cerebral ischemia: neurological outcome and infarct size. *J Neurosurg* 2001; 94:90-96.
6. Zivin JA. Factors determining the therapeutic window for stroke. *Neurology* 1998; 50:599-603.
7. Heiss WD, Thiel A, Grond M, Graf R. Which targets are relevant for therapy of acute ischemic stroke? *Stroke* 1999; 30:1486-1489.
8. Furlan A, Higashida R, Wechsler L, et al. Intra-arterial prourokinase for acute ischemic stroke: the PROACT II study: a randomized controlled trial. *JAMA* 1999; 282:2003-2011.
9. Del Zoppo GJ, Higashida RT, Furlan AJ, et al. PROACT: a phase II randomized trial of recombinant pro-urokinase by direct arterial delivery in acute middle cerebral artery stroke. *Stroke* 1998; 29:4-11.
10. Fieschi C, Argentino C, Lenzi GL, et al. Clinical and instrumental evaluation of patients with ischemic stroke within the first six hours. *J Neurol Sci* 1989; 91:311-321.
11. Wolpert SM, Bruckmann H, Greenlee R, et al. Neuroradiologic evaluation of patients with acute stroke treated with recombinant tissue plasminogen activator. *Am J Neuroradiol* 1993; 14:3-13.
12. Sherman DG, Easton JD, Kagan-Hallet KS. Spectrum of pathology responsible for ischemic stroke. In: Moore WS, ed. *Surgery for cerebrovascular disease.* Philadelphia: W.B. Saunders, 1996: pp 43-47.
13. Bock RW, Lusby RJ. Lesions, dynamics, and pathogenetic mechanisms responsible for ischemic events in the brain. In: Moore WS, ed. *Surgery for cerebrovascular disease.* Philadelphia: W.B. Saunders, 1996: pp 48-71.
14. Rosenblum WI. Histopathologic clues to the pathways of neuronal death following ischemia/hypoxia. *J Neurotrauma* 1997; 14:313-326
15. Lee JM, Zipfel GJ, Choi DW. The changing landscape of ischaemic brain injury mechanisms. *Nature* 1999; 399:Suppl:A7-A14.
16. Kristian T, Siesjo BK. Calcium in ischemic cell death. Stroke 1998, 29:705-718.
17. Nagesh V, Welch KM, Windham JP, et al. Time course of ADCw changes in ischemic stroke: beyond the human eye! *Stroke* 1998; 29:1778-1782.
18. Baron J. Mapping the ischaemic penumbra with PET: implications for acute stroke treatment. *Cerebrovasc Dis* 1999; 9:193-201.
19. Jones TH, Morawetz RB, Crowell RM, et al. Thresholds of focal cerebral ischemia in awake monkeys. *J Neurosurg* 1981; 54:773-782

20. Aronowski J, Strong R, Grotta JC. Reperfusion injury: demonstration of brain damage produced by reperfusion after transient focal ischemia in rats. *J Cereb Blood Flow Metab* 1997; 17:1048-1056.

21. Kawai N, Okauchi M, Morisaki K, Nagao S. Effects of delayed intraischemic and postischemic hypothermia on a focal model of transient cerebral ischemia in rats. *Stroke* 2000; 31:1982–1989.

22. Szabo, C., and Dawson, V.L. Role of poly (ADP-ribose) synthetase inflammation and ischaemia-reperfusion. *Trends Pharmacol. Sci* 1998; 19:287–298.

23. Hamann GF, Okada Y, del Zoppo GJ. Hemorrhagic transformation and microvascular integrity during focal cerebral ischemia/reperfusion. *J Cereb Blood Flow Metab* 1996; 16:1373-1378.

24. Hamann GF, Okada Y, Fitridge R, del Zoppo GJ. Microvascular basal lamina antigens disappear during cerebral ischemia and reperfusion. *Stroke* 1995; 26:2120-2126.

25. Yurchenco PD, Schittny JC. Molecular architecture of basement membranes. *FASEB J* 1990; 4:1577-1590.

26. Del Zoppo GJ, von Kummer R, Hamann GF. Ischaemic damage of brain microvessels: inherent risks for thrombolytic treatment in stroke. *J Neur, Neurosurg & Psych* 1998; 65:1-9.

27. Hamann GF, del Zoppo GJ, von Kummer R. Hemorrhagic transformation of cerebral infarction - possible mechanisms. *Thromb Haemost* 1999; 82 (Suppl.):92-94.

28. Petty MA, Wettstein JG. Elements of cerebral microvascular ischaemia. *Brain Res Rev* 2001; 36:23- 34.

29. Reith J, Jørgensen HS, Pedersen PM, et al. Body temperature in acute stroke: relation to stroke severity, infarct size, mortality, and outcome. *Lancet* 1996; 347:422-425.

30. Naritomi H, Shimizu T, Oe H, et al. Mild hypothermia in acute embolic stroke: a pilot study. *J Stroke and Cereb Dis* 1996; 6:193-196.

31. Shimizu T, Naritomi H, Kakud W, et al. Mild hypothermia is effective for the treatment of acute embolic stroke if induced within 24 hours after onset but not in the later phase. *J Cereb Blood Flow Metab* 1997; 17:42.

32. Krieger DW, DeGeorgia M, Abou-Chebl A, et al. Cooling for acute ischemic brain damage (COOL AID): an open pilot study of induced hypothermia in acute ischemic stroke. *Stroke* 2001; 32:1847-1854.

33. Schwab S, Schwarz S, Spranger M, et al. Moderate hypothermia in the treatment of patients with severe middle cerebral artery infarction. *Stroke* 1998; 29:2461-2466

34. Schwab S, Georgiadis D, Berrouschot J, et al. Feasibility and Safety of Moderate Hypothermia After Massive Hemispheric Infarction. *Stroke* 2001; 32:2033-2035

35. Michenfelder J. Protecting the brain. In: Michenfelder J. ed. *Anesthesia & the Brain. Clinical, Functional, Metabolic and Vascular Correlates.* 1st Ed. Churchill Livingstone, USA, 1988: pp 181-193.

36. Hajat C, Hajat S, Sharma P. Effects of post stroke pyrexia on stroke outcome: a meta-analysis of studies in patients. *Stroke* 2000; 31:410-414.

37. Busto R, Dietrich WD, Globus MY-T et al. Small differences in intraischemic brain temperature critically determine the extent of ischemic neuronal injury. *J Cereb Blood Flow Metab* 1987; 7:729-738.

38. Kammersgaard LP, Rasmussen BH, Jørgensen HS, et al. Feasibility and safety of inducing modest hypothermia in awake patients with acute stroke through surface cooling. *Stroke* 2000; 31:2251-2256.

39. Boysen G, Christensen H. Stroke severity determines body temperature in acute stroke. Stroke 2001; 32:413-417.

40. Naritomi H, Nagatsuka K, Miyashita K, et al. The importance of thermal changes in the pathophysiology of stroke: post-stroke fever and hypothermia therapy. In: Kikuchi H (Ed) *Strategic Medical Science Against Brain Attack*. Springer Verlag, Tokyo 2002: pp 171-185.

41. Zhang Y-H, Hosono T, Yanase-Fujiwara M, et al. Effect of midbrain stimulation on thermoregulatory vasomotor response in rats. *J Physiol* 1997; 503:177–186.

42. He Z, Yamawaki T, Yang S, et al. Experimental model of small deep infarcts involving the hypothalamus in rats. Changes in body temperature and postural reflex. *Stroke* 1999; 30:2743-2751.

43. Dippel DWJ, Van Breda EJ, Van Gemert HMA, et al. Effect of paracetamol (acetaminophen) on body temperature in acute ischemic stroke. A double-blind, randomized phase II clinical trial. *Stroke* 2001; 32:1607-1612.

44. Kasner SE, Wein T, Piriyawat P, et al. Acetaminophen for altering body temperature in acute stroke. A randomized clinical trial. *Stroke* 2002; 33:130-135.

45. Kammersgaard L, Rasmussen B, Jorgensen H, et al. Feasibility and safety of inducing modest hypothermia in awake patients with acute stroke through surface cooling. *Stroke* 2000; 31:2251-2256.

46. Hacke W, Schwab S, Horn M, et al. Malignant middle cerebral artery territory infarction: clinical course and prognostic signs. *Arch Neurol* 1996; 53:309 –315.

47. Frank JI. Large hemispheric infarction, deterioration, and intracranial pressure. *Neurology* 1995; 45:1286-1290.

48. Schwab S, Spranger M, Schwarz S, Hacke W. Barbiturate coma in severe hemispheric stroke: useful or obsolete? *Neurology* 1997; 48:1608-1613.

49. Rieke K, Schwab S, Krieger D, et al. Decompressive surgery in space-occupying hemispheric infarction: results of an open, prospective trial. *Crit Care Med* 1995; 23:1576-1587.

50. Schwab S, Steiner T, Aschoff A, et al. Early hemicraniectomy in patients with complete middle cerebral artery infarction. *Stroke* 1998; 29:1888-1893.

51. Faraday N, Rosenfeld BA. In vitro hypothermia enhances platelet GPIIb-IIIa activation and P-selectin expression. *Anesthesiolog* 1998; 88:1579-1585.

52. Watts DD, Trask A, Soeken K, et al. Hypothermic coagulopathy in trauma: effect of varying levels of hypothermia on enzyme speed, platelet function, and fibrinolytic activity. *J Trauma* 1998; 44:846-854.

53. Yenari MA, Palmer JT, Bracci P, Steinberg GK. Thrombolysis with Tissue plasminogen activator (tpa) is temperature dependent. *Thromb Res* 1995; 77:475-481.

54. Schwarzenberg H, Muller-Hulsbeck S, Brossman J et al. Hyperthermic fibrinolysis with rt-PA: in vitro results. *Cardiovasc Intervent Radiol* 1998; 21:142-145.

55. Meden P, Overgaard K, Pedersen H, Boysen G. Effect of hypothermia and delayed thrombolysis in a rat embolic stroke model. *Acta Neurol Scand* 1994; 90:91-98.

56. Chair KM, Gao DW, Dae MW. Influence of Mild Hypothermia on Tissue Plasminogen Activator-induced Clot Lysis in Carotid Thrombosis. Presentation at TCT 2002, the annual meeting of Transcatheter Cardiovascular Therapeutics.

57. Georgiadis D, Schwarz S, Kollmar R, Schwab S. Endovascular Cooling for Moderate Hypothermia in Patients With Acute Stroke First Results of a Novel Approach. *Stroke* 2001; 32:2550-2553.

58. Dixon SR, Whitbourn RJ, Dae MW, et al. Induction of Mild Systemic Hypothermia With Endovascular Cooling During Primary Percutaneous Coronary Intervention for Acute Myocardial Infarction. *J Am Coll Cardiol* 2002;40:1928–1934.

59. Mokhtarani M, Mahgoub A, Morioka N, et al. Buspirone and meperidine synergistically reduce the shivering threshold. *Anesth Analg* 2001; 93:1233–1239.

60. DeGeorgia M, Krieger DW, Abou-Chebl A, et al. Cooling for Acute Ischemic Brain Damage (COOL AID): A Feasibility Trial of Endovascular Cooling. *Neurology* 2004; 63:312-317.

Chapter 5

TRAUMATIC BRAIN INJURY: LABORATORY STUDIES

Patrick M. Kochanek, MD, Larry W. Jenkins, PhD, Robert S.B. Clark, MD
Safar Center for Resuscitation Research, University of Pittsburgh, Pittsburgh, PA, USA

INTRODUCTION

This chapter will address the use of therapeutic hypothermia in traumatic brain injury (TBI). Hypothermia has a long-standing history of clinical use in the management of patients with severe TBI, specifically as a second tier therapy in the treatment of refractory intracranial hypertension. The resurgence in the interest in the use of mild and moderate hypothermia in experimental cerebral ischemia and cardiac arrest in the late 1980s and early 1990s (culminating in its recent successful translation to clinical use for cardiac arrest) prompted parallel investigation in TBI beginning in 1991. This chapter will focus on that work—specifically, both laboratory and clinical investigation in the use of therapeutic hypothermia in TBI since 1991.

The potential value of therapeutic hypothermia in the treatment of patients with severe TBI was suggested by Charles Phelps as early as 1897 (1), and may have even earlier roots. Phelps, in his classic treatise on "Traumatic Injuries of the Brain and its Membranes" recommended the application of an "ice cap" which, with the exception of trephination, he viewed as the most "directly curative resource." A number of reports in the mid 20th century suggested beneficial effects of hypothermia in patients with severe TBI (2-6) but these were not controlled clinical trials. Rosomoff reported on the use of moderate hypothermia in experimental TBI in a series of studies in dogs in the late 1950s and early 1960s (7-9). Beneficial effects of hypothermia on both mortality rate and specific secondary injury mechanisms, such as local cerebral inflammation, were shown. State-of-the-art reviews by central nervous system (CNS) trauma experts written in the 1960s and early 1970s, such as Langfitt et al (10), clearly document that moderate hypothermia had become part of the routine clinical treatment of patients with severe TBI, particularly those with intracranial hypertension. Even in the classic first report of the use of continuous intracranial pressure (ICP) monitoring in patients with severe TBI, by Lundberg et al (11), moderate hypothermia was already an integral component of the standard treatment regimen. In the early 1980s, moderate hypothermia gradually fell out of favor--likely as a result of infectious complications associated with its prolonged use. Documentation of complications with the prolonged use of moderate hypothermia, although limited, was most convincing in the literature on management of pediatric victims of near-drowning accidents (12, 13). These reports, however, greatly influenced clinicians treating patients with severe TBI, along with other CNS insults, and therapeutic hypothermia was gradually abandoned (14).

STUDIES OF THERAPEUTIC HYPOTHERMIA IN LABORATORY MODELS OF TBI

Following the resurgence of interest in the application of mild hypothermia in experimental incomplete cerebral ischemia in rats and cardiac arrest in dogs, reports began to resurface on the beneficial effects of both moderate and mild hypothermia in experimental TBI. In 1991, Clifton et al (15) studied the effect of moderate (30°C) and mild (33°C) hypothermia after fluid percussion injury in rats. Rats were cooled before injury and maintained at target temperature for only 1 h. Despite this rather brief period of hypothermia, motor deficits -- assessed over several days posttrauma -- were attenuated versus those seen after TBI in normothermic rats. In Clifton's report, mild hypothermia was shown to be effective, but moderate hypothermia was even more beneficial. Mortality rate was reduced by moderate hypothermia vs. that seen in rats treated with either mild hypothermia or normothermia. This publication was followed by a flurry of over 40 reports from numerous laboratories from the early 1990s to the present investigating the effects of hypothermia on cellular and molecular mechanisms, intracranial dynamics, and outcome in experimental TBI. Over 90% of these reports have demonstrated a beneficial effect of hypothermia in experimental TBI (Table 5-1).

Table 5-1. Synopsis of selected studies of therapeutic hypothermia in experimental traumatic brain injury since 1991

Date (Citation)	Species/ Model	Temperature	Outcome parameter(s)	Key Finding(s)
1991 (15)	Rat/[1]FPI	30°C, 33°C	Motor function and mortality	Hypothermia reduced motor deficits and mortality, 30°C better than 33°C
1992 (29)	Rat/FPI	30°C	[2]BBB	Hypothermia reduced BBB injury
1993 (51)	Rat/FPI	30°C	[3]MAP2	Hypothermia reduced MAP2 loss
1993 (52)	Rat/FPI	30°C	Motor function	Hypothermia reduced motor deficits, 30 min treatment window
1993 (16)	Rat/FPI	30°C	[3]CSF [4]ACh levels	Hypothermia reduced the increase in ACh
1993 (47)	Rat/CCI	32-33°C	Histology [5]EAA levels by microdialysis	Hypothermia reduced lesion volume but not EAA levels
1993 (23)	Dog/Epidural balloon	31°C 5 h 35 °C 5-62 h	[6]ICP and histopathology	31°C reduced ICP
1994 (27)	Rat/FPI	30°C	Histopathology	Hypothermia reduced cell loss in CA3 and CA4 loss and contusion volume
1994 (53)	Rat/ Contusion		[7]SOD [8]mRNA	No effect
1995 (43)	Rat/[9]CCI	32°C	[10]IL-1 and [11]NGF mRNA	Increases in both outcome parameters were reduced by hypothermia
1995 (54)	Rat/FPI	30-31.5°C	[12]HSP72	Increase in HSP72 reduced by hypothermia
1995 (17)	Rat/FPI	30°C	Motor and cognitive function	Hypothermia reduced functional deficits
1995 (46)	Rat/FPI	30°C	Glutamate [13]DHBA	Hypothermia reduced the increases in both outcome parameters
1996 (30)	Rat/CCI with hypotension	35.5°C	BBB	Hypothermia reduced BBB damage
1996 (22)	Immature Rat/Weight-drop	32°C	Contusion volume and edema	Hypothermia delayed edema formation but had no effect on contusion volume
1996 (55)	Rat/CCI	32°C, 35.4°C	Mortality	Both 32°C and 35.4°C reduced mortality rates
1996 (33)	Rat/CCI	32°C and/or Tirilizad	Axonal damage	Axonal damage reduced by either therapy but effects were not additive
1997 (40)	Rat/CCI	32°C	[14]PMN accumulation, [15]ICAM-1, [16]E-sel	Hypothermia reduced PMN accumulation

Date (Citation)	Species/ Model	Temperature	Outcome parameter(s)	Key Finding(s)
1997 (31)	Rat/CCI	30°C	Edema and cognitive outcome	Hypothermia reduced edema, no effect on cognitive deficits
1997 (56)	Rat/Weight-drop	32°C	EAA	Hypothermia did not reduce EAA levels
1997 (57)	Rat/Weight-drop	32°C	Nitrite and nitrate levels by microdialysis	Increase totally blocked by hypothermia
1998 (18)	Rat/CCI	32°C	Functional outcome and histopathology	Hypothermia reduced functional deficits; no effect on contusion volume or CA1/CA3 cell counts
1998 (26)	Dog/Epidural balloon	31°C	[17]ICP and herniation	ICP was reduced during cooling
1998 (58)	Rat/Freeze injury	32°C	[18]TUNEL and [19]DNA ladders	Hypothermia attenuated the increase in markers of apoptosis
1998 (48)	Rat/Impact acceleration	32°C	[20]APP levels	Hypothermia reduced APP positive axons
1999 (49)	Rat/FPI	30°C	[21]CBF and [22]CMRglu	After rewarming in the hypothermia group, CMR and CBF were mismatched at 3 h
1999 (45)	Rat/FPI	30°C	[23]cNOS and [24]iNOS	Hypothermia reduced the early increase in cNOS and the delayed increase in iNOS
1999 (37)	Rat/Impact acceleration with hypoxemia/ hypotension	30°C	Histopathology	Hypothermia provided almost complete protection
1999 (34)	Rat/Impact acceleration	32°C	Spectrin proteolysis	Marked reduction by hypothermia
2000 (41)	Rat/FPI	30°C	Myeloperoxidase	Hypothermia reduced the posttraumatic increase
2000 (24)	Rat/CCI with Hypoxemia	32°C	Functional outcome and histopathology	No effect of hypothermia
2000 (19)	Rat/CCI	32°C and/or [25]FGF	Functional outcome and histopathology	Hypothermia or FGF improved functional outcome but effects were not additive
2001 (21)	Rat/CCI	30°C	Functional outcome	Hypothermia was effective but results depended on level of injury severity
2001 (35)	Rat/Impact acceleration	32°C and/or [26]CyA	APP	Rewarming induced axonal injury which was attenuated by CyA
2001 (59)	Rat/Impact acceleration; propofol vs. isoflurane	33-34°C	CBF and ICP	Hypothermia with propofol reduced ICP most effectively

Date (Citation)	Species/ Model	Temperature	Outcome parameter(s)	Key Finding(s)
2001 (36)	Rat/Impact acceleration	32°C and/or FK506	APP	Rewarming induced axonal injury which was attenuated by FK506; implicates calcineurin as a target
2001 (25)	Rat/FPI with hypoxemia	30°C	Contusion volume	Demonstrated importance of rewarming rate
2001 (32)	Rat/CCI	30°C	Functional outcome and edema	60 min therapeutic window for beneficial effect of hypothermia on functional outcome and edema
2001 (60)	Rat/Impact acceleration	32°C	TUNEL and DNA ladders	Hypothermia attenuated TUNEL positivity in CA2 and CA3
2002 (20)	Rat/CCI	30-32°C and/or IL-10	Functional outcome, histopathology and PMN accumulation	Hypo improved functional outcome and CA3 neuron survival
2002 (44)	Rat/FPI	33°C	IL-1 mRNA	Hypo attenuated the posttraumatic increase
2002 (61)	Rat/FPI	30 or 33	Tissue hemoglobin	Hypo attenuated the posttraumatic increase
2003 (50)	Rat/CCI; fentanyl vs. isoflurane anesthesia	32°C,	Histopathology	Lesion volume was expanded by hypothermia on fentanyl anesthesia
2001 (28)	Mouse CCI	32°C	Histopathology, TUNEL, [27]PANT	Hypothermia reduced hippocampal neuronal death and DNA damage

[1]FPI= fluid percussion injury, [2]BBB = blood-brain barrier, [3]MAP2 = microtubule-associated protein-2, [3]CSF = cerebrospinal fluid, [4]ACh = acetylcholine, [5]EAA = excitatory amino acid, [6]ICP = intracranial pressure, [7]SOD = superoxide dismutase, [8]mRNA = messenger ribonucleic acid, [9]CCI = controlled cortical impact, [10]IL = interleukin, [11]NGF = nerve growth factor, [12]HSP-72 = heat-shock protein-72, [13]DHBA = dihydroxybenzoic acid, [14]PMN = polymorphonuclear leukocytes, [15]ICAM-1 = intercellular adhesion molecule-1, [16]E-sel = E-selectin, [17]ICP = intracranial pressure, [18]TUNEL = terminal deoxynucleotidyl transferase-mediated dUTP nick-end labeling, [19]DNA = deoxyribonucleic acid, [20]APP = amyloid precursor protein, [21]CBF= cerebral blood flow, [22]CMRglu = cerebral metabolic rate for glucose, [23]cNOS constitutive nitric oxide synthase, [24]iNOS = inducible nitric oxide synthase, [25]FGF = fibroblast growth factor, [26]CyA = cyclosporin-A, [27]PANT = DNA polymerase I-mediated biotin-dATP nick-translation.

Most of the experimental studies of moderate hypothermia in experimental TBI in the past decade were carried out in rats and a few in dogs and mice. Controlled cortical impact, fluid percussion, and impact acceleration models predominate in the rodent studies. Unlike the resurgence of studies of hypothermia in cardiac arrest models in the late 1980s, where mild hypothermia was the focus of investigation, the studies in experimental TBI have focused predominantly on moderate hypothermia. This is somewhat surprising, and the explanation for this fact is not completely clear. Although the studies in experimental TBI have focused on moderate hypothermia, recent randomized controlled trials (RCTs) of hypothermia in severe TBI have used either moderate or mild hypothermia, as discussed later.

Studies in rodent models of TBI have generally used a transient application (1-4 h) of moderate hypothermia (either 30 or 32°C). These studies have consistently demonstrated that moderate hypothermia attenuates functional deficits after injury (15-21). However, most studies suggest that the time window for the beneficial effect of hypothermia to improve functional outcome is short, between 30 and 60 min (16, 21). This suggests the importance of a direct effect of hypothermia on early secondary injury mechanisms, such as excitotoxicity or oxidative stress, rather than an effect on intracranial hypertension, which takes time to develop after injury. Studies of the effect of moderate hypothermia on histopathology have produced less consistent results than those assessing function. Experimental TBI produced by either controlled cortical impact or lateral fluid percussion generally produces a contusion with underlying hippocampal pathology (CA3, CA1, or hilar neuronal death). In contrast, the impact acceleration model produces minimal neuronal death but diffuse and focal (brainstem) axonal damage. Beneficial effects of hypothermia on contusion volume have been variable (17, 18, 22-26). More consistent effects on delayed hippocampal neuronal death in CA3 and/or CA1 have been reported (27, 28). This may result from the fact that at severe injury levels, necrosis within and around contusions is less amenable to therapies than delayed neuronal death in the hippocampus. In addition, penumbral cell death in CA3 or CA1 is associated with excitotoxicity, oxidative stress, and apoptosis, secondary injury mechanisms that may be specifically mitigated by hypothermia after TBI (discussed later).

A number of studies of experimental TBI have suggested beneficial effects of moderate hypothermia on brain swelling. Moderate hypothermia attenuates blood-brain barrier injury after either contusion or diffuse injury in rats (29, 30). Similarly, reductions in posttraumatic edema by moderate hypothermia have been reported in rodent models of cerebral contusion (22, 31, 32). The effect of moderate hypothermia on intracranial hypertension has been studied most extensively in dogs subjected to local compression ischemia produced by epidural balloon inflation (23, 26). Moderate (31°C) but not mild (35°C) hypothermia dramatically reduced intracranial hypertension compared to controls when applied in this clinically relevant model of severe acute epidural hematoma. However, even when hypothermia was effective, secondary swelling and herniation during re-warming remained problematic.

Studies in multiple rodent models have shown that moderate hypothermia has favorable effects on traumatic axonal injury (33-36). This beneficial effect was demonstrated across multiple markers of axonal injury including assessment of spectrin degradation, amyloid precursor protein accumulation, and neurofilament compaction. Studies of the beneficial effects of moderate hypothermia on traumatic axonal injury have provided the most comprehensive assessment, to date, on the effect of rapid vs. slow re-warming in TBI and also have produced interesting results of combination therapies with hypothermia. Suchiro et al (29) reported more axonal damage when one hour of posttraumatic hypothermia was followed by rewarming over 20 min vs. 90 min. They also reported synergy between moderate hypothermia and either cyclosporin A or tacrolimus (FK 506), suggesting an avenue for combination therapy and implicating an important role for calcineurin in traumatic axonal damage.

SECONDARY INJURY MECHANISMS

Experimental studies have suggested variable effects of moderate hypothermia on TBI followed by a secondary hypotensive and/or hypoxemic insult (24, 25, 30, 37). Secondary insults after TBI often produce severe damage that may be refractory to even the most efficacious therapies. Patients with secondary insults have been generally excluded from the larger controlled clinical trials (38, 39).

Several secondary injury mechanisms are favorably influenced by moderate hypothermia in experimental TBI. It remains unclear, however, as to which of the multifaceted effects of hypothermia is the most important contributor to its therapeutic benefit. Moderate hypothermia has been shown to attenuate several components of the local inflammatory response to cerebral contusion, as evidenced by reductions in neutrophil accumulation (9, 40-42), interleukin-1 (IL-1) messenger ribonucleic acid (mRNA) upregulation (43, 44), and inducible nitric oxide synthase activity (45). Surprisingly, administration of the anti-inflammatory cytokine IL-10 negated the beneficial effects of hypothermia on functional and histological outcome after controlled cortical impact in rats (20). It may be risky to augment the potent anti-inflammatory effects of moderate hypothermia after TBI. Moderate hypothermia can also attenuate posttraumatic excitotoxicity. Moderate hypothermia has been shown to reduce the posttraumatic increase in CSF levels of acetylcholine (16) and brain interstitial levels of glutamate and aspartate (46) in rats. However, a reduction of posttraumatic glutamate levels by moderate hypothermia has not been a consistent finding across experimental models (47, 48). Oxidative stress after TBI is linked to excitotoxicity along with a number of other secondary cascades. Moderate hypothermia has been shown to attenuate posttraumatic oxidative stress after fluid percussion in rats (46). This mirrors recent clinical findings that are discussed latter.

Not all of the studies of the effect of moderate hypothermia in experimental TBI have reported beneficial effects on outcome, and some clues may be derived from the negative studies. There has been little work on the effect of hypothermia on cerebral blood flow (CBF) after experimental TBI. Zhao (49) reported that moderate hypothermia (30°C for 3 h) reduced posttraumatic CBF at 3 h after rewarming in rats but failed to attenuate the increase cerebral metabolic rate for glucose (CMRglu), producing a mismatch between blood flow and metabolic demands. The increase in CMRglu after TBI is believed to result, in large part, from astrocyte-mediated uptake of the massive release in glutamate. Astrocyte uptake of glutamate is dependent entirely on glycolysis. Delayed excitotoxicity after rewarming may have occurred and this was not accompanied by a compensatory increase in CBF, leading to the observed mismatch after rewarming. One could envisage that during rapid rewarming, increases in metabolic demands from enhanced synaptic activity, stimulated glutamate re-uptake, and possibly subclinical status epilepticus, could be substantial and overwhelm the capacity of the injured cerebral circulation to keep pace and adequately vasodilate. Additional study of the effect of hypothermia and rewarming on CBF and CMR is warranted after experimental TBI.

Statler et al (50) recently compared transient moderate (32°C) hypothermia versus normothermia in rats anesthetized with fentanyl. Surprisingly, moderate hypothermia was associated with expansion of the lesion volume at 72 h after injury in rats anesthetized with fentanyl. Aspects of the stress response, such as plasma catecholamine levels were increased by hypothermia in the fentanyl anesthetized rats, suggesting the possibility of an exacerbated stress response by hypothermia. The beneficial effects of moderate hypothermia in most of the studies in Table 5-1 reflect its use in isoflurane-anesthetized rats. Clearly, more studies of the effect of hypothermia in experimental TBI are needed using clinically relevant anesthetic regimens.

EFFECT OF HYPOTHERMIA IN CLINICAL TBI

The resurgence in interest in mild hypothermia related to its beneficial effects in experimental cerebral ischemia and cardiac arrest sparked re-examination of hypothermia in experimental TBI. This rapidly lead to a re-examination of therapeutic hypothermia in clinical TBI, including several RCTs. Remarkably, over 25 clinical reports of the effect of therapeutic hypothermia on outcome, secondary injury mechanisms, or complications have been published since 1992 (Table 5-2). In contrast to the focus of experimental studies of TBI on moderate hypothermia, the studies of hypothermia in clinical TBI are equally mixed between those using mild or moderate levels; however, the vast majority of patients studied to date have been cooled to either 32 or 33°C.

Effect of hypothermia on ICP, physiology and secondary injury mechanisms

Two well-described studies carried out in 1993 evaluated the effect of moderate and mild hypothermia, respectively, on ICP and cerebrovascular physiology in adults after severe TBI. Marion et al (62) randomized 40 consecutive patients to either moderate hypothermia or normothermia and found that moderate hypothermia (maintained for 24 hours) reduced ICP, therapeutic intensity level (TIL), and CBF. The effects on ICP and CBF were limited to the initial 24 h after injury. $CMRO_2$ was not significantly altered. In a separate but concurrent study, Shiozaki et al (63) assessed ICP, cerebral perfusion pressure (CPP), CBF, $CMRO_2$ and mortality rate in 33 patients randomized to mild hypothermia versus normothermia. Hypothermia reduced posttraumatic intracranial hypertension, CBF, and $CMRO_2$, while improving CPP. The mortality rate from refractory intracranial hypertension was reduced from 12 of 17 to 5 of 16 patients in the normothermic vs. hypothermic groups, respectively, suggesting a powerful effect of mild hypothermia. Metz et al (64) reported similar effects on ICP in 10 patients with severe TBI, although a reduction in $CMRO_2$ was observed without an accompanying decrease in CBF with hypothermia. However, there was no concurrent control group. Shiozaki et at (65) reported on the effect of mild hypothermia (34°C) in a second prospective series of 62 patients with severe TBI and persistently raised ICP (> 20 mmHg) despite aggressive medical management. Mild hypothermia reduced ICP in 56.5% of these high-risk patients. In this series, mild hypothermia was most effective in patients with focal lesions. Tateishi et al [66] also evaluated patients with refractory intracranial hypertension after cerebral contusion, but used a titrated approach to both the depth and duration of

Table 5-2. Synopsis of selected clinical trials of therapeutic hypothermia in severe traumatic brain injury (TBI) since 1992

Date (Citation)	Temp	Population	Outcome	Key finding	Comment
1992 (87)	30-32°C	Prospective study of 21 patients undergoing elective craniotomy	Feasibility Complication	Two patients cooled to <32°C experienced ventricular arrhythmias or AV[1] block; no intracranial complications	
1993 (88)	32-33 °C vs. 37°C	Prospective RCT[2] of 46 patients with severe TBI	Phase II study	Trend toward improved GOS[3] in hypothermia group; Seizure incidence was reduced by hypothermia; no complications.	Cooling began within 6 h; 48 h duration
1993 (62)	32-33 °C vs. 37-38°C	Prospective RCT of 40 patients with severe TBI	[4]ICP, [5]TIL, [6]CBF, [7]CMRO$_2$, GOS	Moderate hypothermia reduced ICP, TIL, and CBF vs. normothermia	Target temperature reached in ~10 h; maintained for 24 h
1993 (63)	33.5-34.5 °C vs. normothermia	Prospective RCT in 33 patients with severe TBI	ICP, CPP, mortality, CBF, CMRO$_2$	Mild hypothermia reduced ICP, increased [8]CPP, reduced mortality rate. Mild hypothermia also decreased CBF and CMRO$_2$	CBF and CMRO$_2$ studied in a subgroup of 5 patients
1993 (89)	32-33 °C vs. normothermia	Prospective RCT in 36 patients with severe TBI	Delayed intracerebral hemorrhage; [9]PT, [10]PTT and platelet count	No differences between the two groups for any parameter	Cooling began within 6 h
1994 (68)	34.5-36°C	Case Report	Peritoneal cooling	Peritoneal cooling shown to be fast and effective in severe TBI	
1997 (64)	32.5-33°C; no control group	Prospective study of 10 patients with severe TBI	ICP; CBF; CMRO$_2$; [11]CMRlactate	Hypothermia reduced ICP and CMRO$_2$ and CMRlactate, but did not reduce CBF	Cooling began at a median of 16 h

Date (Citation)	Temp	Population	Outcome	Key finding	Comment
1997 (38)	32-33°C vs. normothermia	Prospective single-center RCT of 82 patients	3, 6, and 12 month GOS	Moderate hypothermia hastened neurologic recovery in patients GCS 5-7 and was associated with reductions in [12]CSF levels of glutamate and [13]IL-1	Target temperature achieved at median of 10 h; cooling for 24 h
1998 (66)	33-35°C; no control group	Prospective study; 9 patients with severe TBI	ICP	Mild hypothermia reduced ICP; Increased C-reactive protein and decreased platelet count	Hypothermia titrated to control ICP
1998 (73)	32-33°C vs. normothermia	Thirty-nine patients with severe TBI; Subgroup of an RCT	CSF levels of quinolinic acid, a macrophage marker	Hypothermia had no effect on CSF quinolinic acid levels	Suggests macrophage accumulation not attenuated by hypothermia
1998 (65)	34°C; no control group	Prospective study of 62 patients with severe TBI and persistent ICP > 20 mm Hg	ICP	Mild hypothermia reduced ICP in 56.5% of the patients whose ICP was > 20 mm Hg despite conventional treatment. Mild hypothermia more effective at controlling ICP in focal vs. diffuse swelling	
1999 (71)	32-33°C vs. normothermia	Prospective study of 23 patients with severe TBI	Jugular venous levels of IL-6	Moderate hypothermia reduced jugular venous levels of IL-6	Hypothermia at 4-9 d after injury
1999 (69)	34°C vs. normothermia	Prospective RCT of 16 patients with severe TBI, ICP<20 mm Hg	GOS; CSF [14]TNFα, IL-1β, IL-6, IL-8, IL-10	Most patients in both groups with good outcome; No reduction in CSF cytokines by hypothermia despite high levels of IL-6, IL-8 and IL-10	

Date (Citation)	*Temp*	*Population*	*Outcome*	*Key finding*	*Comment*
1999 (90)	30-33°C; no control group	Prospective study of 43 patients with severe TBI	Feasibility of prolonged hypothermia	Nosocomial pneumonia seen in 45% but death from sepsis rare (5%); no other complications	Hypothermia maintained a median of 8 d
2000 (84)	33-35°C; no control group	Prospective RCT of 87 patients with severe TBI	12 month GOS	GOS improved by hypothermia; Favorable outcome (GOS 4,5) was 46.5% in hypothermia vs. 27.27% in normothermia; Mortality rate was 25.58% in hypothermia vs. 45.45% in normothermia; ICP lower in the hypothermia group at d 7.	Duration of hypothermia 3-14 d; Hypothermia was stopped when ICP normalized
2000 (91)	32-33°C vs. normothermia	Prospective study of 26 patients with severe TBI	Jugular venous levels of thromboxane and 6-keto-^{15}PGF$_1\alpha$	Moderate hypothermia reduced the increase in jugular venous levels of thromboxane; no effect on 6-keto-PGF$_1\alpha$	
2001 (39)	33°C vs. normothermia	Prospective multi-center RCT of 392 patients	6 month GOS	Hypothermia failed to improve GOS; mortality rate was 28 and 27% in the hypothermia and normothermia groups, respectively; Fewer patients in the hypothermia group had elevated ICP; The hypothermia group had longer hospital stays and more complications	48 h treatment; mean time to target temperature was 8.4 h in hypothermia group

Date (Citation)	Temp	Population	Outcome	Key finding	Comment
2001 (92)	32-33°C vs. normothermia	Prospective study of 22 patients with severe TBI	Plasma phosphate concentration	Reduction in plasma phosphate concentration in hypothermia group that resolved with rewarming	
2001 (82)	33°C vs. normothermia	Further analysis of the multi-center RCT	Assessment of inter-center differences in a variety of parameters	Marginally different inter-center outcomes; wide differences in age, admission temperature, [16]MABP < 70 mmHg, and CPP < 50 mmHg between centers.	Suggests need for a detailed protocol for fluid and hemodynamic management for phase III trials in TBI
2002 (93)	34-36°C	Prospective study in 58 patients, 33 with persistent ICP >20 mmHg treated with hypothermia	Brain temperature monitored (multi-parameter probe)	Brain temperature monitoring is feasible; difference between brain and rectal temperature was directly correlated with outcome	Suggests that low brain vs. rectal temperature is predictive of poor outcome
2002 (94)	34-36°C	Prospective study in 58 patients, 33 with persistent ICP >20 mmHg treated with hypothermia	Brain tissue pO_2, pCO_2, pH; brain interstitial levels of glutamate and lactate	Mild hypothermia reduced brain tissue pO_2 and pCO_2 and increased brain tissue pH. Patients with spontaneous hypothermia on admission had high levels of glutamate and lactate	
2002 (83)	33°C vs. normothermia	Further analysis of the multi-center RCT	Assessment of fluid balance during the 96 h after randomization	Fluid balance varied from −10 L to +20L. A fluid balance lower than −594 mL was associated with poor outcome	Variability in fluid balance for patients with isolated TBI; suggests dehydration therapy in some patients

Date (Citation)	Temp	Population	Outcome	Key finding	Comment
2002 (95)	Not applicable	Meta-analysis of the studies carried up to and including 2001	GOS, ICP, complications	No beneficial effect of hypothermia on any parameter, the only complication significantly influenced was mild prolongation of PTT	Seven studies included; 368 of the 668 patients were part of one study (52)
2002 (96)	34 °C vs. normothermia	Thirty patients with severe TBI divided into two groups	GOS and ICP	GOS did not differ between treatment groups but ICP was reduced by hypothermia	72 h of cooling; European Brain Injury Consortium protocol
2002 (79)	33-35°C vs. normothermia	Thirty five severe TBI patients were treated vs. separate controls	GOS	GOS better in hypothermia group vs. normothermic controls. Age > 50 years was associated with poor outcome	
2002 (98)	33°C vs. normothermia	Further analysis of the multi-center RCT (52)	Assessment of the impact of hypothermia on admission	Hypothermia on admission associated with improved outcome	Suggests possible benefit of early posttraumatic hypothermia
2003 (99)	33°C; no control group	Thirty one severe TBI patients all treated with hypothermia	ICP	ICP decreased at 35-36°C, but no differences seen at temperatures below 35°C; CPP also peaked at 35-36°C; CPP decreased below 35°C	Suggests that mild hypothermia can reduce ICP in some cases
2003 (74)	RCT of 32°C vs. normothermia	Prospective study of 28 infants and children with severe TBI	CSF levels of markers of oxidative stress	Reduction in both lipid peroxidation (F_2-isoprostane) and loss of endogenous antioxidants by moderate hypothermia	

Date (Citation)	Temp	Population	Outcome	Key finding	Comment
2003 (72)	RCT of 32°C vs. normothermia	Prospective study of 28 infants and children with severe TBI	CSF levels of IL-6, IL-8	Marked increase in CSF levels of IL-6 and IL-8 after injury but no difference in hypothermia vs. normothermia	Selective effects of moderate hypothermia on biochemical cascades
2003 (70)	32-33°C vs. normothermia	Sixty eight adults; subset of patients from the multi-center RCT (52)	CSF levels of glutamate, and F_2-isoprostane	Hypothermia reduced both glutamate and F_2-isoprostane; the magnitude of the reduction was greater for glutamate than isoprostane	
2003 (85)	Not applicable	Meta-analysis of 12 trials including 1069 adults with severe TBI	Mortality and neurological outcome	Overall benefit of moderate or mild hypothermia (32-33°C); 19% relative reduction in the risk of death and a 22% relative reduction in the risk of poor neurological outcome vs. normothermia.	Favorable effects of cooling for 24-48 h, or longer, target of 32-33°C, and rewarming duration ≤24 h

[1]AV = atrioventricular, [2]RCT= randomized controlled trial, [3]GOS = Glasgow outcome scale, [4]ICP = intracranial pressure, [5]TIL = therapeutic intensity level, [6]CBF = cerebral blood flow, [7]CMRO$_2$ = cerebral metabolic rate for oxygen, [8]CPP = cerebral perfusion pressure, [9]PT = prothrombin time, [10]PTT = partial thromboplastin time, [11]CMRlactate = cerebral metabolic rate for lactate, [12]CSF = cerebrospinal fluid, [13]IL = interleukin, [14]TNFα = tumor necrosis factor alpha, [15]PGF = prostaglandin-F, [16]MABP = mean arterial blood pressure,

hypothermia. In his series, ICP was controlled in 8 of 9 patients using relatively mild hypothermia—with a temperature range between 33 and 35°C. The mean duration of cooling required to control ICP was 68 h, and some patients were cooled for 4 days. One patient died of septicemia; platelet counts decreased to less than 100,000/μL in 5 of the 9 patients by day 4. A number of other authors (Table 5-2) have reported reductions of ICP in patients with severe TBI treated with either mild or moderate hypothermia, and this finding was confirmed even in the multi-center trial carried out by Clifton (39). Studies in an animal model of TBI suggest that moderate hypothermia is necessary to control intracranial hypertension (23, 26). However, clinical studies indicate that mild hypothermia is often successful at controlling ICP, even in many cases refractory to medical management. Recently, Tokutomi et al (67) confirmed the efficacy of mild hypothermia by carefully evaluating the effect of temperature level on ICP during cooling to 33°C in 31 adults with severe TBI.   Surprisingly, the decrease in ICP and improvement in CPP was greatest at 35.5°C.

In all of these studies hypothermia was induced by surface methods with or without gastric lavage. In a report on a single case, Cancio et al (68) described rapid cooling using peritoneal lavage in a patient with severe TBI. Inotropic and/or pressor agents were required to support hemodynamics, but complications of hypothermia were generally reported as manageable.

The effects of hypothermia on a number of secondary injury mechanisms after severe TBI, have been assessed in CSF, jugular venous blood, or brain interstitial fluid.   Marion et al (38), in a small subset of patients from his single center RCT, reported that moderate hypothermia attenuated the increase in CSF levels of glutamate, suggesting a key beneficial effect of moderate hypothermia on excitotoxicity.   In contrast, Shiozaki et al (69) serially assessed CSF levels of glutamate, aspartate, and glycine in 16 patients randomized to mild hypothermia (34°C) vs. normothermia.   No differences between treatment groups in any of excitatory amino acids was seen in hypothermic versus normothermic groups; however, glutamate levels were only modestly increased on admission, and the other excitatory amino acids were not increased.   Recently, Wagner et al (70) reported a marked reduction of CSF glutamate by moderate hypothermia vs. normothermia in a large study of patients (n = 68) with severe TBI.

Marion et al (38) reported a reduction in CSF levels of IL-1β by moderate hypothermia—although the increases in IL-1β were modest in magnitude.   Nevertheless, this suggested a beneficial effect of hypothermia on posttraumatic inflammation.   Aibiki et al (71) measured levels of the cytokine IL-6 in jugular venous samples from 23 adults randomized to moderate hypothermia (32-33°C) or normothermia after severe TBI. Hypothermia attenuated the increase in IL-6 after injury.   In contrast, Shiozaki et al (69) serially assessed CSF levels of a battery of cytokines (tumor necrosis factor [TNF]α, IL-1β, IL-6, IL-8, and IL-10) in his previously described study of 16 patients with TBI (but without elevated ICP) randomized to mild (34°C) vs. normothermia. No differences between treatment groups were also seen for the cytokines, despite the fact that CSF levels of some cytokines such as IL-6 and IL-8 were dramatically increased after injury.   Similar findings were recently reported by Shore et al (72)— who reported no difference in CSF levels of either IL-6 or IL-8 after severe TBI in infants and children treated with moderate hypothermia vs. normothermia.   Sinz et al (73) studied the effect of moderate hypothermia vs. normothermia on CSF levels of the macrophage marker quinolinic acid in adults with severe TBI. CSF quinolinic acid levels did not differ between treatment groups—suggesting that macrophage accumulation was neither attenuated nor delayed by the use of moderate therapeutic hypothermia. Thus, except for IL-1β in CSF and IL-6 in jugular venous blood, increases in cytokines after severe TBI are not consistently attenuated by mild or moderate hypothermia.

Another dramatic effect of moderate hypothermia on the secondary injury cascade was recently reported by Bayir et al (74) and Wagner et al(70). Bayir et al (74) reported that moderate hypothermia (vs. normothermia) markedly attenuated both lipid peroxidation and consumption of endogenous antioxidants after severe TBI in infants and children. Wagner et al (70) similarly reported that moderate hypothermia attenuated both glutamate and F2-isoprostane levels in adults after severe TBI in adults. The effect of hypothermia was greater on glutamate levels than on F2-isoprostane levels. Since excitotoxicity and oxidative stress are linked in TBI, this suggests that inhibition of excitotoxicity likely contributes substantially to the reduction in oxidative stress by hypothermia. In addition, CSF levels of markers of lipid peroxidation are lower in women than in men after TBI; and the reduction of posttraumatic oxidative stress by moderate hypothermia in adults is easier to demonstrate in males than in females (75). Much additional work is needed to define the secondary injury cascades that are favorably influenced by mild or moderate hypothermia; however, a picture is emerging that mild and moderate hypothermia do not indiscriminately slow all biochemical reactions in the secondary injury cascade, rather they appear to have selective effects, particularly on excitotoxicity and oxidative stress.

Finally, hypothermia is a unique modulator of protein synthesis. Although it depresses overall protein synthesis, it selectively increases the synthesis of stress proteins via cold shock stress (76). Cold stress protein expression is affected by the depth and duration of hypothermia as well as the rate of rewarming. Hypothetically, these parameters could be intentionally manipulated to selectively increase the protein expression of neuroprotective protein effectors. In support of this approach, several studies in experimental brain injury have suggested that mild or moderate hypothermia selectively stimulates production of neuroprotective factors (rather than inhibits deleterious pathways). Brain-derived neurotrophic factor (BDNF) has been suggested to be an example of a neuroprotective molecule stimulated by mild hypothermia after experimental brain ischemia/reperfusion (77). However, recent clinical studies have not demonstrated parallel increases in BDNF in CSF samples from patients randomized to hypothermia vs. normothermia after severe TBI (72). Further study is needed on this interesting hypothesis.

CONCLUSIONS

There is strong evidence that hypothermia is effective in preventing the development of raised ICP and/or controlling refractory intracranial hypertension after TBI. Even mild levels can often achieve this goal. For optimal control of intracranial hypertension, hypothermia should probably be titrated, facilitating application of mild rather than moderate hypothermia whenever possible, and avoiding prolonged application. The success rates for the effect of hypothermia in the treatment of refractory intracranial hypertension appear similar to those reported for other therapies such as barbiturates (78). Mild and moderate hypothermia tend to reduce CBF and $CMRO_2$, but these effects are not consistently observed across studies.

After severe TBI, application of mild or moderate therapeutic hypothermia may have cerebral resuscitative effects that occur independent of a reduction of ICP. Recent clinical studies in cardiac arrest (79-81) certainly support a direct neuroresuscitative effect. Although this is likely in TBI, based on the single center trials presented in this review and the extensive data in experimental models, much of the neurotrauma community remains unconvinced. In addition, the optimal temperature, duration, and other details for its use in this manner remain to be determined. Although the multi-center RCT of Clifton et al (39) failed, the variability in the approach to maintaining a target CPP in that study (fluids vs. pressors, etc) was a recognized problem (82, 83). This problem was avoided in two fairly large single center RCTs (38, 84). Several clinical trials in severe TBI are ongoing including pediatric trials and a new adult trial, although it is likely these will all test moderate hypothermia. A recent meta-analysis demonstrated a positive overall effect of therapeutic hypothermia in severe TBI in adults (85). Hopefully, mild hypothermia will receive further clinical investigation in severe TBI, perhaps including rapid induction of cooling via intravenous administration of cold saline (86). Finally, considerable laboratory evidence supports the deleterious effects of hyperthermia after severe TBI; fever should be rigorously avoided.

Acknowledgement

The authors thank the National Institutes of Health NS 30318 and NS 38087, the CDC/University of Pittsburgh Center for Injury Control and Research, and the United States Army DAMD 17-01-2-0038 for support. We thank the late Dr. Peter Safar for his helpful discussions. This chapter is written in his honor.

REFERENCES

1. Phelps C. Principles of Treatment In: *Traumatic Injuries of the Brain and Its Membranes.* Critchley M, Flamm ES, Goodrich JT, et al (Eds.), D. Appleton and Company, NY, 1897; pp 223-224.
2. Fay T. Observations on generalized refrigeration in cases of severe cerebral trauma. *Assoc Res Nerv Ment Dis Proc* 1943; 24:611-619.
3. Woringer E, Schneider J, Baumgartner J, Thomalske G. Essai critique sur l'effet de l'hibernation artificielle sur 19 cas de souffrance du tronc cerebral après traumatisme sélectionnés pour leur gravité parmi 270 comas postcommotionels. *Anesth Analg (Paris)* 1954; 11:34-45.
4. Sedzimir CB. Therapeutic hypothermia in cases of head injury. *J Neurosurg* 1959; 16:407-414.
5. Lazorthes G, Campan L. Hypothermia in the treatment of craniocerebral traumatism. *J Neurosurg* 1958; 15:162-167.
6. Hendrick EB. The use of hypothermia in severe head injuries in childhood. *Ann Surg* 1959; 79:362-364.
7. Rosomoff HL. Protective effects of hypothermia against pathological processes of the nervous system. *Ann NY Acad Sci* 1959; 80:475-486.
8. Rosomoff HL, Shulman K, Raynor R, et al. Experimental brain injury and delayed hypothermia. *Surg Gynecol Obstet* 1960; 110:27.
9. Rosomoff HL, Clasen RA, Hartstock R, Bebin J. Brain reaction to experimental injury after hypothermia. *Arch Neurol* 1965; 13:337-345.
10. Langfitt TW, Kumar VS, James HE, Miller JD. Continuous recording of intracranial pressure in patients with hypoxic brain damage. In: *Brain Hypoxia.* Brierley JB, Meldrum BS (eds), William Heinemann Medical Books Ltd, London, 1971; chapter 12: pp. 118-135.
11. Lundberg N, Troupp H, Lorin H. Continuous recording of the ventricular fluid pressure in patients with severe acute traumatic brain injury: A preliminary report. *J Neurosurg* 1965; 22:581-590.
12. Bohn DJ, Biggar WD, Smith CR, et al. Influence of hypothermia, barbiturate therapy, and intracranial pressure monitoring on morbidity and mortality after near-drowning. *Crit Care Med* 1986 14:529-534.
13. Biggart MJ and Bohn DJ. Effect of hypothermia and cardiac arrest on outcome of near-drowning accidents in children. *J Pediatr* 1990; 117:179-183.
14. White RJ. Is hypothermia dead? *Surg Neurol.* 1985, 23:324-5.
15. Clifton GL, Jiang JY, Lyeth BG, et al. Marked protection by moderate hypothermia after experimental traumatic brain injury. *J Cereb Blood Flow Metab* 1991; 11:114-121.
16. Lyeth BG, Jiang JY, Robinson SE, et al. Hypothermia blunts acetylcholine increase in CSF of traumatically brain injured rats. *Mol Chem Neuropathol* 1993; 18:247-56.
17. Bramlett HM, Green EJ, Dietrich WD, et al. Posttraumatic brain hypothermia provides protection from sensorimotor and cognitive behavioral deficits. *J Neurotrauma* 1995; 12:289-298.
18. Dixon CE, Markgraf CG, Angileri F, et al. Protective effects of moderate hypothermia on behavioral deficits but not necrotic cavitation following cortical impact injury in the rat. J Neurotrauma 1998; 15:95-103.
19. Yan HQ, Yu J, Kline AE, et al. Evaluation of combined fibroblast growth factor-2 and moderate hypothermia therapy in traumatically brain injured rats. *Brain Res* 2000; 887:134-143.

20. Kline AE, Bolinger BD, Kochanek PM, et al. Acute systemic administration of Interleukin-10 suppresses the beneficial effects of moderate hypothermia following traumatic brain injury in rats. *Brain Res* 2002; 937:22-31.

21. Markgraf CG, Clifton GL, Aguirre M, et al. Injury severity and sensitivity to treatment after controlled cortical impact in rats. *J Neurotrauma* 2001; 18:175-86.

22. Mansfield RT, Schiding JK, Hamilton RL, Kochanek PM. Effects of hypothermia on traumatic brain injury in immature rats. *J Cereb Blood Flow Metab* 1996; 16:244-252.

23. Pomeranz S, Safar P, Radovsky A, et al. The effect of resuscitative moderate hypothermia following epidural brain compression on cerebral damage in a canine outcome model. *J Neurosurg* 1993; 79:241-251.

24. Robertson CL, Clark RSB, Dixon CE, et al. No long term benefit from hypothermia after severe traumatic brain injury with secondary insult in rats. *Crit Care Med* 2000; 28:3218-3223.

25. Matsushita Y, Bramlett HM, Alonso O, Dietrich WD. Posttraumatic hypothermia is neuroprotective in a model of traumatic brain injury complicated by a secondary hypoxic insult. *Crit Care Med* 2001; 29:2060-2066.

26. Ebmeyer U, Safar P, Radovsky A, et al Moderate hypothermia for 48 hours after temporary epidural brain compression injury in a canine outcome model. *J Neurotrauma* 1998; 15:323-336.

27. Dietrich WD, Alonso O, Busto R, et al. Post-traumatic brain hypothermia reduces histopathological damage following concussive brain injury in the rat. *Acta Neuropathol* 1994; 87:250-258.

28. Sullivan R, Alce G, Dixon CE, et al. Therapeutic hypothermia after experimental traumatic brain injury in mice: Effects on DNA damage, histopathology and functional outcome. *Crit Care Med* 2001; 29:A122.

29. Jiang JY, Lyeth BG, Kapasi MZ, et al. Moderate hypothermia reduces blood-brain barrier disruption following traumatic brain injury in the rat. Acta Neuropathol 1992; 84:495-500.

30. Smith SL, Hall ED. Mild pre-and posttraumatic hypothermia attenuates blood-brain barrier damage following controlled cortical impact injury in the rat. *J Neurotrauma* 1996; 13:1-9.

31. Heegaard W, Biros M, Zink J. Effect of hypothermia, dichloroacetate, and deferoxamine in the treatment for cortical edema and functional recovery after experimental cortical impact in the rat. *Acad Emerg Med* 1997; 4:33-39.

32. Markgraf CG, Clifton GL, Moody MR. Treatment window for hypothermia in brain injury. *J Neurosurg* 2001; 95:979-83.

33. Marion DW, White MJ. Treatment of experimental brain injury with moderate hypothermia and 21-aminosteroids. *J Neurotrauma* 1996; 13:139-147.

34. Buki A, Koizumi H, Povlishock JT. Moderate posttraumatic hypothermia decreases early calpain-mediated proteolysis and concomitant cytoskeletal compromise in traumatic axonal injury. *Exp Neurol* 1999; 159:319-328.

35. Suehiro E, Povlishock JT. Exacerbation of traumatically induced axonal injury by rapid posthypothermic rewarming and attenuation of axonal change by cyclosporine A. *J Neurosurg* 2001; 94:493-498.

36. Suehiro E, Singleton RH, Stone JR, Povlishock JT. The immunophilin ligand FK506 attenuates the axonal damage associated with rapid rewarming following posttraumatic hypothermia. *Exp Neurol* 2001; 172:199-210.

37. Yamamoto M, Marmarou CR, Stiefel MF, . Neuroprotective effect of hypothermia on neuronal injury in diffuse traumatic brain injury coupled with hypoxia and hypotension *J Neurotrauma* 1999;16:487-500.

38. Marion DW, Penrod LE, Kelsey SF, et al. Treatment of traumatic brain injury with moderate hypothermia. *N Engl J Med* 1997; 336:540-546.

39. Clifton GL, Miller ER, Choi SC, et al. Lack of effect of induction of hypothermia after acute brain injury *N Engl J Med* 2001 344:556-63.

40. Whalen MJ, Carlos TM, Clark RS, et al. The effect of brain temperature on acute inflammation after traumatic brain injury in rats. *J Neurotrauma* 1997; 14:561-572.

41. Chatzipanteli K, Yanagawa Y, Marcillo AE, et al. Posttraumatic hypothermia reduces polymorphonuclear leukocyte accumulation following spinal cord injury in rats. *J Neurotrauma* 2000; 17:321-32.

42. Chatzipanteli K, Alonso OF, Kraydieh S, Dietrich WD. Importance of posttraumatic hypothermia and hyperthermia on the inflammatory response after fluid percussion brain injury: biochemical and immunocytochemical studies. *J Cereb Blood Flow Metab* 2000; 20:531-42.

43. Goss JR, Styren SD, Miller PD, et al. Hypothermia attenuates the normal increase in interleukin 1 beta RNA and nerve growth factor following traumatic brain injury in the rat. *J Neurotrauma* 1995; 12:159-167.

44. Kinoshita K, Chatzipanteli K, Vitarbo E, et al. Interleukin-1beta messenger ribonucleic acid and protein levels after fluid-percussion brain injury in rats: importance of injury severity and brain temperature. *Neurosurgery* 2002; 51:195-203.

45. Chatzipanteli K, Wada K, Busto R, Dietrich WD. Effects of moderate hypothermia on constitutive and inducible nitric oxide synthase activities after traumatic brain injury in the rat. *J Neurochem* 1999; 72:2047-52.

46. Globus MY, Alonso O, Dietrich WD, et al. Glutamate release and free radical production following brain injury: effects of posttraumatic hypothermia. *J Neurochem* 1995; 65:1704-1711.

47. Palmer A, Marion DW, Botscheller ML, Redd EE. Therapeutic hypothermia is cytoprotective without attenuating the traumatic brain injury-induced elevations in interstitial concentrations of aspartate and glutamate. *J Neurotrauma* 1993; 10:363-372.

48. Koizumi H, Povlishock JT. Posttraumatic hypothermia in the treatment of axonal damage in an animal model of traumatic axonal injury. *J Neurosurg* 1998; 89:303-9.

49. Zhao W, Alonso OF, Loor JY, et al. Influence of early posttraumatic hypothermia therapy on local cerebral blood flow and glucose metabolism after fluid-percussion brain injury. *J Neurosurg* 1999; 90:510-519.

50. Statler KD, Alexander HL, Vagni V,et al. Moderate hypothermia may be detrimental after traumatic brain injury in fentanyl-anesthetized rats. *Crit Care Med* 2003; in press.

51. Taft WC, Yang K, Dixon CE, et al. Hypothermia attenuates the loss of hippocampal microtubule-associated protein 2 (MAP2) following traumatic brain injury. *J Cereb Blood Flow Metab* 1993; 13:796-802.

52. Lyeth BG, Jiang JY, Liu S. Behavioral protection by moderate hypothermia initiated after experimental traumatic brain injury. *J Neurotrauma* 1993; 10:57-64.

53. Fukuhara T, Nishio S, Ono Y, et al. Induction of Cu, Zn-superoxide dismutase after cortical contusion injury during hypothermia. *Brain Res* 1994; 657:333-336.

54. Nakamura M, Tanno H, Fukuda K, Yamaura A. The effects of mild hypothermia on expression of stress protein (HSP72) after experimental brain injury. *No To Shinkei* 1995; 47:484-490.

55. Clark RS, Kochanek PM, Marion D, et al. Mild posttraumatic hypothermia reduces mortality after severe controlled cortical impact in rats. *J Cereb Blood Flow Metab* 1996; 16:253-261.

56. Koizumi H, Povlishock JT. Posttraumatic hypothermia in the treatment of axonal damage in an animal model of traumatic axonal injury. *J Neurosurg* 1998; 89:303-309.

57. Sakamoto KI, Fujisawa H, Koizumi H, et al. Effects of mild hypothermia on nitric oxide synthesis following contusion trauma in the rat. *J Neurotrauma* 1997; 14:349-353.

58. Xu RX, Nakamura T, Nagao S, et al. Specific inhibition of apoptosis after cold-induced brain injury by moderate postinjury hypothermia. *Neurosurgery* 1998; 43:107-115.

59. Kahveci FS, Kahveci N, Alkan T, et al. Propofol versus isoflurane anesthesia under hypothermic conditions: effects on intracranial pressure and local cerebral blood flow after diffuse traumatic brain injury in the rat. *Surg Neurol* 2001; 56:206-214.

60. Lin X, Zhi D, Zhang S. Inhibiting effect of moderate hypothermia on cell apoptosis after diffuse brain injury in rats. *Chin J Traumatol* 2001; 4:14-19.

61. Kinoshita K, Chatzipanteli K, Alonso OF, et al. The effect of brain temperature on hemoglobin extravasation after traumatic brain injury. *J Neurosurg* 2002; 97:945-53

62. Marion DW, Obrist WD, Carlier PM, et al. The use of moderate therapeutic hypothermia for patients with severe head injuries: a preliminary report. *J Neurosurg* 1993; 79:354-362.

63. Shiozaki T, Sugimoto H, Taneda M, et al. Effect of mild hypothermia on uncontrollable intracranial hypertension after severe head injury. *J Neurosurg* 1993; 79:363-368.

64. Metz C, Holzschuh M, Bein T, et al. Moderate hypothermia in patients with severe head injury: cerebral and extracerebral effects. *J Neurosurg* 1996; 85:533-541.

65. Shiozaki T, Sugimoto H, Taneda M, et al. Selection of severely head injured patients for mild hypothermia therapy. *J Neurosurg* 1998; 89:206-211.

66. Tateishi A, Soejima Y, Taira Y, et al. Feasibility of the titration method of mild hypothermia in severely head-injured patients with intracranial hypertension. *Neurosurgery* 1998; 42:1065-1070.

67. Tokutomi T, Morimoto K, Miyagi T, et al. Optimal temperature for the management of severe traumatic brain injury: effect of hypothermia on intracranial pressure, systemic and intracranial hemodynamics, and metabolism. Neurosurgery 2003; 52:102-112.

68. Cancio LC, Wortham WG, Zimba F. Peritoneal dialysis to induce hypothermia in a head-injured patient: case report. *Surg Neurol* 1994; 42:303-307.

69. Shiozaki T, Kato A, Taneda M, et al. Little benefit from mild hypothermia therapy for severely head injured patients with low intracranial pressure. *J Neurosurg* 1999; 91:185-191.

70. Wagner AK, Bayır H, Ren D, et al. Relationships between cerebrospinal fluid markers of excitotoxicity, ischemia, and oxidative stress after severe TBI: The impact of gender, age, and hypothermia. *J Neurotrauma* 2004; 21:125-136.

71. Aibiki M, Maekawa S, Ogura S, et al. Effect of moderate hypothermia on systemic and internal jugular plasma IL-6 levels after traumatic brain injury in humans. *J Neurotrauma* 1999; 16:225-232.

72. Shore PM, Jackson EK, Clark RSB, et al. Therapeutic hypothermia does not affect markers of injury, cellular energetics, inflammation, and regeneration in cerebrospinal fluid after severe traumatic brain injury in infants and children. *Pediatr Crit Care Med* 2003; 4:A143 (Suppl).

73. Sinz EH, Kochanek PM, Heyes MP, et al. Quinolinic acid is increased in CSF and associated with mortality after traumatic brain injury in humans. *J Cereb Blood Flow Metab* 1998; 18:610-615.

74. Bayir H, Adelson PD, Kagan VE, et al. Therapeutic hypothermia attenuates oxidative stress after traumatic brain injury in infants and children. *Crit Care Med Suppl* 2002; 30:A7.

75. Bayır H, Marion DW, Kagan VE, et al. Marked gender effect on lipid peroxidation after severe traumatic brain injury in adult patients. *J Neurotrauma* 2004; 21:1-8.

76. Sonna, LA, Fujita, J, Gaffin, SL and Lilly, CM. Invited review: Effects of heat and cold stress on mammalian gene expression. *J Appl Physiol* 2002; 92:1725-42.
77. D'Cruz BJ, Fertig KC, Filiano AJ, et al. Hypothermic reperfusion after cardiac arrest augments brain-derived neurotrophic factor activation. *J Cereb Blood Flow Metab* 2002; 22:843-851.
78. Pittman T, Bucholz R, Williams D. Efficacy of barbiturates in the treatment of resistant intracranial hypertension in severely head-injured children. *Pediatr Neurosci* 1989;15:13-7.
79. Hypothermia after Cardiac Arrest Study Group. Mild therapeutic hypothermia to improve the neurologic outcome after cardiac arrest. *N Engl J Med* 2002; 346:549-56.
80. Bernard SA, Gray TW, Buist MD, et al. Treatment of comatose survivors of out-of-hospital cardiac arrest with induced hypothermia. *N Engl J Med* 2002; 346:557-563.
81. Nolan JP, Morley PT, Vanden Hoek TL, et al. International Liaison Committee on Resuscitation. Therapeutic hypothermia after cardiac arrest: an advisory statement by the advanced life support task force of the International Liaison Committee on Resuscitation. *Circulation* 2003; 108:118-121.
82. Clifton GL, Miller ER, Choi SC, Levin HS. Fluid thresholds and outcome from severe brain injury. *Crit Care Med* 2002; 30:739-45.
83. Clifton GL, Choi SC, Miller ER, et al. Intercenter variance in clinical trials of head trauma--experience of the National Acute Brain Injury Study: Hypothermia. *J Neurosurg* 2001; 95:751-5.
84. Jiang J, Yu M, Zhu C. Effect of long-term mild hypothermia therapy in patients with severe traumatic brain injury: 1-year follow-up review of 87 cases. *J Neurosurg* 2000 93:546-9.
85. McIntyre LA, Fergusson DA, Hebert PC, et al. Prolonged therapeutic hypothermia after traumatic brain injury in adults: a systematic review. *JAMA* 2003; 289:2992-9.
86. Bernard S, Buist M, Monteiro O, Smith K. Induced hypothermia using large volume, ice-cold intravenous fluid in comatose survivors of out-of-hospital cardiac arrest: a preliminary report. *Resuscitation* 2003; 56:9-13.
87. Clifton GL, Allen S, Berry J, Koch SM. Systemic hypothermia in treatment of brain injury. *J Neurotrauma* 1992; 9:S487-495.
88. Clifton GL, Allen S, Barrodale P, et al. A phase II study of moderate hypothermia in severe brain injury. *J Neurotrauma* 1993; 10:263-273.
89. Resnick DK, Marion DW, Darby JM. The effect of hypothermia on the incidence of delayed traumatic intracerebral hemorrhage. *Neurosurgery* 1994; 34:252-256.
90. Bernard SA, MacC Jones B, Buist M: Experience with prolonged induced hypothermia in severe head injury. *Crit Care* 1999; 3:167-172.
91. Aibiki M, Maekawa S, Yokono S: Moderate hypothermia improves imbalances of thromboxane A and prostaglandin I2 production after traumatic brain injury in humans. *Crit Care Med* 2000; 28:3902-3906.
92. Aibiki M, Kawaguchi S, Maekawa N. Reversible hypophosphatemia during moderate hypothermia therapy for brain-injured patients. *Crit Care Med* 2001; 29:1726-1730.
93. Soukup J, Zauner A, Doppenberg EM, et al. The importance of brain temperature in patients after severe head injury: relationship to intracranial pressure, cerebral perfusion pressure, cerebral blood flow, and outcome. *J Neurotrauma* 2002; 19:559-571.
94. Soukup J, Zauner A, Doppenberg EM, et al. Relationship between brain temperature, brain chemistry and oxygen delivery after severe human head injury: the effect of mild hypothermia. *Neurol Res* 2002; 24:161-168.
95. Harris OA, Colford JM Jr, Good MC, Matz PG. The role of hypothermia in the management of severe brain injury: a meta-analysis. *Arch Neurol* 2002; 59:1077-1083.

96. Gal R, Cundrle I, Zimova I, Smrcka M. Mild hypothermia therapy for patients with severe brain injury. *Clin Neurol Neurosurg* 2002; 104:318-321.
97. Yamamoto T, Mori K, Maeda M. Assessment of prognostic factors in severe traumatic brain injured patients treated by mild therapeutic cerebral hypothermia. *Neurol Res* 2002; 24:789-795.
98. Clifton GL, Miller ER, Choi SC, et al. Hypothermia on admission in patients with severe brain injury. *J Neurotrauma* 2002; 19:293-301.
99. Tokutomi T, Morimoto K, Miyagi T, et al. Optimal temperature for the management of severe traumatic brain injury: effect of hypothermia on intracranial pressure, systemic and intracranial hemodynamics, and metabolism. *Neurosurgery* 2003; 52:102-112.

Chapter 6

TRAUMATIC BRAIN INJURY: CLINICAL STUDIES

Donald W. Marion, MD
The Brain Trauma Foundation, New York, New York, USA

The treatment of traumatic brain injury (TBI) using hypothermia was first described by Temple Fay in 1943 (1). In the 1950s, Sedzimir noted "better than expected" outcomes in several patients with TBI after lowering their body temperatures to between 27° and 30°C for 1 to 5 days (2). Reports of contemporaneous research suggest that this pioneering use of hypothermia was based on the premise that TBI causes a hypermetabolic state, and that an increase in cerebral blood flow in response to the increased metabolic demand is responsible for the brain swelling associated with TBI. In uninjured dogs, for example, Rosomoff found that both cerebral blood flow and the cerebral metabolic rate for oxygen fell 6.7% for every 1°C reduction in body temperature between 35° and 25°C (3, 4). Stone and co-workers reported that cooling to 30°C in a primate model produced a 50% reduction in the cerebral metabolic rate for oxygen and a significantly lower rate of adenosine triphosphate depletion (5). According to Lundberg in 1959, hypothermia was as effective as osmotic diuretics for reducing elevated intracranial pressure (ICP) and had a more prolonged ICP-reducing effect than hyperventilation (6). James and colleagues found that hypothermia lowered the ICP in 20 of 40 patients with severe TBI; the ICP reduction averaged 51% (7).

Hypothermia did not gain wide acceptance, however, because it was not tested against normothermia in prospective clinical trials, nor was the optimal depth and duration of cooling established. Moreover, an increased incidence of hemorrhage and other complications after cerebral aneurysm surgery was attributed to the intraoperative use of hypothermia for neuroprotection. Extracerebral complications of hypothermia were also noted. The risk of cardiac arrhythmias and coagulopathy was unacceptable with body temperatures below 30°C. Cooling for several days or more was associated with a high incidence of pneumonia and other infections. Consequently, by the mid 1960s, most neurosurgeons had abandoned hypothermia.

Pre-clinical studies conducted during the past two decades have clearly established the efficacy of therapeutic hypothermia, fueling renewed interest in its use after TBI. This research points to several mechanisms by which hypothermia may limit secondary brain injury and has shown how such effects translate into tissue preservation and improved functional and cognitive outcomes. Among the most important pre-clinical discoveries was that efficacy does not require moderate hypothermia (below 32°C) and that hypothermia can be effective if administered after the injury. Most of the earlier studies had examined the effects of hypothermia administered during the injury, a paradigm that is not clinically relevant. In 1991, Clifton and associates reported on a series of experiments in rodents in which TBI was induced by a controlled cortical contusion device (8). They showed that 4 hours of hypothermia at 32°C, beginning 30 minutes after injury, significantly preserved tissue as compared to normothermia. Others consistently have found that treatment with mild to moderate hypothermia after a TBI results in reduced levels of excitatory amino acids and inflammatory cytokines, (9, 10) a diminished cellular inflammatory response, (11) and decreased edema (12). In addition, studies showed that hypothermia leads to preservation of tissue (13, 14) and of energy reserves, (15) as well as improved functional outcomes (16).

Given the promising results of these and other experimental studies, more than 20 clinical trials of therapeutic moderate hypothermia to treat patients with a severe TBI have been conducted over the past 15 years. Although some of these studies have not found the dramatic improvement seen in the pre-clinical studies, they have produced increasing evidence that therapeutic moderate hypothermia can help reduce elevated ICP and minimize secondary brain injury (Table 6-1). They also suggest that this treatment may benefit only certain subgroups of patients with a TBI and actually may harm others.

CLINICAL TRIALS

The first controlled, randomized clinical trial of therapeutic moderate hypothermia to treat severe TBI was reported in 1993 (17). The study enrolled 40 subjects, 20 of whom were cooled to 32°C as soon as possible after injury and kept at that temperature for 24 hours, using surface-cooling techniques. The temperatures of the 20 control subjects were kept at 37° to 38°C. Outcomes 3 months after injury, defined by the Glasgow Outcome Scale (GOS) and Disability Rating Scale, did not differ significantly between the two groups. However, hypothermia significantly lowered ICP and cerebral blood flow during the period of cooling and improved cerebral metabolism for at least 5 days after injury. Later that same year Clifton and co-workers (18) and Shiozaki and associates (19) also reported on clinical trials of hypothermia for severe TBI. Both studies used longer periods of hypothermia, Clifton, et al., cooling 24 of their 46 subjects to 32° to 33°C for 48 hours, Shiozaki, et al., using "mild hypothermia" of "approximately34°C" for up to 4-5 days in 16 of their 33 subjects. In Clifton's protocol, hypothermia treatment was initiated as soon as possible after injury, but Shiozaki and co-workers did not enroll subjects into their study unless they already had intracranial hypertension refractory to conventional treatment. Both studies showed a trend toward improved outcomes in the hypothermia groups. All three studies found that therapeutic hypothermia used in this way did not cause cardiac arrhythmias or clinically significant coagulopathies. When hypothermia was limited to 48 hours or less, the incidence of pneumonia or other infectious complications did not increase.

Table 6-2. Effect of hypothermia on ICP in clinical TBI studies.

Author (year)	PRCT*	n	Duration	Effect on ICP
Shiozaki (1993)[19]	Y	33	48 hrs	Decrease
Clifton (1993)[18]	Y	46	48 hrs	No change
Metz (1996)[478]	N	10	25 hrs	Decrease
Marion (1997)[20]	Y	82	24 hrs	Decrease
Nara (1998)[49]	N	23	?	Decrease
Tateishi (1998)[50]	N	9	1-6 days	Decrease
Clifton (2001)[23]	Y	392	48 hrs	"Decreased % of patients with ICP >20 mm Hg"
Takahashi (2000)[51]	N	9 (peds)*	3-21 days	Decrease
Jiang (2000)[21]	Y	87	3-14 days	Decrease
Biswas (2002)[512]	Y	21 (peds)	48 hrs	Decrease
Gal (2002)[53]	Y	30	72 hrs	Decrease
Tokutomi (2003)[32]	N	31	48-72 hrs	Decrease

*PRCT = prospective randomized clinical trial; ICP = intracranial pressure; Peds = pediatric subjects

In 1997, Marion and co-investigators reported the findings of a clinical trial examining therapeutic moderate hypothermia (32°C) in 82 patients with severe TBI (20). The experimental subjects (n=40) were cooled within 10 hours of injury and kept at 32° C for 24 hours. The 42 control patients were kept at 37° to 38°C. Outcomes in the hypothermia group were significantly better than in the normothermia group at 3 and 6 months after injury, but not at 12 months, in those with an initial Glasgow Coma Scale (GCS) score of 5-

7. Subjects, whose initial GCS score was 3 or 4 did not benefit from the treatment. Although both the experimental and control groups had similar mortality rates, the hypothermia group had a significantly larger proportion of subjects with mild or no disability. As in their 1993 study, they found a significant decrease in the ICP in the hypothermia group, and the treatment was associated with no significant medical complications.

In a subsequent study Jiang and associates compared outcomes after severe TBI between a group of 43 patients who received hypothermia (33° to 35°C) for 3 to 14 days and a group of 44 patients assigned to normothermia (21). One year after injury, good outcomes, defined as a GOS score of 4 or 5, were seen in 46.5% of the hypothermia group and only 27.3% of the normothermia group (p<0.05). The hypothermia group also had significantly lower ICPs and a lower incidence of hyperglycemia during their acute care, although subjects kept hypothermic for more than 3 days had a higher incidence of pneumonia and other infections.

In 2000, Signorini and Alderson published a meta-analysis of eight clinical trials of therapeutic moderate hypothermia for severe TBI conducted during the previous decade. They concluded that the odds of death or severe disability were significantly lower for patients treated with hypothermia than for those kept normothermic (22). They found 61% less death and severe disability in the hypothermia group, with an odds ratio of 0.39, a confidence interval of 0.02-0.74, and a p value of 0.004.

Two large clinical trials of therapeutic moderate hypothermia for severe TBI were completed in 2001. Clifton, et al., conducted a multi-center prospective randomized trial, which enrolled 392 subjects, aged 16-65 years (23). Patients assigned to hypothermia were cooled to between 32° and 33°C as soon as possible after injury and slowly rewarmed 48 hours later. The normothermia group was kept at 37° to 38°C. The severity of injury at enrollment and medical management were similar in both groups. Among the 368 patients for whom 6-month follow-up data were available, no significant differences in neurologic outcomes were found between the hypothermia and normothermia groups. Approximately 57% of the patients in both groups were severely disabled, vegetative, or had died, and 43% had good outcomes. Subjects who received hypothermia had a significantly lower incidence of intracranial hypertension during their acute care. Hypothermia was associated with a trend toward better outcomes among subjects 45 years of age and younger.

Zhi, et al., also conducted a prospective clinical trial of hypothermia (24). Of the 396 subjects enrolled, 198 were cooled within 24 hours and kept at 32° to 35°C for 1 to 7 days after injury, while the control group was kept at 36.5° to 37°C. Subjects ranged in age from 15 to 65 years (mean, 42.5 years). Both groups had similar initial GCS scores, and all patients were cared for at the same trauma center (Tianjin Huanhu Hospital), where they received similar initial medical treatment. The hypothermia group had significantly better outcomes than the normothermia group: a good outcome (GOS score of 4 or 5) was attained in 62% of the hypothermia group compared with 38% of the normothermia subjects. Mortality rates were 26% and 36%, respectively, in the hypothermia and normothermia groups, and ICP in the hypothermia group fell significantly during hypothermia.

A review of all clinical studies examining the use of therapeutic mild-moderate hypothermia for severe TBI was published in July 2002 (25). Harris and co-investigators identified 445 publications by carefully searching the six most comprehensive medical-literature databases. Only those reports that met the following predetermined criteria were included in their final meta-analysis: [1] randomized clinical trial comparing the efficacy of hypothermia with normothermia in patients with TBI, [2] all subjects at least 10 years old, and [3] results available to enable the calculation of relative risks (odds ratios, cumulative incidence, or incidence density measures) and 95% confidence intervals, or weighted mean differences and 95% confidence intervals. They found that only 7 of the 445 publications met these criteria. They then calculated the odds ratios and confidence intervals for the GOS scores and several medical complications in hypothermia patients vs. normothermia patients in these seven studies and found that therapeutic moderate hypothermia did not improve outcomes after severe TBI, nor was it associated with a significant decrease in ICP. They also found that hypothermia did not cause an increased incidence of pneumonia or cardiac arrhythmias, but that it did cause an increase in the partial thromboplastin time.

Several important flaws in their methodology cast doubt on these conclusions, however. Most important was the fact that the protocols for application of hypothermia had significant differences between studies. The validity of a meta-analysis relies on the similarity of study characteristics that are likely to affect the results. To their credit, Harris, et al., statistically analyzed the homogeneity of the studies included in their meta-analysis. The rapidity of cooling was variable; duration of cooling ranged from 24 hours to 7 or more days; and the target temperature ranged from 32° C to 35° C. Another major issue was that the meta-analysis of outcomes actually included only four studies, one of which (Clifton, et al.), (23) had four times as many subjects as the next largest study (20) and twice as many as the other three combined. Thus, Clifton's study was far over-represented in the meta-analysis of outcomes and the resultant conclusions. Harris, et al., also considered only the crude overall results of the seven studies, which can be misleading. For example, in the study of 82 patients by Marion, et al., they did not account for the fact that only those with an initial GCS score of 5 to 7 benefited from hypothermia. Others also have concluded that hypothermia may be beneficial only for subgroups of patients with a severe TBI. In a study of 91 patients, Shiozaki and colleagues found that therapeutic hypothermia did not improve outcomes for patients who did not have intracranial hypertension (26). Likewise, Harris, et al., did not consider the effects of age. Among Clifton's subjects who were older than 45 years, those who received hypothermia had worse outcomes than those assigned to normothermia (27). Yamamoto, et al., examined the effect of age in 35 patients who were cooled to between 33° and 35°C for several days after a severe TBI (28). Those who achieved a good outcome (mild, moderate or no disability) had a mean age of 30.2 years, whereas those with a poor outcome (severe disability, vegetative, or dead), averaged 45.2 years of age, and all subjects older than 50 years had a poor outcome.

The insensitivity of the analytic methods of the meta-analysis by Harris, et al., had an even greater influence on their conclusions regarding hypothermia's effect on ICP. As noted above, there were significant differences in the hypothermia protocols between studies. Also, the methods used to measure ICP were variable. They found significant heterogeneity among the studies used to determine the effect of hypothermia on ICP ($p<0.001$). Furthermore, most of the studies in this meta-analysis evaluated the effect of hypothermia on ICP values averaged over 5 or more days, thus including measurements obtained after hypothermia subjects were rewarmed. The ICP-reducing effect of hypothermia has been noted for nearly 50 years (6) and occurs during the period of cooling in most patients with severe TBI if hypothermia is initiated soon after injury. ICP usually increases upon rewarming of the patient and may slightly exceed average levels in normothermic patients, emphasizing a need to control the rewarming rate, as well as the cooling rate. Thus, the reduced ICP values during hypothermia are masked when averaged with post-rewarming measurements.

Finally, this meta-analysis did not include all of the important clinical trials. Some studies, though valid, were excluded because the published results omitted certain statistical details (21). Their inclusion may have altered the authors' conclusions. In addition, the previously described study by Zhi, et al., had not been published when the meta-analysis was conducted, but it is one of the largest to date and found a significant benefit from therapeutic hypothermia in patients with a TBI (24).

The conflicting results of the clinical trials by Clifton and Zhi have several possible explanations. Clifton's study was multi-center; significant inter-center differences occurred that may have confounded the results (29). These differences included the incidence of mean arterial blood pressures below 70 mm Hg ($p<0.001$), the percentage of patients who were dehydrated (p<0.001), and the incidence of cerebral perfusion pressures below 50 mm Hg (p<0.05) during the first 5 days after injury in the hypothermia patients. This study and several others have shown that a cerebral perfusion pressure of less than 50 mm Hg is a powerful independent predictor of poor outcomes. The centers also differed significantly in their use of vasopressor agents and morphine. In contrast, Zhi, et al., conducted a single-center study in which all these variables were well controlled and optimized.

UNANSWERED QUESTIONS

Although a relatively large number of clinical trials already have been completed (Table 6-2), some with rather disappointing results, the efficacy of therapeutic hypothermia remains uncertain. Among the questions still to be answered is whether the spontaneous hypothermia that often occurs after a severe TBI is protective. If so, how quickly should such patients be rewarmed after they arrive at the trauma center. Gentilello, et al., examined this issue in a randomized prospective study of 57 hypothermic (body temperature ≤34.5°C), critically injured patients who required pulmonary artery catheterization (30). One group underwent a technique of rapid continuous arteriovenous rewarming, the other group, standard (surface) rewarming. Although the rapid rewarming group required less fluid for resuscitation, the rate of survival to hospital discharge was not different between groups. However, only a small proportion of all subjects had a severe TBI, and outcome assessment did not include a GOS score or any other determination of functional outcomes. Soukup and associates studied the effect of body temperature at hospital admission on outcomes in 58 patients with a severe TBI. They found that this temperature was strongly related to outcome: the lower the body temperature, the worse the outcome (31). This study was not designed to determine if outcomes would be altered by rapidly raising body temperature, however. In a subanalysis of Clifton's multi-center study, the speed of rewarming seemed to affect outcomes, i.e., rapidly rewarmed patients had worse outcomes than did those who were allowed to rewarm passively over 12 or more hours. The chance of a poor outcome was 78% for subjects who arrived with a temperature of 35°C or less and were assigned to the normothermia group but 52% for those who were normothermic on admission and assigned to the normothermia group (p<0.004) (27). Conversely, among patients hypothermic upon admission, those assigned to the hypothermia group had a 61% risk of a poor outcome, although this risk was not significantly different from that for those assigned to normothermia.

Table 6-3. Prospective randomized clinical trials of therapeutic moderate hypothermia for severe traumatic brain injury.

Author (year)	n	Good outcome (GOS 4,5)		Significant differences
		Hypothermia	Normothermia	
Shiozaki (1993)[19]	33	38%	6%	No
Clifton (1993)[18]	46	52%	36%	No
Marion (1997)[20]	82	56%	33%	Yes
Shiozaki (2001)[26]	91	23%	30%	No
Jiang (2000)[21]	87	46.5%	27%	Yes
Clifton (2001)[23]	368	43%	43%	No
Zhi (2003)[24]	396	62%	38%	Yes

GOS = Glasgow Outcome Scale

Hypothermia that occurs spontaneously after a severe TBI may simply reflect a particularly severe brain injury. Studies have shown that patients who arrive at the trauma center with brain temperatures of less than 36°C have significantly higher levels of brain extracellular glutamate and lactate, well-known mediators of secondary brain injury, compared to those who arrive with normal brain temperatures (31). Moreover, the findings of the Clifton study are insufficient to determine if maintaining hypothermia in those who arrive hypothermic will necessarily improve outcomes. To clarify this issue, Clifton has organized a new multi-center clinical trial focusing on patients who arrive at the trauma center hypothermic after a severe TBI. This trial will compare 6-month outcomes between a group left hypothermic for 48 hours and a group that is slowly rewarmed over 12 hours.

Cooling to as low as 32° to 33°C may not be necessary to improve outcome from severe TBI. Mild hypothermia (35° to 36°C) may provide maximum benefit while avoiding adverse systemic and cerebral metabolic sequelae of the treatment. Tokutomi, et al., investigated the physiologic and metabolic consequences of cooling to various brain temperatures in 31 adults with a severe TBI (32). They found that ICP dropped significantly from 37° to 35°C but fell no further when the temperature was reduced below this level. The cerebral perfusion pressure peaked at 35° to 36°C and decreased with lower temperatures. Cerebral oxygen delivery and oxygen consumption also decreased when temperatures were reduced below 35°C. Gupta, et al., directly measured the partial pressure of oxygen (PO_2) of the brain tissue in 30 patients with a severe TBI who were cooled to as low as 33°C (33). Although this measurement fell with cooling of any degree, the greatest reduction occurred when the brain temperature was reduced below 35°C.

Another question to be resolved is whether fever during the first several days after a TBI is detrimental. Pre-clinical studies have clearly established that brain temperatures greater than 39°C are harmful to ischemic regions of the brain (34). This effect is evident even with fever at 24 hours after injury (35). In a meta-analysis of 3790 stroke victims, Hajat and co-workers found that fever had a highly significant correlation with increased morbidity and mortality (36). Others have found a similar relationship between fever and poor outcomes in patients with spontaneous intracerebral hemorrhage and subarachnoid hemorrhage (37, 38). Thus, the beneficial effects attributed to hypothermia in some of the earlier studies may instead have been due to the prevention of febrile episodes, which are common in the neurosurgical intensive care unit (ICU). We measured rectal temperatures every 4 hours in 428 consecutive patients in our neurosurgical ICU after a stroke, subarachnoid hemorrhage, or TBI (39). We noted febrile episodes in 47% of these patients; the rate increased to 93% for those in the ICU for at least 14 days. This finding is of particular concern given that brain temperatures commonly are 1° to 2°C higher than rectal temperatures after a severe TBI (40).

Laboratory studies suggest that some of the mechanisms of action of hypothermia include reduction of the levels of excitatory amino acids, oxygen free radicals, and inflammatory cytokines. At least in rodent models, these mediators reach peak levels within minutes after the initial injury. Most of the clinical trials of hypothermia have used surface cooling techniques, which require a minimum of 4-6 hours to reduce the body temperature from 37° to 32°C, a delay that may undermine the effectiveness of hypothermia. In fact, studies of rodents have shown that hypothermia is not effective if induced more than 1 hour after a controlled cortical contusion injury (41, 42). Several companies have developed heat-exchange indwelling venous catheters that can reduce body temperature rapidly; future hypothermia trials will likely include their use. This technique of temperature modulation already has been used successfully to prevent fever in the ICU (43).

The optimal treatment for severe TBI ultimately may involve a combination of therapies, including hypothermia. In this regard, we agree with the conclusions of Bayir, Clark, and Kochanek, that multiple mechanisms cause secondary brain injury, and that successful future treatment strategies must target several, if not all, of those mechanisms (44). Pre-clinical studies already have investigated the combination of hypothermia with 21-aminosteroids, (42) fibroblast growth factor-2, (45) cyclosporin A, (46) and interleukin-10 (47). None of these studies found the combination therapy more efficacious than hypothermia alone, however.

SUMMARY

Laboratory studies of mild-moderate hypothermia following TBI have consistently shown benefit. In clinical trials, however, therapeutic hypothermia can decrease ICP, but effects on neurologic outcome are variable. Multiple explanations for the variability include details of patient selection, timing and duration of hypothermia, and target temperature. Future clinical trials should focus on the speed of cooling, perhaps with the use of intravascular heat-exchange devices. Trials investigating the effect of fever and the combination of hypothermia with other therapies are also needed.

REFERENCES

1. Fay T. Observations on generalized refrigeration in cases of severe cerebral trauma. *Assoc Res Nerv Ment Dis Proc* 1943; 24:611-619.
2. Sedzimir CB. Therapeutic hypothermia in cases of head injury. *J Neurosurg* 1959; 16:407-414.
3. Rosomoff HL, Holaday DA. Cerebral blood flow and cerebral oxygen consumption during hypothermia. *Am J Physiol* 1954; 179:85-88.
4. Rosomoff HL. Relationship of metabolism to hypothermia. *Res Publ Assoc* 1966; 41:116-126.
5. Stone HH, Donnelly C, Frobese AS. The effect of lowered body temperature on the cerebral hemodynamics and metabolism of man. *Surg Gynecol Obstet* 1956; 103:313-322.
6. Lundberg N, Kjallquist A, Bien C. Reduction of increased intracranial pressure by hyperventilation. *Acta Psychiatr Scand* 1959; 34:4-64.
7. James HE, Langfitt TW, Kumar VS, Ghostine SY. Treatment of intracranial hypertension. Analysis of 105 continuous recordings of intracranial pressure. *Acta Neurochir (Wien)* 1977; 36:189-200.
8. Clifton GL, Jiang JY, Lyeth BG, et al. Marked protection by moderate hypothermia after experimental traumatic brain injury. *J Cereb Blood Flow Metab* 1991; 11:114-121.
9. Busto R, Globus MYT, Dietrich WD, et al. Effect of mild hypothermia on ischemia-induced release of neurotransmitters and free fatty acids in rat brain. *Stroke* 1989; 7:904-910.
10. DeKosky ST, Miller PD, Styren S, O'Malley M, Marion DW. Interleukin-1B elevation in CSF following head injury in humans is attenuated by hypothermia. *J Neurotrauma* 1994; 11:106.
11. Chatzipanteli K, Alonso OF, Kraydieh S, Dietrich WD. Importance of posttraumatic hypothermia and hyperthermia on the inflammatory response after fluid percussion brain injury: biochemical and immunocytochemical studies. *J Cereb Blood Flow Metab* 2000; 20:531-42.
12. Kawai N, Nakamura T, Okauchi M, Nagao S. Effects of hypothermia on intracranial pressure and brain edema formation: studies in a rat acute subdural hematoma model. *J Neurotrauma* 2000; 17:193-202.
13. Busto R, Dietrich WD, Globus MY, et.al. Postischemic moderate hypothermia inhibits CA1 hippocampal ischemic neuronal injury. *J Cereb Blood Flow Metab* 1989; 9:S266.
14. Dietrich WD, Alonso O, Busto R, et al. Post-traumatic brain hypothermia reduces histopathological damage following concussive brain injury in the rat. *Acta Neuropathol* 1994; 87:250-258.
15. Kramer RS, Sanders AP, Lesage AM. The effect of profound hypothermia on preservation of cerebral ATP content during circulatory arrest. *J Thorac Cardiovasc Surg* 1968; 56:699-709.
16. Dixon CE, Markgraf CG, Angileri F, et al. Protective effects of moderate hypothermia on behavioral deficits but not necrotic cavitation following cortical impact injury in the rat. J Neurotrauma. 1998; 15:95-103.
17. Marion DW, Obrist WD, Carlier PM, Penrod LE, Darby JM. The use of moderate therapeutic hypothermia for patients with severe head injuries: A preliminary report. *J Neurosurg* 1993; 79:354-362.
18. Clifton GL, Allen S, Barrodale P et al. A phase II study of moderate hypothermia in severe brain injury. *J Neurotrauma* 1993; 10:263-271.

19. Shiozaki T, Sugimoto H, Taneda M, et al. Effect of mild hypothermia on uncontrollable intracranial hypertension after severe head injury. *J Neurosurg* 1993; 79:363-368.

20. Marion DW, Penrod LE, Kelsey SF, et al. Treatment of traumatic brain injury with moderate hypothermia. *N Engl J Med* 1997; 336:540-546.

21. Jiang J, Yu M, Zhu C. Effect of long-term mild hypothermia therapy in patients with severe traumatic brain injury: 1-year follow-up review of 87 cases. *J Neurosurg* 2000; 93:546-549.

22. Signorini DF, Alderson P. Therapeutic hypothermia for head injury. *Cochrane Database Syst Rev* 2000; CD001048.

23. Clifton GL, Miller ER, Choi SC, et al. Lack of effect of induction of hypothermia after acute brain injury. *N Engl J Med* 2001; 344:556-563.

24. Zhi D, Zhang S, and Lin X. Study on the therapeutic mechanism and clinical effect of mild hypothermia in patients with severe head injury. *Surg Neurol.* 2003; 59:381-385.

25. Harris OA, Colford JM, Jr., Good MC, Matz PG. The role of hypothermia in the management of severe brain injury: a meta-analysis. *Arch Neurol* 2002; 59:1077-1083.

26. Shiozaki T, Hayakata T, Taneda M, et al. A multicenter prospective randomized controlled trial of the efficacy of mild hypothermia for severely head injured patients with low intracranial pressure. Mild Hypothermia Study Group in Japan. *J Neurosurg* 2001; 94:50-54.

27. Clifton GL, Miller ER, Choi SC, et al. Hypothermia on admission in patients with severe brain injury. *J Neurotrauma* 2002; 19:293-301.

28. Yamamoto T, Mori K, Maeda M. Assessment of prognostic factors in severe traumatic brain injury patients treated by mild therapeutic cerebral hypothermia therapy. *Neurol Res* 2002; 24:789-795.

29. Clifton GL, Choi SC, Miller ER, et al. Intercenter variance in clinical trials of head trauma--experience of the National Acute Brain Injury Study: Hypothermia. *J Neurosurg* 2001; 95:751-755.

30. Gentilello LM, Jurkovich GJ, Stark MS, Hassantash SA, O'Keefe GE. Is hypothermia in the victim of major trauma protective or harmful? A randomized, prospective study. *Ann Surg* 1997; 226:439-447.

31. Soukup J, Zauner A, Doppenberg EM, et al. Relationship between brain temperature, brain chemistry and oxygen delivery after severe human head injury: the effect of mild hypothermia. *Neurol Res* 2002; 24:161-168.

32. Tokutomi T, Morimoto K, Miyagi T, et al. Optimal temperature for the management of severe traumatic brain injury: effect of hypothermia on intracranial pressure, systemic and intracranial hemodynamics, and metabolism. *Neurosurg* 2003; 52:102-112.

33. Gupta AK, Al Rawi PG, Hutchinson PJ, Kirkpatrick PJ. Effect of hypothermia on brain tissue oxygenation in patients with severe head injury. *Br J Anaesth* 2002; 88:188-192.

34. Dietrich WD, Alonso O, Halley M, Busto R. Delayed posttraumatic brain hyperthermia worsens outcome after fluid percussion brain injury: A light and electron microscopic study in rats. *Neurosurg* 1996; 38:533-541.

35. Baena RC, Busto R, Dietrich WD, Globus MY, Ginsberg MD. Hyperthermia delayed by 24 hours aggravates neuronal damage in rat hippocampus following global ischemia. *Neurologyl* 1997; 48:768-773.

36. Hajat C, Hajat S, Sharma P. Effects of poststroke pyrexia on stroke outcome : a meta-analysis of studies in patients. *Stroke* 2000;31 :410-414.

37. Schwarz S, Hafner K, Aschoff A, Schwab S. Incidence and prognostic significance of fever following intracerebral hemorrhage. *Neurology* 2000 ; 54:354 -361.

38. Oliveira-Filho J, Ezzeddine MA, Segal AZ, et al. Fever in subarachnoid hemorrhage: relationship to vasospasm and outcome. *Neurology* 2001; 56:1299-1304.
39. Kilpatrick MM, Lowry DW, Firlik AD, Yonas H, Marion DW. Uncontrolled hyperthermia in the neurosurgical intensive care unit. *Neurosurg* 2000; 47:850-856.
40. Henker RA, Brown SD, Marion DW. Comparison of brain temperature with bladder and rectal temperatures in adults with severe head injury. *Neurosurg* 1998; 42:1071-1075.
41. Markgraf CG, Clifton GL, Moody MR. Treatment window for hypothermia in brain injury. *J Neurosurg* 2001; 95:979-983.
42. Marion DW, White MJ. Treatment of experimental brain injury with moderate hypothermia and 21-aminosteroids. *J Neurotrauma* 1996; 13:139-147.
43. Diringer MN. Treatment of fever in the neurologic intensive care unit with a catheter-based heat exchange system. *Crit Care Med* 2004; 32:559-564.
44. Bayir H, Clark RS, Kochanek PM. Promising strategies to minimize secondary brain injury after head trauma. *Crit Care Med* 2003; 31:S112-S117.
45. Yan HQ, Yu J, Kline AE, et al. Evaluation of combined fibroblast growth factor-2 and moderate hypothermia therapy in traumatically brain injured rats. *Brain Res* 2000; 887:134-143.
46. Li PA, He QP, Siesjo BK. Effects of intracarotid arterial injection of cyclosporin A and spontaneous hypothermia on brain damage incurred after a long period of global ischemia. *Brain Res* 2001; 890:306-313.
47. Kline AE, Bolinger BD, Kochanek PM, et al. Acute systemic administration of interleukin-10 suppresses the beneficial effects of moderate hypothermia following traumatic brain injury in rats. *Brain Res* 2002; 937:22-31.
48. Metz C, Holzschuh M, Bein T, et al. Moderate hypothermia in patients with severe head injury: cerebral and extracerebral effects. *J Neurosurg* 1996; 85:533-541.
49. Nara I, Shiogai T, Hara M, Saito I. Comparative effects of hypothermia, barbiturate, and osmotherapy for cerebral oxygen metabolism, intracranial pressure, and cerebral perfusion pressure in patients with severe head injury. *Acta Neurochir Suppl (Wien)* 1998; 71:22-26.
50. Tateishi A, Soejima Y, Taira Y, et al. Feasibility of the titration method of mild hypothermia in severely head-injured patients with intracranial hypertension. *Neurosurg* 1998; 42:1065-1069.
51. Takahashi I, Kitahara T, Endo M, Ohwada T. Clinical analysis of hypothermia in children with severe head injury. *No Shinkei Geka* 2000; 28:983-989.
52. Biswas AK, Bruce DA, Sklar FH, Bokovoy JL, Sommerauer JF. Treatment of acute traumatic brain injury in children with moderate hypothermia improves intracranial hypertension. *Crit Care Med* 2002; 30:2742-2751.
53. Gal R, Cundrle I, Zimova I, Smrcka M. Mild hypothermia therapy for patients with severe brain injury. *Clin Neurol Neurosurg* 2002; 104:318-321.

Chapter 7

SPINAL CORD ISCHEMIA AND TRAUMA

James D. Guest, MD, PhD, W. Dalton Dietrich, III, PhD
University of Miami, Miami, FL, USA

INTRODUCTION

Therapeutic hypothermia as a potential treatment for spinal cord injury (SCI) has a long history. In early studies by Albin and colleagues (1-3), selective spinal cord cooling to approximately 12°C resulted in marked neurological and functional recovery after SCI. In a study by Green and colleagues (4), regional hypothermia (6-18°C) in cats initiated 1 hr post-injury decreased edema formation and hemorrhage. In studies by Wells and Hansebout (5), local cooling to 6°C was also reported to be effective in minimizing functional deficits in dogs, even when initiated 4 hr after spinal cord compression. Taken together, these early investigations support the use of profound hypothermia as a therapeutic strategy to protect the spinal cord after injury. Nevertheless, producing profound local hypothermia of the injured spinal cord presents various technical problems, and the alternative use of systemic hypothermia can lead to potentially serious complications. Because the beneficial effects of hypothermia have been somewhat inconsistent in laboratory experiments, and some clinical studies lacked adequate controls, it is currently difficult to determine the degree of benefit with hypothermic therapy after SCI.

A resurgence in the use of therapeutic hypothermia in experimental models of brain and SCI occurred in the 1980s when relatively small variations in intraischemic brain temperature were discovered to critically determine whether neurons died after a transient global ischemic insult (6). Since that discovery, laboratories throughout the world have reported the benefits of moderate to mild hypothermia in cerebral ischemia and brain trauma models (7-11). Success with mild therapeutic hypothermia has also been seen in a variety of clinical studies, including cardiac arrest, traumatic brain injury (TBI), and stroke (12-16). Although more work is required to understand how to best use hypothermia in specific targeted patient populations, the potential use of hypothermia to protect the brain after injury is being investigated worldwide.

For SCI, questions remain regarding whether mild systemic hypothermia or local cooling represents the best strategy for protecting the spinal cord after injury (17). In terms of focal spinal cord cooling, the advantages of epidural vs. subarachnoid cooling remain to be clarified. The purpose of this report is to review and summarize the potential use of therapeutic hypothermia as a neuroprotective strategy in experimental and clinical SCI investigations. Mechanisms underlying the benefits of hypothermia are also discussed, as well as novel cooling techniques that are undergoing clinical evaluation. Finally, questions regarding future directions for the use of therapeutic hypothermia will be addressed.

MECHANISMS OF PROTECTION

The pathogenesis of SCI is complex, and is composed of the primary injury and various secondary injury mechanisms that lead to cell death, axotomy, and neurological deficits (18-20). Pathophysiologic mechanisms, including ischemia, excitotoxicity, free radical production, inflammatory and apoptotic processes, are believed to significantly contribute to cell injury. Various studies have investigated potential mechanisms contributing to hypothermic protection. Pathophysiologic mechanisms sensitive to temperature alterations following ischemic and traumatic injury include glutamate release, stabilization of the blood-brain barrier, oxygen radical production, intracellular signaling conduction, protein synthesis, reduced cerebral metabolism, membrane stabilization, inflammation, activation of protein kinases, cytoskeletal breakdown, and early gene expression (21, 22). Because the pathophysiology of ischemic and traumatic injury is complex, the fact that many injury mechanisms have been reported to be temperature-sensitive may account for the dramatic effects of temperature on outcome in various injury models. Similar to brain injury, hypothermic protection in models of SCI is felt to involve inhibiting the release of excitatory amino acids, as well as apoptotic cell death and inflammation (23, 24).

In addition to neuronal vulnerability, an important component of SCI is widespread axonal injury. Studies from various laboratories have demonstrated that moderate post-traumatic hypothermia reduces the extent of traumatic axonal injury (10, 25). Although hypothermia is believed to exert its beneficial effects on traumatic axonal injury through its membrane-protective properties, the mechanism of axonal protection is not well understood. Recently, several studies have implicated calcium-induced calpain-mediated proteolysis in the pathogenesis of ischemic and traumatic neuronal injury (26, 27). Focal calpain-mediated spectrin proteolysis takes place and is associated with classic pathological markers of traumatic axonal injury, including local axolemmal permeability changes, neurofilament compaction, and mitochondrial damage (28). In this regard, recent studies have shown that post-traumatic hypothermia decreases early calpain-mediated proteolysis and concomitant cytoskeletal compromise following traumatic axonal injury (27). In that study, moderate hypothermia (32°C) for 90 min dramatically reduced the number of damaged axons displaying calpain-mediated spectrin proteolysis and reduced neurofilament compaction. In SCI, hypothermia may improve axonal function by inhibiting axonal/cytoskeletal damage.

EFFECT OF COOLING ON PERIPHERAL NERVE INJURY AND WALLERIAN DEGENERATION

Mechanisms relevant to the survival and subsequent repair of peripheral axons may provide important information about how recovery from SCI may be enhanced. It is known that the distal segments of severed myelinated axons undergo Wallerian degeneration within 1-2 days *in vivo* at normal mammalian temperatures. Distal segments of several mammalian PNS axons can survive for longer periods under cooled conditions (29-32). Sea and colleagues (31) assessed the histological and ultrastructural structures of severed axons of the ventral tail nerve of rats at 32, 23, and 13°C. Distal (anucleate) portions of severed myelinated axons degenerated within 3 days at 32°, and within 6 days at 23°C. When tail cuff temperature was reduced to 13°C, the nerve did not degenerate for 10 days.

In a recent study by Tsao and colleagues (33), isolated sciatic nerve segments from wild-type and C57BL/Wld mice (which carry a gene that slows Wallerian degeneration) were maintained at 25°C and 35°C. The degeneration rate of wild-type axons was slowed dramatically at 25°C, with the compound action potential preserved up to 7 days post-transection compared to 2 days at 37°C. When temperature was raised to 37°C after 24-72 hr at 25°C, degeneration occurred within the subsequent 24 hr. This finding suggests that cooling delays a "final" stage of the induction of Wallerian degeneration, but when that stage commences, it progresses rapidly to completion. It is possible that hypothermia can extend the window of opportunity to treat compressed or severed axons, with other techniques currently employed to repair severed axons (34, 35).

EXPERIMENTAL INVESTIGATIONS

Laboratory Studies

Laboratory studies of spinal cord ischemia and trauma are summarized in tables 7-1 and 7-2.

Table 7-1. Effects of spinal cord cooling in experimental spinal cord trauma.

.First author (ref)	Species	Level	Method	Cooling Start	°C, Duration	Other	Outcome
Albin (1)	Dog	T10	WD	0 h	12 SC, 2.5 h	DO	Positive
Albin (2)	Dog	T10	WD	0 h	5 SOL, 2.5 h		Positive
Albin (3)	Monkey	T10	WD	4 h post	10 SC, 3 h	DO	Positive
Ducker (46)	Dog	T11	WD	3 h post	3 SOL, 3 h	DO	Positive
Kelly (103)	Dog	T10	WD	0 h	12 SC, 2.5 h	DO	Positive
Black (47)	Monkey	T10	WD	1 h post	4-8 SOL, 5 h	±DO	Negative
Tator (61)	Monkey	T9-10	ICD	3 h post / 3 h post	5, 3 h / 36, 3h	±DO / ±DO	Positive / Positive
Campbell (48)	Cat	T9	WD	3 h post	4 SOL, 3 h	DO	Positive
Hansebout (65)	Dog	T13	ICD	0 h	4 EP, 4 h		Positive
Kuchner (49)	Dog	T13	ICD	15' post	6 SOL, 4 h		Positive
Eidelberg (50)	Ferret	Mid-T	SWL	1 h post	10 EP, 3 h		Positive
Wells (5)	Dog	T13	ICD	4 h post	6 EP, 1-18 h		Positive
Green (4)	Cat	T10	WD	1,4 h post	6-18°C, 3 h	DO	Positive
Martinez (63)	Rat	T8	WD	Pre & post	31-32°C, 4 h	DI	Positive
Yu (53)	Rat	T10	WD	Post	33°C, 4 h	DI	Positive
Chatzipanteli (23)	Rat	T10	WD	Post	33°C, 4 h	DI	Positive

Methods: WD = weight drop, ICD = inflatable compression device, SWL = static weight load
Temperatures: SC = spinal cord, SOL = solution, EP = epidural
Other: DO = dura open, DI = dura intact.

Table 7-2. Hypothermia in experimental spinal cord ischemia.

First author (ref)	Species	Cooling	°C, Duration	Outcome Measures
Vacanti (36)	Rabbit	During	34.0-36.8°C, 25 min	Behavior/24 h
Robertson (37)	Rabbit	During	30°C, 25-50 min	SSEPs, Behavior, 48 h
Berguer (44)	Dog	During	19-12°C, 45 min	Behavior/Pathology, 24 h
Naslund (76)	Rabbit	During	30°C, 21 min	Behavior/Pathology, 5 d
Vanicky (39)	Rabbit	During	<15°C, 20-60 min	Behavior/Pathology, 2 d
Marsala (102)	Dog	During	28.5°C, 40 min	Behavior/SSEP, Pathology, 2d
Westergren (40)	Rat	After	30°C, 2 hr	Motor, behavior, 14 days
Yu (53)	Rat	After	30°C, 20 min	MAP, behavior, 24 hr
Westergren (109)	Rat	After	30°C	Blood flow
Westergren (52)	Rat	After	30°C, 20 min	Axonal changes, 24 hr
Yu (51)	Rat	After	30°C, 20 min	Plasma protein extravasation
Kakinohana (38)	Rat	After	34, 30, 27°C, 2 hr	Motor dysfunction, pathology, 2-3 d

SSEP = somatosensory evoked potential, MAP = mean arterial pressure

In the early studies by Vacanti and Ames (36), a temperature reduction of 3°C during temporary occlusion of the abdominal aorta increased the duration of spinal cord ischemia that could still allow normal recovery. In 1986, Robinson and colleagues showed that moderate hypothermia (30°C) applied systemically also increased the duration of ischemia required to produce neurological deficits (37). In that study, hypothermia allowed a high percentage of rabbits to demonstrate persistent spinal somatosensory evoked potentials (SSEP) and retain normal motor function up to 48 hr after injury. Other experimental studies have indicated that the therapeutic window for spinal cord neuroprotection from ischemia may be as short as 5 minutes (38). Other ischemic studies have reported positive findings under a variety of experimental conditions (39, 40).

In a more recent study by Dimar and colleagues (41), the effects of precisely controlled hypothermia (19°C) to the area of SCI was reported. Following spinal cord contusion and sustained compression, two hours of hypothermia improved the Basso, Beattie, Bresnahan (BBB) motor scores (42) and transcranial magnetic motor-evoked potential responses compared to normothermic (37°C) rats. In contrast, no improvement with hypothermia was seen following severe SCI produced by weight drop injury.

Different methods of cooling have been attempted by SCI investigations (43). These include perfusion of the spinal cord vasculature with a chilled physiologic fluid, perfusion of the spinal subarachnoid space, perfusion of the spinal epidural space, and cooling of tissues adjacent to the spinal cord. Berguer and colleagues (44), used an extracorporeal perfusion device consisting of a heat exchanger and pumps to infuse cooled saline into the subarachnoid space at L6. Albin and colleagues (3, 45) also used selective cooling to about 12°C that resulted in a marked neurological and functional recovery 2 months after injury. Ducker and Hamit (46) used local cooling to 3°C for 3 hr and reported improvement in recovery and neurological function when begun 3 hr after injury. In a study by Kakinohana and colleagues (38), a technique of selective spinal cord cooling in the rat utilizing a small copper heat exchanger implanted into the subcutaneous space overlying the lumbosacral spinal cord segments was used. These investigators reported that decreases in dorsal or ventral spinal cord surface temperatures to 27°C resulted in improved motor recovery following spinal cord ischemia. Local cooling has been conducted in other models of spinal cord trauma, with varying results (47-50).

In contrast to local cooling, the potential benefits of mild or moderate systemic hypothermia on outcome following SCI have recently been investigated (51-53). Yu and colleagues (51) reported that systemic hypothermia (30°C) for 20 min following compression injury led to reduction of plasma protein extravasation in rats. In a study by Westergren and colleagues (52), systemic hypothermia (30°C) for 20 minutes decreased the number of damaged axons as assessed immunohistochemically using β-amyloid precursor protein, ubiquitin, and protein gene product 9.5. Because reductions in systemic temperature to 30°C can lead to serious complications such as cardiac arrhythmia, the beneficial effects of milder degrees of hypothermia have recently been investigated.

Following spinal cord contusion (at T10) in adult rats, systemic hypothermia was induced by cooling to 32-33°C beginning 30 min post-injury and continued for 4 hr (53). Over the 6 week survival period, an assessment of locomotor function was performed twice weekly, utilizing the BBB locomotive scale. Rats were also perfusion-fixed for histopathological analysis of tissue damage. Modest changes in the temperature recorded from the epidural space were associated with significantly improved locomotive deficits and reduced areas of tissue damage at both 7 and 44 days after injury. These studies demonstrated the benefits of mild systemic hypothermia and supported the potential use of this strategy in the treatment of acute SCI. Subsequent studies using the same injury model have shown that systemic hypothermia reduces the extent of migration of polymorphonuclear leukocytes into injured spinal cord tissue (23). These inflammatory cells are believed to contribute to the propagation of the secondary injury through the generation of free oxygen radicals and nitric oxide-induced cytotoxic products. Whether local cooling can also achieve this alteration in the inflammatory response should be studied.

CLINICAL STUDIES OF LOCAL HYPOTHERMIA FOR TRAUMATIC SCI

Experience with the ability of moderate to deep hypothermia to increase the brain's ischemic tolerance developed from cerebrovascular neurosurgery (54) and from other surgical disciplines such as cardiac surgery. Clinical trials with SCI were begun in the 1960s after the promising experimental reports by Albin, et al (1-3). These trials were facilitated by the clinical practice of laminectomy and durotomy for acute SCI during the 1960s and 1970s (Table 7-3). Because patients were undergoing surgical decompression, including exposure of the spinal cord, soon after their injuries, techniques of local cooling were facilitated. In several non-randomized trials, some benefits of hypothermia were reported (61, 62). In these studies, the spinal cord was locally cooled by irrigating the exposed cord with cold saline following laminectomy. These studies are particularly difficult to evaluate because they included only a few patients, lacked randomized control groups (63, 64), and included adjunctive therapeutic measures such as spinal cord decompression and the use of steroids (methylprednisolone) (65), treatments that remain controversial.

Table 7-3. Local spinal cord cooling in human spinal cord injury.

First author (ref)	n, Level	Cooling Start	°C, Duration	Steroids	Improved	Mortality
Selker (55)	2, C 2, T	3 h	4-5, 3 h	-	50%	50%
Meacham (56)	12, C	4-8 h	4, 3 h	Yes	70%	29%
Koons (57)	3, C 4, T	3-8 h	1.5, 30 min	Yes	40%	0%
Negrin (58)	1, C 2, T	5 h-1 yr	Uncertain	-	0%	0%
Bricolo (59)	4, C	7-26 h	5, 1.5 h – 8 d	Yes	50%	38%
Tator (60)	7, C 4, T	3-8 h	5 or 36, 3 h	-	27%	38%
Hansebout (65)	4, C 6, T	8 h	6, 4 h	Yes	43%	10%

C = cervical, T = thoracic

The most substantial objection to inducing systemic hypothermia following SCI has been the need for associated anesthesia to prevent a shivering response. With the patient anesthetized for a prolonged period, one can not monitor neurologic function clinically and the risk of complications such as pneumonia is increased. With intravascular heat-exchange catheters it may now be possible to cause mild systemic hypothermia and maintain the conscious state. These devices could be combined with the drug meperidine, which is known to lower the shivering threshold (66).

INTRAOPERATIVE HYPOTHERMIA

The most compelling clinical evidence for hypothermic neuroprotection of the spinal cord comes from studies involving thoracoabdominal aneurysm repair in which the spinal cord was actively rendered hypothermic at the time of the ischemia or compression (67-73) (Table 7-4). Neurologic deficits including lower limb paralysis can occur as a result of ischemia during these procedures (75-78), which often require a period of clamping of the aortic region that gives rise to the vessels that supply the spinal cord. In this setting, hypothermia may inhibit ischemic cell processes, including excitotoxicity, free radical production, oxidative stress, and apoptosis. The methods that have been employed are systemic hypothermia, perfusion of the vessels taking off from the cross-clamped aortic segment with cooled physiologic fluid, and perfusion of either the epidural or subarachnoid spaces with cooled physiologic fluid. The latter method is relatively simple and analogous to insertion of an epidural catheter for anesthesia. It should be noted that such studies have also reported that removal of CSF improves the spinal cord's tolerance to ischemia. This implies that attention should be directed to the pressure that perfusion procedures create within the spinal cord and surrounding subarachnoid and epidural spaces. In a randomized study, Svensson and colleagues (79) demonstrated that utilizing cooling with aortofemoral bypass to between 29°C and 32°C combined with CSF drainage significantly reduced the occurrence of postoperative lower limb deficits. Other studies that have used deep hypothermia and circulatory arrest on a selective basis for high risk complex repairs have not reported good results (68, 70).

Table 7-4. Intraoperative hypothermia for thoracic and thoracoabdominal aorta repair.

First author (ref)	*# Patients*	*Temperature*	*Outcome*
Crawford (68)	25	18°C or 4-6°C RT	Satisfactory
Svensson (79)	31	29-31° BT	Positive
Cambria (74)	70	24°C CSFT, 34°C CT	Positive
Safi (70)	409	PHCA	Positive
Kouchoukos (73)	161	11-16°C NT; 22°C BT	Positive
Svensson (80)	132	29-32°C or <20°C BT	Positive

RT = rectal temperature, BT = bladder temperature, CSFT = cerebrospinal fluid temperature, CT = core temperature, PHCA = profound hypothermic circulatory arrest, NT = nasopharyngeal temperature

Recently, the effects of mild (36.5°C), moderate (29-32°C), or deep (<20°C) hypothermia on the development of neurologic defects after aortic surgery were compared (80). In this retrospective case-comparison of prospectively collected data, moderate or deep hypothermia resulted in fewer transient neurologic deficits. Thus, actively cooling patients with aortofemoral or cardiopulmonary bypass offered more protection than mild passive hypothermia. The aforementioned evidence and also evidence from the practice of deep hypothermia for procedures requiring cerebral circulatory arrest has lead some spinal surgeons to cool patients during surgical procedures that involve a risk of injury to the spinal cord such as the removal of spinal cord tumors. The merits of pre-emptive protective cooling in these non-ischemic applications are unknown and the risks of exposing the patient to hypothermia must be considered.

A mild degree of hypothermia usually follows anesthetic induction due to a core-to-peripheral heat redistribution (81). Temperature continues to fall until systemic vasoconstriction is activated and an equilibrium is established between metabolic heat production, heat loss and warming. A useful variable to define hypothermia is the temperature at which a physiologic response such as skin vasoconstriction, or shivering, occurs. It should be noted that these levels vary with different anesthetic conditions and with the age of the patients. The risk of cardiac arrhythmia is increased with deeper levels of cooling, but even mild hypothermia has been linked to wound or pulmonary infections (82). The association of mild hypothermia with wound infection in neurosurgery is somewhat controversial (83-86). In addition, some data indicates that blood loss is increased during mild hypothermia (87, 88) but this issue is also controversial (89). Other concerns include the potential for post-operative shivering thermogenesis to cause myocardial ischemia (90). Our own experience indicates that the risk of wound infection is linked to the extent of exposure to hypothermia and that mild hypothermia does not significantly increase blood loss (91).

Other factors of importance to the clinical use of hypothermia include the rates at which cooling and warming can be achieved. Passive cooling may be too slow to provide the desired spinal cord temperature during the period of risk and re-warming is notoriously difficult in the presence of systemic vasoconstriction. Because neurophysiological monitoring is frequently used during spinal cord surgery the extent of change in the latency and amplitude of monitored potentials attributable to cooling should be considered (43, 92). Based on our clinical and experimental experience and review of the literature we believe that systemic cooling to mild degrees such as 33°C may improve the ability of the spinal cord to tolerate reversible ischemia or transient mechanical deformation such as tension or compression. However, we and others emphasize the importance of titrating the hypothermic exposure to the period of risk and making provisions for rewarming to normothermia prior to termination of anesthesia (93).

METHODS OF INDUCING HYPOTHERMIA

One of the major obstacles in evaluating the potential benefits of therapeutic hypothermia is identifying strategies to produce the hypothermia itself. In models of cerebral ischemia and traumatic brain injury (TBI), systemic hypothermia has been used predominantly in both experimental and clinical investigations (7, 8, 11, 14, 94). In these cases, systemic hypothermia is necessary because of diffuse patterns of brain injury following ischemic, hypoxic, or traumatic insults. In addition, local cooling procedures (selective head cooling) can only achieve mild brain temperature reductions (<1.5°C) (95-97).

In contrast to TBI, SCI commonly results in a well-demarcated area of contusion or ischemic damage that can be targeted by local cooling techniques (18). Following contusion or compression injury, local approaches to cooling can be conducted through the use of laminectomy or other surgical approaches (98). Following laminectomy, cool saline can be infused over the overlying dura or directly around the surface of the spinal cord if the dura is opened. Alternatively, adjacent tissues may be cooled so that heat transfer occurs away from the spinal cord. A limitation of such techniques that involve cooling through an intact dura is that temperature gradients can exist in the spinal cord (38, 64). White matter, for example, may be adequately cooled with such procedures, but deeper areas of the spinal cord, such as gray matter may not be cooled to the hypothermic levels required for neuroprotection. Alternative methods to achieve local cooling are the placement of input and output catheters into the subarachnoid space. The extent to which this simple method could adequately cool injured spinal cord tissue in the presence of co-existing compression is unknown. In experimental studies, it is important to record intrinsic spinal cord temperature to appropriately correlate temperature with the magnitude of the decrease in SCI (2). Recently, intravascular heat-exchange catheters have been developed that create well-controlled systemic hypothermia (99, 100). Some advantages of these catheters are that the degree of temperature variation can be tightly controlled and the devices can provide much more rapid rates of cooling or warming than the alternative devices such as forced-air devices and water jackets.

SPINAL CORD BLOOD FLOW DURING HYPOTHERMIA

Mild to moderate hypothermia (30-34°C) provides protection against transient spinal cord ischemia (36, 37, 101, 102). Regional ischemia to the spinal cord can occur during thoracoabdominal aneurysm repair, following compression-induced injury, as well as during surgery of the spinal cord or vertebral column, e.g., scoliosis correction. Significant reductions in spinal cord blood flow (SCBF) have been documented following traumatic SCI (103-105). In this regard, cooling of the spinal cord might improve the survival of post-traumatic or post-ischemic hypoperfused spinal cord tissue (106).

Some studies have shown SCBF to be increased in phenobarbital-anesthetized rats during systemic hypothermia (27-28°C) (107). In contrast, local cooling of the spinal cord has been reported to actually decrease SCBF in the 32-58% range (106, 108). Although increases in spinal cord perfusion associated with local spinal cord cooling have been reported (109, 110), most studies have indicated that the perfusion decreases. In terms of hypothermic protection, the effects of temperature on local spinal cord perfusion are critical in regards to outcome. If profound levels of hypothermia induce reduced perfusion in ischemic areas, for example, this would be expected to potentially worsen outcome. This variable could explain some of the inconsistencies in the literature regarding the effects of local cooling on outcome following SCI.

SUMMARY AND CONCLUSIONS

Mild, moderate, and deep hypothermia have been shown to be neuroprotective in various animal models of SCI (111). In contrast, small elevations in brain temperature over normothermic (hyperthermia) levels have been shown to worsen traumatic outcome (112, 113). Since temperature fluctuations can have a profound effect on outcome following SCI, careful attention to the core and spinal cord temperature is required. Indeed, a vast literature indicates that hypothermia of varying degrees induced locally or systemically can have a benefit on outcome. Future studies are required to determine optimal levels of hypothermia as well as durations for hypothermic therapy. In the area of acute SCI, the determination of the therapeutic window for hypothermia requires additional study (114). In addition, the rewarming phase following the hypothermic period appears to be an extremely important variable in some clinical and experimental studies. New methods of cooling, including advanced external cooling devices as well as endovascular cooling catheters may facilitate the precision of temperature control in future investigations. The potential synergy between mild hypothermia and various neuroprotective agents should also continue to be investigated in both the laboratory and clinical settings (115-119). Continued investigations into this important research area should improve how therapeutic hypothermia is used and identify which patient population can benefit most.

REFERENCES

1. Albin M, White R, Locke G. Treatment of spinal cord trauma by selective hypothermic perfusion. *Surg Forum* 1965; 16:423-424.
2. Albin M, White R, Locke G, et al. Localized spinal cord cooling-Anesthetic effects and applications to spinal cord injury. *Anesth Analg* 1967; 46:8-16.
3. Albin MS, White RJ, Acosta-Rua G, Yashon D. Study of functional recovery produced by delayed localized cooling after spinal cord injury in primates. *J Neurosurg* 1968; 29:113-120.
4. Green B, Khan T, Raimondi A. Local hypothermia as treatment of experimentally induced spinal cord contusion: quantitative analysis of beneficent effect. *Surg Forum* 1973; 24:436-438.
5. Wells JD, Hansebout RR. Local hypothermia in experimental spinal cord trauma. *Surg Neurol* 1978; 10:200-204.
6. Busto R, Dietrich WD, Globus MY, et al. Small differences in intraischemic brain temperature critically determine the extent of ischemic neuronal injury. *J Cereb Blood Flow Metab* 1987; 7:729-738.
7. Dietrich W, Alonso O, Busto R, Globus MT, Ginsberg M. Post-traumatic brain hypothermia reduces histopathological damage following contusive brain injury in the rat. *Acta Neuropathol* (Berl) 1994; 87:250-258.
8. Busto R, Dietrich WD, Globus MY, Ginsberg MD. The importance of brain temperature in cerebral ischemic injury. *Stroke* 1989; 20:1113-1114.
9. Colbourne F, Corbett D. Delayed and prolonged post-ischemic hypothermia is neuroprotective in the gerbil. *Brain Res* 1994; 654:265-272.
10. Koizumi H, Povlishock JT. Posttraumatic hypothermia in the treatment of axonal damage in an animal model of traumatic axonal injury. *J Neurosurg* 1998; 89:303-309.
11. Leonov Y, Sterz F, Safar P, et al. Mild cerebral hypothermia during and after cardiac arrest improves neurologic outcome in dogs. *J Cereb Blood Flow Metab* 1990; 10:57-70.
12. Marion DW, Penrod LE, Kelsey SF, et al. Treatment of traumatic brain injury with moderate hypothermia. *N Engl J Med* 1997; 336:540-6.
13. Jiang J, Yu M, Zhu C. Effect of long-term mild hypothermia therapy in patients with severe traumatic brain injury: 1-year follow-up review of 87 cases. *J Neurosurg* 2000; 93:546-549.
14. Schwab M, Schwarz S, Spranger M, et al. Moderate hypothermia in the treatment of patients with severe middle cerebral artery infarction. *Stroke* 2000; 29:2461-2466.
15. Bernard S, Gray T, Buist M, et al. Treatment of comatose survivors of out-of-hospital cardiac arrest with induced hypothermia. *N Engl J Med* 2002; 346:557-563.
16. The Hypothermia After Cardiac Arrest Study Group. Mild therapeutic hypothermia to improve the neurologic outcome after cardiac arrest. *N Engl J Med* 2002; 346:549-556.
17. Inamasu J, Ichikizaki K. Mild hypothermia in neurologic emergency: an update. *Ann Emerg Med* 2002; 40:220-230.
18. Tator C, Update on the pathophysiology and pathology of acute spinal cord injury. *Brain Pathol* 1995; 5:407-413.
19. Anderson D, Hall E. Pathophysiology of spinal cord trauma. *Ann Emerg Med* 1993; 22:987-992.
20. Bethea JR, Dietrich WD. Targeting the host inflammatory response in traumatic spinal cord injury. *Curr Opin Neurol* 2002; 15:355-360.
21. Dietrich WD, Busto R, Globus MY, Ginsberg MD. Brain damage and temperature: cellular and molecular mechanisms. *Adv Neurol* 1996; 71:177-194.

22. Colbourne F, Sutherland G, Corbett D. Postischemic hypothermia. A critical appraisal with implications for clinical treatment. *Mol Neurobiol* 1997; 14:171-201.

23. Chatzipanteli K, Yanagawa Y, Marcillo AE, et al. Posttraumatic hypothermia reduces polymorphonuclear leukocyte accumulation following spinal cord injury in rats. *J Neurotrauma* 2000; 17: 321-332.

24. Wakamatsu H, Matsumoto M, Nakakimura K, Sakabe T. The effects of moderate hypothermia and intrathecal tetracaine on glutamate concentrations of intrathecal dialysate and neurologic and histopathologic outcome in transient spinal cord ischemia in rabbits. *Anesth Analg* 1999; 88:56-62.

25. Marion DW, White MJ. Treatment of experimental brain injury with moderate hypothermia and 21- aminosteroids. *J Neurotrauma* 1996; 13:139-147.

26. Banik NL, Shields DC, Ray S, et al. Role of calpain in spinal cord injury: effects of calpain and free radical inhibitors. *Ann N Y Acad Sci* 1998; 844:131-137.

27. Buki A, Koizumi, H, Povlishock JT. Moderate posttraumatic hypothermia decreases early calpain-mediated proteolysis and concomitant cytoskeletal compromise in traumatic axonal injury. *Exp Neurol* 1999; 159:319-328.

28. Buki A, Siman R, Trojanowski JQ, Povlishock JT. The role of calpain-mediated spectrin proteolysis in traumatically induced axonal injury. *J Neuropathol Exp Neurol* 1999; 58:365-375.

29. Gamble H, Goldby F, Smith G. Effect of temperature on the degeneration of nerve fibers. *Nature* 1957; 179:527.

30. Gamble H, Jha B. Some effect of temperature upon the rate and progress of Wallerian degeneration in mammalian nerve fibers. *J Anat* 1958; 92:171-177.

31. Sea T, Ballinger M, Bittner G. Cooling of peripheral myelinated axons retards Wallerian degeneration. *Exp Neurol* 1995; 13:85-95.

32. Marzullo TC, Britt JM, Stavisky RC, Bittner GD. Cooling enhances in vitro survival and fusion-repair of severed axons taken from the peripheral and central nervous systems of rats. *Neurosci Lett* 2002; 327:9-12.

33. Tsao JW, George EB, Griffin JW. Temperature modulation reveals three distinct stages of Wallerian degeneration. *J Neurosci* 1999; 19:4718-4726.

34. Shi R, Borgens RB, Blight AR. Functional reconnection of severed mammalian spinal cord axons with polyethylene glycol. *J Neurotrauma* 1999; 16:727-738.

35. Sunio A, Bittner GD. Cyclosporin A retards the wallerian degeneration of peripheral mammalian axons. *Exp Neurol* 1997; 146:46-56.

36. Vacanti FX, Ames A, 3rd. Mild hypothermia and Mg++ protect against irreversible damage during CNS ischemia. *Stroke* 1984; 15:695-698.

37. Robertson CS, Foltz R, Grossman RG, Goodman JC. Protection against experimental ischemic spinal cord injury. *J Neurosurg* 1986; 64:633-642.

38. Kakinohana M, Taira Y, Marsala M. The effect of graded postischemic spinal cord hypothermia on neurological outcome and histopathology after transient spinal ischemia in rat. *Anesthesiology* 1999; 90:789-798.

39. Vanicky I, Marsala M, Galik J, Marsala J: Epidural perfusion cooling protection against protracted spinal cord ischemia in rabbits. J Neurosurg 1998; 79:736-741.

40. Westergren H, Farooque M, Olsson Y, Holtz A: Motor function changes in the rat following severe spinal cord injury. Does treatment with moderate systemic hypothermia improve functional outcome? Acta Neurochir (Wien) 2000; 142:567-573.

41. Dimar JR, Shields CB, Zhang YP, et al. The role of directly applied hypothermia in spinal cord injury. *Spine* 2000; 25:2294-2302.

42. Basso DM., Beattie MS, Bresnahan JC. A sensitive and reliable locomotor rating scale for open field testing in rats. *J Neurotrauma* 1995; 12:1-21.

43. Jou IM. Effects of core body temperature on changes in spinal somatosensory-evoked potential in acute spinal cord compression injury: an experimental study in the rat. *Spine* 2000; 25:1878-1885.

44. Berguer R, Porto J, Fedoronko B, Dragovic L. Selective deep hypothermia of the spinal cord prevents paraplegia after aortic cross-clamping in the dog model. *J Vasc Surg* 1992; 15:62-71.

45. Albin MS, White RJ, Locke GE, Kretchmer HE. Spinal cord hypothermia by localized perfusion cooling. *Nature* 1966; 210: 1059-1060.

46. Ducker TB, Hamit HF. Experimental treatments of acute spinal cord injury. *J Neurosurg* 1969; 30: 693-697.

47. Black P, Markowitz RS: Experimental spinal cord injury in monkeys: Comparison of steroids and local hypothermia. Surg Forum 1971; 22:409-411.

48. Campbell JB, DeCrescito V, Tomasula JJ, et al: Experimental treatment of spinal cord contusion in the cat. Surg Neurol 1972; 1:102-106.

49. Kuchnor EF, Hansebout RR: Combined steroid and hypothermia treatment of experimental spinal cord injury. Surg Neurol 1976; 6:371-376.

50. Eidelberg E, Staten E, Watkins CJ, Smith JS: Treatment of experimental spinal cord injury in ferrets. Surg Neurol 1976; 6:243-246.

51. Yu WR, Westergren H, Farooque M, Holtz A, Olsson Y. Systemic hypothermia following compression injury of rat spinal cord: reduction of plasma protein extravasation demonstrated by immunohistochemistry. *Acta Neuropathol* (Berl) 1999; 98:15-21.

52. Westergren H, Yu WR, Farooque M, Holtz A, Olsson Y. Systemic hypothermia following spinal cord compression injury in the rat: axonal changes studied by beta-APP, ubiquitin, and PGP 9.5 immunohistochemistry. *Spinal Cord* 1999; 37:696-704.

53. Yu CG, Jimenez O, Marcillo AE, et al. Beneficial effects of modest systemic hypothermia on locomotor function and histopathological damage following contusion-induced spinal cord injury in rats. *J Neurosurg* 2000;93(1 Suppl):85-93.

54. Uihlein A, MacCarty CS, Michenfelder JD, Terry HR, Jr, Daw EF. Deep hypothermia and surgical treatment of intracranial aneurysms. A five-year survey. *JAMA* 1966; 195:639-641.

55. Selker RG: Icewater irrigation of the spinal cord. *Surg Forum* 1971; 22:411-413.

56. Meacham WF, McPherson WF: Local hypothermia in the treatment of acute injuries of the spinal cord. *South Med J* 1973; 66:95-97.

57. Koons DD, Gildenberg PL, Dohn DF, Henoch M: Local hypothermia in the treatment of spinal cord injuries. Report of seven cases. *Cleve Clin Q* 1972; 39:109-117.

58. Negrin J: Spinal cord hypothermia. NY State J Med 1975; 75:23987-2392.

59. Bricolo A, Galleore G, DaPian R, Faccioli F Local cooling in spinal cord injury. *Surg Neurol* 1976; 6:101-106.

60. Tator CH: Spinal cord cooling and irrigation for treatment of acute cord injury, In: *Neural Trauma*. AJ Popp (ed). Raven Press: New York, 1979; pp 363-370.

61. Tator CH, Deecke L. Value of normothermic perfusion, hypothermic perfusion, and durotomy in the treatment of experimental acute spinal cord trauma. *J Neurosurg* 1973; 39:52-64.

62. Negrin J, Jr. Spinal cord hypothermia in the neurosurgical management of the acute and chronic post-traumatic paraplegic patient. *Paraplegia* 1973; 10:336-343.

63. Martinez-Arizala A, Green BA. Hypothermia in spinal cord injury. *J Neurotrauma* 1992; 9 Suppl 2:S497-505.

64. Westergren H, Holtz A, Farooque M, Yu WR, Olsson Y. Systemic hypothermia after spinal cord compression injury in the rat: does recorded temperature in accessible organs

reflect the intramedullary temperature in the spinal cord? *J Neurotrauma* 1998; 15:943-954.

65. Hansebout RR, Tanner JA, Romero-Sierra C. Current status of spinal cord cooling in the treatment of acute spinal cord injury. *Spine* 1984; 9:508-511.

66. Kurz A, Ikeda T, Sessler DI, et al. Meperidine decreases the shivering threshold twice as much as the vasoconstriction threshold. *Anesthesiology* 1997; 86:1046-1054.

67. Pontius R, Brockman H, Hardy E, Cooley D, DeBakey M. The use of hypothermia in the prevention of paraplegia following temporary aortic occlusion: experimental observations. *Surgery* 1954; 36:33-38.

68. Crawford E, Coselli J, Safi H. Partial cardiopulmonary bypass, hypothermic circulatory arrest, and posterolateral exposure for thoracic aortic aneurysm operation. *J Thorac Cardiovasc Surg* 1987; 94:824-827.

69. Sun J, Hirsch D, Svensson G. Spinal cord protection by papaverine and inthathecal cooling during aortic crossclamping. *J Cardiovasc Surg* 1998; 39: 839-842.

70. Safi HJ, Campbell MP, Ferreira ML, Azizzadeh A, Miller CC. Spinal cord protection in descending thoracic and thoracoabdominal aortic aneurysm repair. *Semin Thorac Cardiovasc Surg* 1998; 10:41-44.

71. Downey C. Epidural cooling for spinal cord protection during thoracoabdominal aortic aneurysm repair (a case study). *Can Oper Room Nurs J* 2000; 18:9-14.

72. Fernandez Suarez F, Sanchez Buron J, et al. Cerebrospinal fluid drainage and deep systemic hypothermia with total absence of circulation for spinal cord protection during surgery on the thoracic aorta. *Rev Esp Anestesiol Reanim* 2001; 48:192-195.

73. Kouchoukos NT, Masetti P, Rokkas CK, Murphy SF, Blackstone EH. Safety and efficacy of hypothermic cardiopulmonary bypass and circulatory arrest for operations on the descending thoracic and thoracoabdominal aorta. *Ann Thorac Surg* 2001; 72:699-707.

74. Cambria RP, Davison JK, Zanetti S, et al: Clinical experience with epidural cooling for spinal cord protection during thoracic and thoracoabdominal aneurysm repair. *J Vasc Surg* 1997; 25:234-243.

75. Moore WM, Jr, Hollier LH. The influence of severity of spinal cord ischemia in the etiology of delayed-onset paraplegia. *Ann Surg* 1991; 213:427-431.

76. Naslund TC, Hollier LH, Money SR, Facundus EC, Skenderis BS, 2nd. Protecting the ischemic spinal cord during aortic clamping. The influence of anesthetics and hypothermia. *Ann Surg* 1992; 215:409-415.

77. Coselli JS, LeMaire SA, Miller CC, 3rd, et al. Mortality and paraplegia after thoracoabdominal aortic aneurysm repair: a risk factor analysis. *Ann Thorac Surg* 2000; 69:409-414.

78. Estrera AL, Miller CC, 3rd, Huynh TT, Porat E, Safi HJ. Neurologic outcome after thoracic and thoracoabdominal aortic aneurysm repair. *Ann Thorac Surg* 2001; 72:1225-1230.

79. Svensson LG, Hess KR, D'Agostino RS, et al. Reduction of neurologic injury after high-risk thoracoabdominal aortic operation. *Ann Thorac Surg* 1998; 66:132-138.

80. Svensson LG, Khitin L, Nadolny EM, Kimmel WA. Systemic temperature and paralysis after thoracoabdominal and descending aortic operations. *Arch Surg* 2003; 138:175-179.

81. Sessler DI. Perianesthetic thermoregulation and heat balance in humans. *FASEB J* 1993; 7:638-644.

82. Kurz A, Sessler DI, Lenhardt R. Perioperative normothermia to reduce the incidence of surgical-wound infection and shorten hospitalization. Study of Wound Infection and Temperature Group. *N Engl J Med* 1996; 334:1209-1215.

83. Winfree CH, Baker KZ, Connolly ES. Perioperative normothermia and surgical-wound infection. *N Engl J Med* 1996; 335:749.
84. Gerszten PC, Albright AL, Pollack IF, Adelson PD. Intraoperative hypothermia and ventricular shunt infections. *Acta Neurochir* 1998; 140:591-594.
85. Baker KZ, Young WL, Stone JG, et al. Deliberate mild intraoperative hypothermia for craniotomy. *Anesthesiology* 1994; 81:361-367.
86. Clifton GL, Christensen ML. Use of moderate hypothermia during elective craniotomy. *Tex Med* 1992; 88:66-69.
87. Kahn HA, Faust GR, Richard R, Tedesco R, Cohen JR. Hypothermia and bleeding during abdominal aortic aneurysm repair. *Ann Vasc Surg* 1994; 8:6-9.
88. Bernabei AF, Levison MA, Bender JS. The effects of hypothermia and injury severity on blood loss during trauma laparotomy. *J Trauma* 1992; 33: 835-839.
89. Johansson T, Lisander B, Ivarsson I. Mild hypothermia does not increase blood loss during total hip arthroplasty. *Acta Anaesthesiol Scand* 1999; 43:1005-1010.
90. Sessler DI. Complications and treatment of mild hypothermia. *Anesthesiology* 2001; 95:531-543.
91. Guest J, Vanni S, Silbert L. Mild hypothermia, blood loss and complications in spinal surgery. *The Spine Journal* 2003; 4:130-137.
92. Lang M, Welte M, Syben R, Hansen D. Effects of hypothermia on median nerve somatosensory evoked potentials during spontaneous circulation. *J Neurosurg Anesthesiol* 2002; 14:141-145.
93. Insler SR, O'Connor MS, Leventhal MJ, Nelson DR, Starr NJ. Association between postoperative hypothermia and adverse outcome after coronary artery bypass surgery. *Ann Thorac Surg* 2000; 70:175-181.
94. Clifton GL, Miller ER, Choi SC, et al. Lack of effect of induction of hypothermia after acute brain injury. *N Engl J Med* 2001; 344:556-563.
95. Tooley JR, Satas S, Porter H, Silver IA, Thoresen M. Head cooling with mild systemic hypothermia in anesthetized piglets is neuroprotective. *Ann Neurol* 2003; 53:65-72.
96. Laptook AR, Shalak L, Corbett RJ. Differences in brain temperature and cerebral blood flow during selective head versus whole-body cooling. *Pediatrics* 2001; 108:1103-1110.
97. Battin MR, Penrice J, Gunn TR, Gunn AJ. Treatment of term infants with head cooling and mild systemic hypothermia (35.0 degrees C and 34.5 degrees C) after perinatal asphyxia. *Pediatrics* 2003; 111:244-251.
98. Meylaerts SA, Kalkman CJ, de Haan P, Porsius M, Jacobs MJ. Epidural versus subdural spinal cord cooling: cerebrospinal fluid temperature and pressure changes. *Ann Thorac Surg* 2000; 70:222-227.
99. Inderbitzen B, Yon S, Lasheras J, et al. Safety and performance of a novel intravascular catheter for induction and reversal of hypothermia in a porcine model. *Neurosurgery* 2002; 50:364-370.
100. Mack WJ, Huang J, Winfree C, et al. Ultrarapid, Convection-Enhanced Intravascular Hypothermia. Feasibility Study in Nonhuman Primate Stroke. *Stroke* 2003; 34:1994-1999.
101. Allen BT, Davis CG, Osborne D, Karl I. Spinal cord ischemia and reperfusion metabolism: the effect of hypothermia. *J Vasc Surg* 1994; 19:332-339.
102. Marsala M, Vanicky I, Galik J, et al. Panmyelic epidural cooling protects against ischemic spinal cord damage. *J Surg Res* 1993; 55:21-31.
103. Kelly DL, Jr, Lassiter KR, Calogero JA, Alexander E, Jr. Effects of local hypothermia and tissue oxygen studies in experimental paraplegia. *J Neurosurg* 1970; 33:554-563.
104. Sandler A, Tator C. Review of the effects of spinal cord trauma on the vessels and blood flow in the spinal cord. *J Neurosurg* 1976; 45:638-646.

105. Ducker TB, Salcman M, Perot PL, Jr, Ballantine D. Experimental spinal cord trauma, I: Correlation of blood flow, tissue oxygen and neurologic status in the dog. *Surg Neurol* 1978; 10:60-63.

106. Sakamoto T, Iwai A, Monafo W, Regional blood flow in transected rat spinal cord during hypothermia. *Am J Physiol* 1990; 259:H1649-H1654.

107. Sakamoto T, Monafo W. The effect of hypothermia on regional spinal cord blood flow in rats. *J Neurosurg* 1989; 70:780-784.

108. Hansebout RR, Lamont RN, Kamath MV. The effects of local cooling on canine spinal cord blood flow. *Can J Neurol Sci* 1985; 12: 83-87.

109. Westergren H, Farooque M, Olsson Y, Holtz A. Spinal cord blood flow changes following systemic hypothermia and spinal cord compression injury: an experimental study in the rat using Laser-Doppler flowmetry. *Spinal Cord* 2001; 39:74-84.

110. Zielonka JS, Wagner FC, Jr, Dohrmann GJ. Alterations in spinal cord blood flow during local hypothermia. *Surg Forum* 1974; 25:434-6.

111. White R, Albin M. Spinal cord cooling. *J Neurosurg* 2001; 94:183-184.

112. Dietrich WD, Alonso O, Halley M, Busto R. Delayed posttraumatic brain hyperthermia worsens outcome after fluid percussion brain injury: a light and electron microscopic study in rats. *Neurosurgery* 1996; 38:533-541.

113. Yu CG, Jagid J, Ruenes G, et al. Detrimental effects of systemic hyperthermia on locomotor function and histopathological outcome after traumatic spinal cord injury in the rat. *Neurosurgery* 2001; 49:152-158.

114. Albin M, White R. Therapeutic window after spinal cord trauma is longer than after spinal cord ischemia. *Anesthesiology* 2000: 92:281-282.

115. Tetik O, Islamoglu F, Goncu T, Cekirdekci A, Buket S. Reduction of spinal cord injury with pentobarbital and hypothermia in a rabbit model. *Eur J Vasc Endovasc Surg* 2002; 24:540-544.

116. Miyamoto TA, Miyamoto KJ. Alternate explanation of the additive protective effects of regional infusion of hypothermic saline and adenosine solutions. *J Thorac Cardiovasc Surg* 2000; 119:631-632.

117. Kuchner EF, Hansebout RR, Pappius HM: Effects of dexamethasone and of local hypothermia on early and late tissue electrolyte changes in experimental spinal cord injury. *J Spinal Disord* 2000; 13:391-398.

118. Parrino PE, Kron IL, Ross SD, et al. Retrograde venous perfusion with hypothermic saline and adenosine for protection of the ischemic spinal cord. *J Vasc Surg* 2000; 32:171-178.

119. Hansebout RR, Kuchner EF, Romero-Sierra C. Effects of local hypothermia and of steroids upon recovery from experimental spinal cord compression injury. *Surg Neurol* 1975 4:531-536.

Chapter 8

ASPHYXIA

Robert W. Hickey, MD, Clifton W. Callaway, MD, PhD
University of Pittsburgh, Pittsburgh, PA, USA

INTRODUCTION

The first resuscitation societies, founded in the mid-18th century, were organized networks of rescuers responding primarily to drowning victims. In the 19th century, the development of general anesthesia and its attendant airway mishaps generated additional enthusiasm for preventing, understanding, and treating asphyxia. Thus, asphyxia was the main focus of early resuscitation science. More recently however, sudden collapse, primarily as a result of cardiac arrhythmia, has become the focus of resuscitation research and interventions. Reasons for focusing on sudden arrhythmic death include: 1) arrhythmia is more common than asphyxia as a cause of death in adults, 2) when the collapse is sudden and witnessed there is a precise epidemiologic definition for start and duration of ischemia, and 3) defibrillators for treatment of ventricular fibrillation (VF) or ventricular tachycardia (VT) have been developed and deployed worldwide. In addition, prospective clinical trials are strengthened by the selection of relatively homogenous patient populations and the use of discrete, measurable outcomes (e.g. defibrillation). Accordingly, the recently performed clinical trials of induced hypothermia following cardiac arrest (discussed in Chapter 2) excluded asphyxial arrest and limited enrollment to a highly-selected population of patients resuscitated from VF/VT.

In contrast to the carefully designed clinical trials of induced hypothermia for VF/VT, there is a limited experience with induced hypothermia for asphyxial arrest. Thus, a key question is, "Can the results from the studies demonstrating benefit of induced hypothermia for treatment of resuscitation from VF/VT be generalized to patients resuscitated from asphyxial cardiac arrest?" The objective of this chapter is to address this question by 1) comparing and contrasting the brain injury from VF/VT arrest with asphyxial cardiac arrest, 2) reviewing data from animal experiments of hypothermic treatment for asphyxial arrest, and 3) reviewing the clinical experience with hypothermic treatment of asphyxia.

EXTENT OF THE PROBLEM

Asphyxia can be clinically defined as airway obstruction or inadequate ventilation leading to hypoxemia and hypercarbia. Some examples include drowning, choking, and coma accompanied by loss of airway patency. The typical progression of untreated asphyxia is hypertension and increased work of breathing (where possible) followed by bradycardia, hypotension, pulseless electrical activity (PEA), and eventually asystole (reviewed by Safar et al. [1]).

It is well established that the most common cause of non-traumatic cardiopulmonary arrest in children is airway compromise (2-4). It is more difficult to ascertain the contribution of asphyxia to adult cardiopulmonary arrest because, for the reasons detailed above, most studies of adult arrest are limited to sudden cardiac deaths. However, a study published by Kuisma et al *designed* to determine the prevalence of cardiac vs. non-cardiac causes of arrest reported that 1/3 of 800 out-of-hospital adult arrests were non-cardiac in origin and 12% of these patients survived to hospital discharge (5). The most common causes of non-cardiac arrest in this study were trauma, non-traumatic bleeding, intoxication, near drowning, and pulmonary embolism. Thus, asphyxia and other non-cardiac causes of cardiac arrest are not rare in children or adults. Victims of these insults represent a potentially salvageable patient population.

VF/VT VS. ASPHYXIAL CARDIAC ARREST

An essential feature of clinical cardiac arrest and laboratory-induced cardiac arrest (by induced VF, potassium chloride injection, great vessel occlusion, or asphyxia) is that the insult involves the entire organism. Thus, each ischemic organ may have effects upon other organs. For example, cardiac arrest is accompanied by a transient opening of the blood brain barrier (6-8) which allows molecules (cytokines, reactive oxygen species, etc.) produced in one compartment to diffuse into the other. Clinically, this is manifested as a "post-resuscitation syndrome" involving multisystem organ dysfunction (9-11). The post-resuscitation syndrome is an important consideration for testing therapies that can have variable treatment effects on more than one dysfunctional organ. Thus, all cardiac arrest models (including asphyxial arrest) are clinically relevant models of combined, global brain and body ischemia. In contrast, cerebral vascular occlusion models of global brain ischemia do not cause ischemic injury to non-cerebral organs and thus, are less clinically relevant.

While both VF and asphyxial cardiac arrest result in global body/brain ischemia, the pattern of the ischemic insult differs. VF causes an abrupt cessation of cardiac output, whereas asphyxia causes an initial hypertension followed by a gradual decrease in flow until PEA and finally asystole occur. Paradoxically, while low cerebral blood flow (CBF) is better than no flow, a "trickle" of flow can be worse than no flow. This is demonstrated in a study by Bottiger et al. showing worse post resuscitation cerebral reperfusion in rats with 12 min untreated VF plus 5 min VF treated with CPR compared with rats subjected to 17 min untreated VF (12). Theories for the damaging effect of trickle flow include: 1) continued delivery of substrate during conditions of anaerobic metabolism causing worse tissue acidosis, and 2) continued delivery of platelets and coagulation factors causing worse microvascular plugging that will impair reperfusion during resuscitation. Asphyxia, but not VF/VT, has an interval of trickle CBF accompanied by profound hypoxemia.

The histology of cerebral injury following asphyxia differs from that seen in VF. Safar et al have shown that brain damage from asphyxial cardiac arrest in dogs is worse than the damage found after equivalent periods of circulatory arrest from VF (13, 14). After both VF and asphyxia, there is a pattern of delayed neuronal death occurring in selectively vulnerable brain regions. After asphyxia, however, there are scattered microinfarcts not seen in VF animals. Thus, laboratory experiments demonstrate the severity and pattern of cerebral injury following asphyxial cardiac arrest differs from VF arrest. Clinical evidence of a difference in injury patterns is suggested by a report from Morimoto et al (15) describing increased prevalence of brain edema (diagnosed by head CT) in adults remaining comatose following respiratory-induced cardiac arrest compared with cardiac arrhythmia-induced cardiac arrest.

ANIMAL STUDIES OF HYPOTHERMIA AND ASPHYXIAL CARDIAC ARREST

A variety of preclinical studies have examined the influence of hypothermia on mechanisms and outcome after asphyxial cardiac arrest.

Because a well-developed rat model of asphyxial cardiac arrest exists and rats are useful for mechanistic studies, there are also data about specific mechanisms whereby therapeutic hypothermia can improve neurological recovery after asphyxia. This discussion focuses primarily on asphyxial cardiac arrest in mature or immature animals, excluding neonatal hypoxia-ischemia (discussed separately in Chapter 9).

There are several limitations to available data. Specifically, studies of therapeutic hypothermia after asphyxia are limited to studies in rodents or piglets and have used limited assessments of functional outcome. The neurological deficit scores that are used in most studies are gross measures that may not detect significant impairments of memory or learning. Limited data regarding open-field activity (16), and Morris Water Maze (17) are available for asphyxia models. On the positive side, outcomes from animal studies of asphyxial cardiac arrest correlate with available clinical data and that the beneficial effects of hypothermia are of sufficient magnitude that they can be easily detected with gross neurological scoring.

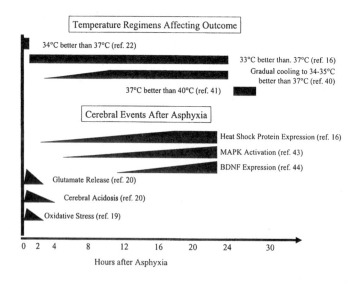

Figure 8-1. Temporal representation of proven beneficial hypothermia regimens and potential therapeutic targets after asphyxial arrest. MAPK = mitogen-activated protein kinase, BDNF = brain-derived neurotrophic factor.

It is important to emphasize the duration of hypothermia used in preclinical studies. Brain temperature affects multiple metabolic pathways. It is likely that induced hypothermia interacts with different components in the cascade of events leading to cell death depending upon the time window of application. Energy failure, loss of ionic homeostasis, intracerebral acidosis, oxidative stress, altered intracellular signaling, transcription control, and new gene expression are all potential targets for hypothermia. The time when each of these pathophysiological processes occurs during or after asphyxia provides clues to the therapeutic targets of induced hypothermia (see Figure 8-1).

Brief Hypothermia

Induction of brief (<4 hours) hypothermia *beginning immediately after reperfusion* improves neurological outcome in animals. However, the efficacy of brief hypothermic treatment declines if it is delayed for 15 minutes or more after reperfusion from VF cardiac arrest in dogs (18). The delay-sensitive benefit of brief hypothermia may suggest that brief, early hypothermia reduces the oxidative stress (19) or the increased excitatory amino acid release (20, 21) that occur during the first hour after reperfusion.

A brief (one-hour) period of hypothermia also improves behavioral and histological outcome after asphyxial cardiac arrest in rats (22). Just as with VF cardiac arrest and arterial occlusion, this regimen is less beneficial when hypothermia begins after resuscitation, than when hypothermia starts during asphyxia. In a separate laboratory, using the same rat model, one hour of mild hypothermia and induced hypertension, beginning immediately after reperfusion, improved survival but did not alter long-term neurological outcome (23). Similarly, brief periods of hypothermia (1-2 hours) may delay but not prevent ischemic neuronal death in arterial occlusion models (24). This narrow therapeutic window and the technical difficulties with rapid induction of hypothermia make brief hypothermia difficult to apply clinically (25).

Therapeutic targets of brief hypothermia *during ischemia* and early reperfusion include energy failure, loss of ionic gradients and cerebral acidosis. For example, in studies using piglets, the depletion of high energy phosphates during cardiac arrest is slowed by 5.3% per degree reduction in temperature (26). Anoxic depolarization, manifested primarily as a rise in extracellular potassium, occurs separately from energy failure. Hypothermia during cerebral arterial occlusion in rats can delay the onset of anoxic depolarization (27), perhaps related to a decrease in cerebral oxygen utilization (28). However, these therapeutic targets are short-lived. Extracellular potassium recovers within a few minutes after reperfusion (29) and brain pH and intracellular stores of high energy phosphates are restored within a few minutes after reperfusion (30, 31). Thus, therapeutic hypothermia induced *after resuscitation* has little opportunity to affect energy failure, ionic gradients or cerebral acidosis.

The time window for the maximal efficacy of brief hypothermia does correspond to the time of maximal excitatory amino acid release. The peak extracellular levels of glutamate and aspartate occur at the end of ischemia in arterial occlusion models (32) and immediately after reperfusion in the rat asphyxial cardiac arrest model (20). Extracellular glutamate levels return towards normal over the next two hours after asphyxia (20). Thus, the impact of a brief bout of hypothermia on excitatory amino acid levels will decline with each minute delay after reperfusion. Furthermore, the protective effects of hypothermia during arterial occlusion in rodents are reduced if rewarming occurs at the onset of reperfusion (33), suggesting that hypothermia influences events that occur during immediate reperfusion. It is tempting to speculate that hypothermia reduces glutamate release. However, measurement of brain glutamate using microdialysis in a rat arterial occlusion model suggests that hypothermia during and after ischemia does not alter glutamate release but may accelerate glutamate reuptake (34). Further studies are needed to relate this mechanism to the observed beneficial effects of cooling on outcome.

Prolonged Hypothermia

Induction of *prolonged* (preferably >12 hours), mild hypothermia after reperfusion reduces neuronal death in rodents after arterial occlusion, even if hypothermia is delayed for up to 6 hours (35, 36). Conversely, *hyper*thermia after global brain ischemia can worsen neurological recovery even if induced 24 hours after reperfusion (37). This sensitivity of the post-ischemic brain to temperature during the first 24-48 hours after reperfusion was observed in the recent clinical trials. In those trials, induction of hypothermia several hours after resuscitation from cardiac arrest improved survival and outcome (38), whereas fever during the first 48 hours after resuscitation was associated with worse outcome (39).

The interaction of hypothermia with asphyxial brain injury in rats has a therapeutic time window similar to that of induced hypothermia in human cardiac arrest. After asphyxia, prolonged (24 hours), mild hypothermia improves mortality, neurological recovery and histological signs of brain injury, whether initiated immediately or one hour after reperfusion (16). In that study, eight minutes of asphyxia and cardiac arrest followed by normothermia resulted in 25% mortality and 50% loss of hippocampal CA1 neurons after two weeks. Induction of hypothermia immediately after asphyxia or one hour after reperfusion and lasting for 24 hours reduced mortality to 0% and CA1 neuronal loss to 25% after two weeks. Because asphyxial cardiac arrest produces large behavioral deficits, rats without active temperature control become spontaneously hypothermic during the first day of their recovery period.   Gradual development of spontaneous hypothermia over 4-6 hours after resuscitation also improves survival and behavioral recovery (40). The histological improvement with this gradual-onset hypothermia is evident for at least 6 weeks after resuscitation. Likewise, hyperthermia can worsen neurological outcome after asphyxial cardiac arrest in rats if it occurs within the first 24 hours of recovery, but has little impact if it occurs after 48 hours (41).

Because prolonged mild hypothermia improves outcome after asphyxia even when delayed by one hour (16) or several hours (40), this regimen is unlikely to act through a reduction in acute oxidative stress. Measurement of tissue antioxidant reserve in brains of rats during and after asphyxial cardiac arrest suggests that oxidative stress is most pronounced during early reperfusion (19).   In that study, the reducing activity of ascorbate, tocopherol, glutathione and other thiol antioxidants was measured in the hippocampus from rats subjected to 8 minutes of asphyxia and cardiac arrest. Activity of these endogenous antioxidants was minimally decreased after asphyxia without resuscitation, but declined by as much as 50% after 10 minutes of reperfusion.   Antioxidant activity had returned to normal by 2 hours after resuscitation. A brief bout of hypothermia may interact with this oxidative stress that occurs during early reperfusion, and the brief nature of oxidative stress may explain why a one-hour bout of cooling is less effective when delayed (18, 22, 23).

POTENTIAL MECHANISMS FOR THE BENEFICIAL EFFECTS OF PROLONGED HYPOTHERMIA

Alternative possibilities for mechanisms mediating the beneficial effects of prolonged hypothermia include altered control of gene expression, altered intracellular signaling and increased expression of neurotrophic factors. New gene expression observed after asphyxia includes stress-associated proteins such as the heat shock proteins. Other data implicate at least two signaling pathways in the effects of prolonged hypothermia after asphyxia: brain-derived neurotrophic factor (BDNF) and the extracellular-signal regulated kinase (ERK). BDNF is a member of the neurotrophin family of polypeptides that signal between cells and promote neuronal survival. ERK is a member of the mitogen-activated protein kinase (MAPK) family. Both neurotrophin signaling and MAPK signaling control gene expression. Both BDNF and ERK have been associated with cell survival.

Hypothermia induced after resuscitation from asphyxia reduces certain markers of cell stress. Heat shock proteins are gene products that are under transcriptional control and that are expressed in response to many types of stress. In particular, the 70-KDa heat shock protein (Hsp70) has been studied extensively as a chaperone molecule that participates in control of intracellular traffic of other proteins, as well as protein folding. Hsp70 is induced during ischemia and helps promote cell survival by counteracting the protein degradation and impaired synthesis that occurs following ischemic injury (42). Accordingly, levels of hsp70 messenger ribonucleic acid (mRNA) and Hsp70 protein are increased during the first 24 hours after asphyxial cardiac arrest in rats (16). However, a 24-hour bout of mild hypothermia beginning one hour after resuscitation from asphyxia can reduce the levels of Hsp70 (16). Thus, the neuroprotective effects of hypothermia may be attenuated by an inappropriate down-regulation of Hsp 70. An alternative explanation for these observations is that the neuroprotective actions of hypothermia result in a less stressed brain that is less of a stimulus for Hsp 70 induction.

Asphyxial cardiac arrest causes activation of both ERK and a separate MAPK, the Jun-N-terminal kinase (JNK), between 6 and 24 hours after reperfusion (43). MAPK activity was measured in protein extracted from rat hippocampus using specific antibodies for the active (phosphorylated) forms of these kinases. Both ERK activation and JNK activation increase over the first 24 hours after asphyxial cardiac arrest. ERK activation increases more when hypothermia is induced between 1 and 24 hours after resuscitation, according to the same regimen shown to improve neurological outcome. Activation of JNK was less affected by hypothermia. Importantly, increased activation of hippocampal ERK in rats subjected to hypothermia is minimal after 3 or 6 hours but pronounced after 12 or 24 hours of cooling. These data suggest that increased ERK activation required prolonged rather than brief bouts of hypothermia. Thus, the timing of hypothermia-induced ERK activation corresponded to the timing of hypothermia-induced improvements in behavioral and histological outcomes.

Several transcription factors that are downstream in the ERK signaling pathway have increased activation after resuscitation from asphyxia. In particular, increased phosphorylation of activating transcription factor (ATF)-2 and p90Rsk were observed after hypothermic reperfusion. ATF-2 is often considered a substrate of JNK rather than ERK. However, we noted that treatment with the specific ERK kinase inhibitor SL327 reduced ATF-2 phosphorylation, indicating that activation of ATF-2 is at least partially dependent upon ERK. SL327 did not alter JNK activity in the same extracts. (43). While p90Rsk is itself a kinase that can be activated by ERK, one of its substrates is the cyclic adenosine mono-phosphate (cAMP) response element binding protein (CREB). Consistent with p90Rsk activation after hypothermic reperfusion, CREB phosphorylation also increases.

Activation of ERK substrates after cardiac arrest follows the anatomical distribution of ERK activation. For example, phosphorylation of the transcription factor ATF-2 appears to require ERK activation in our model. In the hippocampus, active ERK is most prominent in the cellular processes of the ischemic-vulnerable CA1 region, with less immunoreactivity in the relatively ischemia-resistant CA2 and CA3 regions (43). Phosphorylated ATF-2 immunoreactivity is also detected in nuclei of the CA1 region, with relative sparing of CA2 and CA3.

Hypothermia after resuscitation increases BDNF levels (44). We examined neurotrophin activity in the hippocampus of rats 12 and 24 hours after resuscitation from asphyxial cardiac arrest. BDNF levels in whole-cell homogenates of hippocampus increase after resuscitation, more so after hypothermic reperfusion. Increased phosphorylation of the BDNF receptor, TrkB, confirms that these increased levels of BDNF are producing cellular effects. ERK phosphorylation was increased in the same extracts. Separate experiments failed to observe any increase in nerve growth factor or neurotrophin-3, suggesting that the effect on BDNF is specific. Because exogenous BDNF can improve recovery after brain injury (45-47), these data prompt speculation that some of the beneficial effects of post-resuscitation hypothermia are mediated by increased BDNF activity.

Hypothermia and new gene expression

Some data suggest that the beneficial effects of induced hypothermia are associated with altered transcription of particular genes. Many new gene products are expressed after asphyxial cardiac arrest despite the active inhibition of translation that occurs during the first 12 hours or so after resuscitation (48). Specifically, synthesis of Hsp70, TrkB and BDNF occurs after asphyxial cardiac arrest in rats (16, 43). Furthermore, ERK-related and hypothermia-related control of transcription factors may influence gene expression for over 24 hours, when protein synthesis is expected to have recovered. Thus, the pattern of message that has been transcribed into RNA is relevant to the overall functioning of the brain after cardiac arrest and resuscitation.

In arterial occlusion models, transcription of subunits of the AMPA glutamate receptor as well as of the NMDA receptor is decreased in vulnerable regions of the hippocampus after reperfusion. Intraischemic hypothermia preserves expression of these subunits, although a 3-hour bout of post-ischemic hypothermia does not (49). In contrast, prolonged mild hypothermia preserves transcription of glutamate receptor subunits (50).

Likewise, a 3-hour bout of hypothermia after carotid artery occlusion in gerbils can increase transcription of the endoplasmic reticulum-based heat shock protein 78 kDa glucose regulated protein (GRP78) (51). Causal relationships between these changes and improved neurological outcome remain to be established, as well as whether these same gene products are affected after asphyxia.

Summary of Preclinical Data

The therapeutic window for prolonged mild hypothermia after asphyxia (1-24 hours after resuscitation) is after the peaks of oxidative stress (19), excitatory amino acid release, and brain acidosis (20). Thus, we speculate that these processes, which may be affected by brief bouts of hypothermia during or immediately after resuscitation, are not involved in the therapeutic effect of prolonged hypothermia. In contrast, prolonged hypothermia is associated with increased activation of certain signaling pathways (43), increased expression of neurotrophic factors (44), and decreased production of stress-related proteins (16). These processes may result in altered patterns of new gene expression, although the causal connection between these molecular changes and outcome remains to be established.

CLINICAL EXPERIENCE

Patients with brain injury from stroke, trauma, and cardiac arrest frequently develop temperature instability (reviewed by Ginsberg et al [52, 53]). Data specifically restricted to temperature following *asphyxial cardiac arrest* are more limited. However, we have recently described the temperature response in children resuscitated from cardiac arrest, most of whom suffered a respiratory cause of arrest (54). These children typically had an initial period of hypothermia followed by a delayed (approximately 24 hours) development of fever (see Figure 8-2 for a temperature plot from a representative patient). Thus, patients after asphyxial arrest have a temperature pattern that is similar to that produced in the animal experiments of asphyxial arrest (discussed above) which demonstrate early, spontaneous hypothermia-mediated neuroprotection followed by hyperthermia-mediated injury.

There is strong clinical evidence for a neuroprotective effect of hypothermia with onset prior to or during an asphyxial arrest. Specifically, there are numerous case reports of normal neurologic recovery following prolonged hypoxia-ischemia (>60 min arrest time) from ice-water drowning or avalanche asphyxia (55-58). Although case reports are usually considered "low level" evidence, the prolonged periods of cardiac arrest documented in some of the reports and the absence of case reports describing similar outcomes in patients without hypothermia strengthen their significance. Importantly, these "miraculous" saves from intra-ischemic hypothermia occurred in patients with asphyxia suggesting that asphyxial injury can be manipulated by temperature modulation.

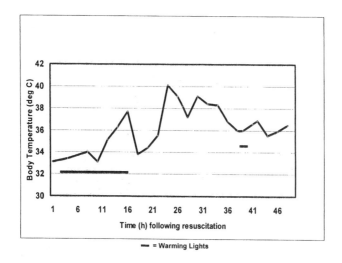

Figure 8-2. Temperature from a child resuscitated from asphyxial cardiac arrest (described in Ref. 54).

Induced hypothermia was used in the late 70's and early 80's as a component of brain-targeted therapy for pediatric patients in coma from near-drowning, traumatic brain injury, or Reye's syndrome. Brain-targeted therapy included combinations of hypothermia, intracranial pressure (ICP) monitoring, hyperventilation, barbiturate coma, mannitol, and fluid restriction. In the early 80's, several studies failed to show improved patient outcomes with this brain-targeted therapy (59-63). Unfortunately, these studies were not rigorously designed. Each was underpowered (sample size ranged from 11 to 24) and was either uncontrolled or used historic controls. Furthermore, we now know that some components of the brain-targeted therapy used in the 70's - 80's have the potential to cause harm (hyperventilation and fluid restriction). Also, the hypothermia protocols were more aggressive (30°C for 72 h) than is currently recommended and may have increased the infectious complications of hypothermia. Nevertheless, hypothermia (and measurement of ICP) fell out of favor for management of children resuscitated from asphyxial cardiac arrest.

There are ongoing trials of induced hypothermia for treatment of neonatal asphyxia (discussed in Chapter 9). To date, the data suggests that the therapy is safe and feasible but long-term outcome has not been reported (64).

SUMMARY

Asphyxia is the common pathway for many non-cardiac causes of cardiac arrest including trauma, intoxication, and drowning. A key question is whether therapeutic hypothermia, which improves survival and neurologic outcome in adults after VF/VT cardiac arrest, can similarly improve outcome after asphyxial arrest. Similar to arrhythmic arrest, asphyxia causes an ischemic injury to the entire body and brain (global ischemia). While the brain injury is somewhat similar after asphyxial or arrhythmic arrest, asphyxia tends to cause more severe injury, which includes microinfarcts. Even so, animal models of asphyxial arrest demonstrate a strong neuroprotective effect of induced hypothermia. Hypothermia appears to affect particular molecular events and changes in cellular signaling after asphyxia. Clinical experience with induced hypothermia for treatment of asphyxia is limited and controlled clinical trials are lacking. Some clinicians will require additional clinical evidence before accepting hypothermia as a treatment of asphyxia. Others will conclude that the adult VF/VT trials combined with animal trials of asphyxia provide sufficient evidence to justify induced hypothermia treatment of asphyxial cardiac arrest.

REFERENCES

1. Safar P, Paradis NA. Asphyxial Cardiac Arrest. In: Paradis NA, Halperin HR, Nowak RM, editors. *Cardiac Arrest: The Science and Practice of Resuscitation Medicine.* Baltimore: Williams and Wilkins, 1999: 702-726.
2. Kuisma M, Suominen P, Korpela R. Paediatric out-of-hospital cardiac arrests-- epidemiology and outcome. *Resuscitation* 1995; 30:141-150.
3. Sirbaugh PE, Pepe PE, Shook JE, et al. A prospective, population-based study of the demographics, epidemiology, management, and outcome of out-of-hospital pediatric cardiopulmonary arrest. *Ann Emerg Med* 1999; 33:174-184.
4. Young KD, Seidel JS. Pediatric cardiopulmonary resuscitation: a collective review. *Ann Emerg Med* 1999; 33:195-205.
5. Kuisma M, Alaspaa A. Out-of-hospital cardiac arrests of non-cardiac origin. Epidemiology and outcome. *Eur Heart J* 1997; 18:1122-1128.
6. Arai T, Watanabe T, Nagaro T, Matsuo S. Blood-brain barrier impairment after cardiac resuscitation. *Crit Care Med* 1981; 9:444-448.
7. Schleien CL, Koehler RC, Shaffner DH, et al. Blood-brain barrier disruption after cardiopulmonary resuscitation in immature swine. *Stroke* 1991; 22:477-483.
8. Pluta R, Lossinsky AS, Wisniewski HM, Mossakowski MJ. Early blood-brain barrier changes in the rat following transient complete cerebral ischemia induced by cardiac arrest. *Brain Res* 1994; 633:41-52.
9. Negovsky VA. Postresuscitation disease. *Crit Care Med* 1988; 16:942.
10. Cerchiari EL, Safar P, Klein E. Cardiovascular function and neurologic outcome after cardiac arrest in dogs. The cardiovascular post-resuscitation syndrome. *Resuscitation* 1993; 25:9.
11. Safar P. Effects of the postresuscitation syndrome on cerebral recovery from cardiac arrest. *Crit Care Med* 1988; 13:932.
12. Bottiger BW, Krumnikl JJ, Gass P, et al. The cerebral 'no-reflow' phenomenon after cardiac arrest in rats-- influence of low-flow reperfusion. *Resuscitation* 1997; 34:79-87.
13. Vaagenes P, Safar P, Diven W, et al. Brain enzyme levels in CSF after cardiac arrest and resuscitation in dogs: markers of damage and predictors of outcome. *J Cereb Blood Flow Metab* 1988; 8:262-275.
14. Vaagenes P, Safar P, Moossy J, et al. Asphyxiation versus ventricular fibrillation cardiac arrest in dogs. Differences in cerebral resuscitation effects--a preliminary study. *Resuscitation* 1997; 35:41-52.
15. Morimoto Y, Kemmotsu O, Kitami K, et al. Acute brain swelling after out-of-hospital cardiac arrest: pathogenesis and outcome. *Crit Care Med* 1993; 21:104-110.
16. Hicks SD, DeFranco DB, Callaway CW. Hypothermia during reperfusion after asphyxial cardiac arrest improves functional recovery and selectively alters stress-induced protein expression. *J Cereb Blood Flow Metab* 2000; 20:520-530.
17. Hickey RW, Akino M, Strausbaugh S, De Courten-Myers GM. Use of the Morris water maze and acoustic startle chamber to evaluate neurologic injury after asphyxial cardiac arrest in rats. *Pediatr Res* 1996; 39:77-84.
18. Kuboyama K, Safar P, Radovsky A, et al. Delay in cooling negates the beneficial effect of mild resuscitative cerebral hypothermia after cardiac arrest in dogs: a prospective, randomized study. *Crit Care Med* 1993; 21:1348-1358.
19. Katz LM, Callaway CW, Kagan VE, Kochanek PM. Electron spin resonance measure of brain antioxidant activity during ischemia/reperfusion. *Neuroreport* 1998; 9:1587-1593.
20. Katz LM, Wang Y, Rockoff S, Bouldin TW. Low-dose Carbicarb improves cerebral outcome after asphyxial cardiac arrest in rats. *Ann Emerg Med* 2002; 39:359-365.

21. Ooboshi H, Ibayashi S, Takano K, et al. Hypothermia inhibits ischemia-induced efflux of amino acids and neuronal damage in the hippocampus of aged rats. *Brain Res* 2000; 884:23-30.

22. Xiao F, Safar P, Radovsky A. Mild protective and resuscitative hypothermia for asphyxial cardiac arrest in rats. *Am J Emerg Med* 1998; 16:17-25.

23. Hachimi-Idrissi S, Corne L, Huyghens L. The effect of mild hypothermia and induced hypertension on long term survival rate and neurological outcome after asphyxial cardiac arrest in rats. *Resuscitation* 2001; 49:73-82.

24. Dietrich WD, Busto R, Alonso O, et al. Intraischemic but not postischemic brain hypothermia protects chronically following global forebrain ischemia in rats. *J Cereb Blood Flow Metab* 1993; 13:541-549.

25. Callaway CW, Tadler SC, Katz LM, et al. Feasibility of external cranial cooling during out-of-hospital cardiac arrest. *Resuscitation* 2002; 52:159-165.

26. Laptook AR, Corbett RJ, Sterett R, et al. Quantitative relationship between brain temperature and energy utilization rate measured in vivo using 31P and 1H magnetic resonance spectroscopy. *Pediatr Res* 1995; 38:919-925.

27. Katsura K, Minamisawa H, Ekholm A, et al. Changes of labile metabolites during anoxia in moderately hypo- and hyperthermic rats: correlation to membrane fluxes of K+. *Brain Res* 1992; 590:6-12.

28. Astrup J, Rehncrona S, Siesjo BK. The increase in extracellular potassium concentration in the ischemic brain in relation to the preischemic functional activity and cerebral metabolic rate. *Brain Res* 1980; 199:161-174.

29. Ekholm A, Katsura K, Kristian T, et al. Coupling of cellular energy state and ion homeostasis during recovery following brain ischemia. *Brain Res* 1993; 604:185-191.

30. Lamanna JC, Griffith JK, Cordisco BR, et al. Rapid recovery of rat brain intracellular pH after cardiac arrest and resuscitation. *Brain Res* 1995; 687:175-181.

31. Hoxworth JM, Xu K, Zhou Y, et al. Cerebral metabolic profile, selective neuron loss, and survival of acute and chronic hyperglycemic rats following cardiac arrest and resuscitation. *Brain Res* 1999; 821:467-479.

32. Globus MY, Busto R, Lin B, et al. Detection of free radical activity during transient global ischemia and recirculation: effects of intraischemic brain temperature modulation. *J Neurochem* 1995; 65:1250-1256.

33. Nakane M, Kubota M, Nakagomi T, et al. Rewarming eliminates the protective effect of cooling against delayed neuronal death. *Neuroreport* 2001; 12:2439-2442.

34. Asai S, Zhao H, Kohno T, et al. Quantitative evaluation of extracellular glutamate concentration in postischemic glutamate re-uptake, dependent on brain temperature, in the rat following severe global brain ischemia. *Brain Res* 2000; 864:60-68.

35. Coimbra C, Wieloch T. Moderate hypothermia mitigates neuronal damage in the rat brain when initiated several hours following transient cerebral ischemia. *Acta Neuropathol (Berl)* 1994; 87:325-331.

36. Colbourne F, Li H, Buchan AM. Indefatigable CA1 sector neuroprotection with mild hypothermia induced 6 hours after severe forebrain ischemia in rats. *J Cereb Blood Flow Metab* 1999; 19:742-749.

37. Baena RC, Busto R, Dietrich WD, et al. Hyperthermia delayed by 24 hours aggravates neuronal damage in rat hippocampus following global ischemia. *Neurology* 1997; 48:768-773.

38. Hypothermia after Cardiac Arrest Study Group. Mild therapeutic hypothermia to improve the neurologic outcome after cardiac arrest. *N Engl J Med* 2002; 346:549-556.

39. Zeiner A, Holzer M, Sterz F, et al. Hyperthermia after cardiac arrest is associated with an unfavorable neurologic outcome. *Arch Intern Med* 2001; 161:2007-2012.

40. Hickey RW, Ferimer H, Alexander HL, et al. Delayed, spontaneous hypothermia reduces neuronal damage after asphyxial cardiac arrest in rats. *Crit Care Med* 2000; 28:3511-3516.
41. Hickey RW, Kochanek PM, Ferimer H, et al. Induced hyperthermia exacerbates neurologic neuronal histologic damage after asphyxial cardiac arrest in rats. *Crit Care Med* 2003; 31:531-535.
42. Kelly S, Zhang ZJ, Zhao H, et al. Gene transfer of HSP72 protects cornu ammonis 1 region of the hippocampus neurons from global ischemia: influence of Bcl-2. *Ann Neurol* 2002; 52:160-167.
43. Hicks SD, Parmele KT, DeFranco DB, et al. Hypothermia differentially increases extracellular signal-regulated kinase and stress-activated protein kinase/c-Jun terminal kinase activation in the hippocampus during reperfusion after asphyxial cardiac arrest. *Neuroscience* 2000; 98:677-685.
44. D'Cruz BJ, Fertig KC, Filiano AJ, et al. Hypothermic reperfusion after cardiac arrest augments brain-derived neurotrophic factor activation. *J Cereb Blood Flow Metab* 2002; 22:843-851.
45. Beck T, Lindholm D, Castren E, Wree A. Brain-derived neurotrophic factor protects against ischemic cell damage in rat hippocampus. *J Cereb Blood Flow Metab* 1994; 14:689-692.
46. Han BH, Holtzman DM. BDNF protects the neonatal brain from hypoxic-ischemic injury in vivo via the ERK pathway. *J Neurosci* 2000; 20:5775-5781.
47. Kiprianova I, Freiman TM, Desiderato S, et al. Brain-derived neurotrophic factor prevents neuronal death and glial activation after global ischemia in the rat. *J Neurosci Res* 1999; 56:21-27.
48. White BC, Grossman LI, O'Neil BJ, et al. Global brain ischemia and reperfusion. *Ann Emerg Med* 1996; 27:588-594.
49. Friedman LK, Ginsberg MD, Belayev L, et al. Intraischemic but not postischemic hypothermia prevents non-selective hippocampal downregulation of AMPA and NMDA receptor gene expression after global ischemia. *Brain Res Mol Brain Res* 2001; 86:34-47.
50. Colbourne F, Grooms SY, Zukin RS, et al. Hypothermia rescues hippocampal CA1 neurons and attenuates down-regulation of the AMPA receptor GluR2 subunit after forebrain ischemia. *Proc Natl Acad Sci* USA 2003; 100:2906-2910.
51. Aoki M, Tamatani M, Taniguchi M, et al. Hypothermic treatment restores glucose regulated protein 78 (GRP78) expression in ischemic brain. *Brain Res Mol Brain Res* 2001; 95:117-128.
52. Ginsberg MD, Sternau LL, Globus MY, et al. Therapeutic modulation of brain temperature: relevance to ischemic brain injury. *Cerebrovasc Brain Metab Rev* 1992; 4:189-225.
53. Ginsberg MD, Busto R. Combating hyperthermia in acute stroke: a significant clinical concern. *Stroke* 1998; 29:529-534.
54. Hickey RW, Kochanek PM, Ferimer H.N., Graham SH. Hypothermia and hyperthermia in children following resuscitation from cardiac arrest. *Pediatrics* 2000;106:118-122.
55. Siebke H, Rod T, Breivik H, Link B. Survival after 40 minutes; submersion without cerebral sequeae. *Lancet* 1975; 1:1275-1277.
56. Schmidt U, Fritz KW, Kasperczyk W, Tscherne H. Successful resuscitation of a child with severe hypothermia after cardiac arrest of 88 minutes. *Prehospital Disaster Med* 1995; 10:60-62.
57. Young RS, Zalneraitis EL, Dooling EC. Neurological outcome in cold water drowning. *JAMA* 1980; 244:1233.

58. Walpoth BH, Walpoth-Aslan BN, Mattle HP, et al. Outcome of survivors of accidental deep hypothermia and circulatory arrest treated with extracorporeal blood warming. *N Engl J Med* 1997; 337:1500-1505.
59. Dean JM, McComb JG. Intracranial pressure monitoring in severe pediatric near-drowning. *Neurosurgery* 1981; 9:627-630.
60. Frewen TC, Swedlow DB, Watcha M, et al. Outcome in severe Reye syndrome with early pentobarbital coma and hypothermia. *J Pediatr* 1982; 100:663-665.
61. Oakes DD, Sherck JP, Maloney JR, Charters AC, III. Prognosis and management of victims of near-drowning. *J Trauma* 1982; 22:544-549.
62. Bruce D, Shut L, Sutton LN. Brain resuscitation in children: Fact or fantasy? *Concepts Pediatr Neurosurg* 4, 219-229. 1983.
63. Bohn DJ, Biggar WD, Smith CR, et al. Influence of hypothermia, barbiturate therapy, and intracranial pressure monitoring on morbidity and mortality after near-drowning. *Crit Care Med* 1986; 14:529-534.
64. Battin MR, Penrice J, Gunn TR, Gunn AJ. Treatment of term infants with head cooling and mild systemic hypothermia (35.0 degrees C and 34.5 degrees C) after perinatal asphyxia. *Pediatrics* 2003; 111:244-251.

Chapter 9

NEONATAL ASPHYXIA

Alistair J. Gunn, MBChB, PhD, Laura Bennet, PhD
University of Auckland, Auckland, NZ

INTRODUCTION

Moderate to severe hypoxic-ischemic encephalopathy continues to be an important cause of acute neurologic injury at birth, occurring in approximately 1 to 2 cases per 1000 term live births (1). The possibility that hypothermia might be able to alleviate neonatal brain injury is a 'dream revisited'. Early experimental studies, mainly in altricial species such as kittens, demonstrated that hypothermia greatly extended the 'time to last gasp' and improved outcomes (2). These findings led to a series of small uncontrolled studies in the 1950s and 1960s where infants not breathing spontaneously at five minutes after birth were immersed in cold water until respiration resumed (3-7). Although outcomes were said to be better than for historical controls, this experimental approach was overtaken by two major developments: the introduction of active ventilation of infants exposed to asphyxia and the recognition that even mild hypothermia is associated with increased oxygen requirements and greater mortality in the premature newborn (8). Thus resuscitation guidelines for the newborn exposed to asphyxia have, until very recently, simply emphasized prevention of hypothermia.

The early experimental studies noted above focused entirely on the effects of cooling *during* severe hypoxia, which is well known to be associated with potent, dose-related, long-lasting neuroprotection (9). The real clinical issue of course is whether cooling *after* asphyxial or hypoxic-ischemic injury is beneficial. The present chapter reviews recent developments, which helped delineate the experimental parameters that are likely to be required for successful post-resuscitation cooling.

PATHOPHYSIOLOGICAL PHASES OF CEREBRAL INJURY

The critical advance in ischemic-anoxic encephalopathy was the clinical and experimental observation in term fetuses, newborns and in adults, that injury to the brain is not a single 'event' occurring at, or just after the insult, but an evolving process that leads to cell death well after the initial insult (10). This delay raised the tantalizing possibility that asphyxial cell death could be prevented even well after reperfusion.

Pathophysiologically, several phases of cellular injury have been identified as illustrated in figures 9-1 and 9-2. The hypoxic ischemic event is the *primary* phase of cell injury. During this phase there is progressive hypoxic depolarization of cells leading to severe cytotoxic edema, with failure of reuptake of neurotransmitters leading to extracellular accumulation of excitatory amino acids ('excitotoxins') (11). Excessive levels of excitatory amino acids cause activation of their ion channels, promoting further excessive entry of salt and water, and calcium into the cells (12). Following reperfusion (Figure 9-2) or return of cerebral circulation during resuscitation from an asphyxial insult, the initial hypoxia-induced cytotoxic edema may transiently resolve over approximately 30 to 60 minutes (13), with at least partial recovery of cerebral oxidative metabolism, in a *'latent'* phase, only to secondarily deteriorate many hours later (approximately 6 to 15 h), in a phase that may extend over many days (14, 15). At term, this so called *secondary* phase is marked by the delayed onset of seizures (16, 17), secondary cytotoxic edema (Figure 9-2) (13), accumulation of excitotoxins (11), failure of cerebral oxidative energy metabolism (15), and, ultimately, neuronal death (17, 18). In asphyxiated infants there is a close correlation between the degree of delayed energy failure and neurodevelopmental impairment at 1 and 4 years of age (14).

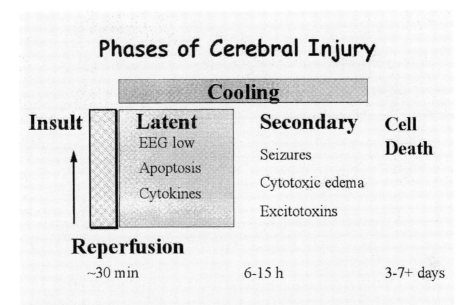

Figure 9-1. Flow diagram illustrating the relationship between the phases of cerebral injury after a severe reversible hypoxic-ischemic insult. During the *reperfusion* period after the insult, there is a period of approximately 30 minutes during which cellular energy metabolism is restored, with progressive resolution of the acute cell swelling secondary to hypoxic-depolarization. This is followed by a *latent* phase, with near-normalization of oxidative cerebral energy metabolism as shown by magnetic resonance spectroscopy, but depressed electroencephalogram (EEG) activity, and typically a delayed interval of reduced cerebral blood flow (CBF). During this phase the intracellular components of apoptosis are activated, and the early inflammatory reaction is initiated, with induction of cytokines. This may be followed by *secondary* deterioration with delayed seizures and cytotoxic edema, extracellular accumulation of potential cytotoxins (such as the excitatory neurotransmitters), and 6 to 15 hours after the asphyxia, failure of oxidative metabolism and damage. The acute changes in this phase may take 3 days or more to resolve. As indicated by the gray bar, treatment with cerebral hypothermia needs to be initiated in the latent phase before the onset of secondary deterioration, and then continued for over 48 hours for long lasting neuroprotection.

This consistent pattern across species and a variety of experimental models and clinical observations suggest that the effectiveness of intervention would be highly dependent on the timing of both initiation and continuation. As discussed in detail below experimental studies of hypothermia have confirmed this hypothesis.

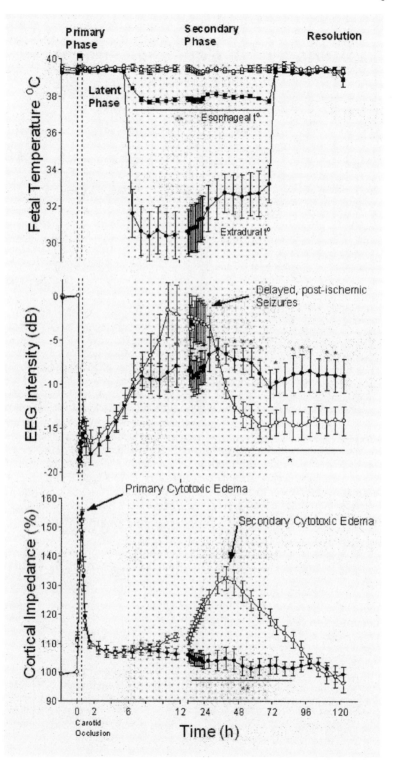

Figure 9-2. The effect of hypothermia started 5.5 hours after reperfusion from 30 min cerebral ischemia in near term fetal sheep. The period of ischemia is shown by dotted lines, while cooling is shown by the bar. The top panel shows changes in extradural (●) and esophageal (■) temperature in the hypothermia group and extradural (O) and esophageal (□) temperature in the sham cooled group. The lower two panels show changes in EEG intensity, and cortical impedance (expressed as percentage of baseline) in the hypothermia (●) and sham cooled (O) groups. Impedance is a measure of cytotoxic edema (cell swelling). The hypothermia group shows greater recovery of EEG intensity after resolution of delayed seizures, and complete suppression of the secondary rise in impedance. Mean ± SEM, * $p<0.05$, ** $p<0.001$ hypothermia vs sham cooled fetuses, for individual time points or intervals (solid bars). Data derived from Gunn et al (42).

FACTORS DETERMINING EFFECTIVE NEUROPROTECTION WITH HYPOTHERMIA

Cooling during resuscitation / reperfusion

Brief hypothermia, for one to two hours, during acute reperfusion appears to be modestly neuroprotective, provided that it is initiated immediately. For example, after 15 minutes of reversible ischemia in the piglet, mild hypothermia (decreasing temperature by 2 to 3°C) for one hour significantly improved recovery and reduced neuronal loss 3 days later (19). Similar data have been reported in the neonatal rat and adult dog (20-23). However, protection was lost if brief hypothermia was delayed by as little as 15 to 45 minutes after the primary insult (24-27). This extreme sensitivity to delay is consistent with the hypothesis that resuscitative hypothermia can suppress oxygen free radical release during reperfusion (28, 29). Alternatively, however, this strategy may simply represent intervention at the tail-end of the primary phase, when cerebrovascular perfusion has not yet been fully re-established and levels of excitatory amino acids are still high (30).

Regardless of the effectiveness or otherwise of immediate cooling during resuscitation, its effectiveness is almost impossible to test in practice. It is simply not possible at present to reliably identify during resuscitation the few infants who subsequently develop significant encephalopathy.

Longer is better

The observations discussed above, namely, that the secondary phase can continue for days after injury, suggest that it would be desirable to maintain hypothermia throughout the course of the secondary phase. Such extended periods of cooling, e.g., between 5 and 72 hours, appear to be more consistently effective (21, 22, 31, 32). For example, in unanesthetized infant rats subjected to moderate hypoxia-ischemia mild hypothermia (2 to 3°C decrease in brain temperature) for 72 hours from the end of hypoxia prevented cortical infarction, while 6 hours of cooling only had intermediate, non-significant effects (22). Similarly, in anesthetized piglets exposed to either hypoxia with bilateral carotid ligation or to hypoxia with hypotension, either 12 hours of mild whole body hypothermia (35°C) or 24 hours of head cooling (to deep brain temperature ~30°C) with mild systemic hypothermia (35°C) started immediately after hypoxia prevented delayed energy failure (31), reduced neuronal loss (33, 34) and suppressed post-hypoxic seizures (34).

How late is too late?

At present, the window of opportunity for treatment can only be determined empirically, however several key principles may be distinguished. The initiation of neuronal degeneration is accelerated by more severe insults. For example, deoxyribonucleic acid (DNA) fragmentation in the hippocampus can be detected as early as 10 hours after a 60 minute hypoxic-ischemic injury in the rat, whereas DNA fragmentation in the hippocampus is only detectable 3 to 5 days after a 15 minute hypoxic-ischemic injury (18). However, the appearance of DNA fragmentation and classic ischemic cell change can represent only the terminal events of this cascade. It is likely that cell death is effectively irreversible well before that stage.

While the precise mechanisms of neuroprotection by hypothermia are not fully understood, there are increasing data to suggest that hypothermia has a particular role in suppressing apoptosis, particularly in the developing brain. In the piglet, hypothermia started after severe hypoxic-ischemic reduced apoptotic cell death, but not necrotic cell death (33). Similarly, moderate hypothermia showed specifically inhibited apoptotic cell death and cellular DNA fragmentation after cold-induced brain injury in rats (35). In the adult rodent, post-ischemic hypothermia reduced both the number of terminal deoxynucleotidyl transferase (TdT) and digoxigenin-11-dUTP nick-end labelling (TUNEL) positive cells and expression of the pro-apoptotic factor Bax (36).

The process of programmed or apoptotic cell death involves both "latent" and active or "execution" phases (37). The latent phase is characterized by caspase activation within the cytoplasm (a large family of enzymes which mediate and amplify apoptosis [38]). In contrast, the active phase involves factors downstream from the caspases that can induce DNA fragmentation and chromatin condensation when injected into previously normal nuclei. These data suggest that activation of intranuclear factors is the critical event that occurs at the transition from the latent to the execution phases of programmed neuronal death (37). In principle it also seems likely that it is this transition which represents the onset of irreversible injury, even though it still precedes terminal DNA fragmentation and cell death. Consistent with this, effective neuroprotection with post-insult hypothermia is associated with potent suppression of activated caspase 3 (39-41).

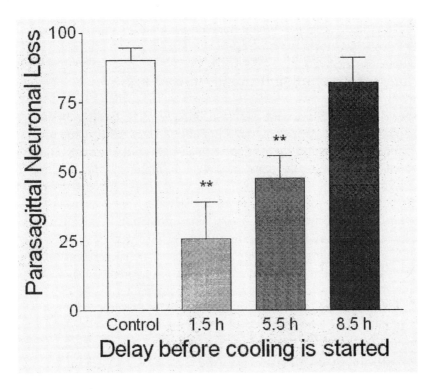

Figure 9-1. The effect of cerebral cooling in the fetal sheep started at different times after reperfusion and continued until 72 h, on neuronal loss in the parasagittal cortex after 5 days recovery from 30 minutes of cerebral ischemia (17, 42, 43). Compared with the sham cooled group (n=13) cooling started 90 minutes after reperfusion (n=7) was protective, whereas cooling started shortly after the start of the secondary phase (8.5 hours after reperfusion, n=5) was not. Cooling started just before the end of the latent phase (5.5 hours after reperfusion, n=11) was partially protective. Only cooled fetuses in which the extradural temperature was successfully maintained below 34°C have been included. *p<0.005 compared with sham-cooled (control) fetuses; data are Mean ± SEM.

Systematic *in vivo* studies support the central importance of starting treatment as early as possible in the latent phase. For example, in the near-term fetal sheep, moderate hypothermia induced 90 minutes after reperfusion, in the early latent phase, and continued until 72 hours after ischemia, prevented secondary cytotoxic edema, and improved electroencephalographic recovery (17). There was a concomitant substantial reduction in parasagittal cortical infarction and improvement in neuronal loss scores in all regions. When the start of hypothermia was delayed until just before the onset of secondary seizures in this paradigm (5.5 hours after reperfusion) partial neuroprotection was seen (Figures 9-2 and 9-3) (42). With further delay until after seizures were established (8.5 hours after reperfusion), there was no electrophysiological or overall histological protection with cooling (Figure 9-3) (43).

How long is long enough for delayed cooling?

There is evidence that optimal protection with delayed initiation of hypothermia requires periods of cooling longer than 12 h. Colbourne & Corbett found in the adult gerbil that with a slightly more severe insult (5 minutes of global ischemia compared with 3 minutes), the duration of moderate hypothermia had to be extended from 12 to 24 hours to provide neuroprotection (44). When the delay before initiating the 24 hour period of cooling was increased from 1 to 4 hours, neuroprotection in the CA1 region of the hippocampus after six months recovery fell from 70 to 12% (45). Subsequent studies using models of both focal and global cerebral ischemia in adult rodents demonstrated that this chronic loss could be prevented by extending the duration of moderate (32 to 34°C) hypothermia to 48 hours or more, even when the start of cooling was delayed until 6 hours after reperfusion (46, 47).

Is neuroprotection maintained long-term?

There have been reports that hypothermia only delayed, rather than prevented, neuronal degeneration after global ischemia in the adult rat (48-50) and severe hypoxia-ischemia in the 7 day old rat (51). These findings were likely related to two factors. First, rebound hyperthermia in the secondary phase can occur after ischemia. Even short periods of hyperthermia, induced 24 hours after either global or brief focal ischemia in the adult rat exacerbate injury (52, 53). When moderate hypothermia from two to nine hours after global ischemia in the rat was combined with prevention of spontaneous delayed pyrexia with antipyretics, histological protection was seen after 2 months recovery (50). Each intervention alone had essentially short-term benefit only.

Alternatively, the duration of hypothermia may have simply been inadequate. Seventy two hours of very mild cooling in the infant rat after carotid occlusion and hypoxia was associated with long-term improvement whereas 6 hours was not (22). Subsequent studies both in the 7 day rat and in adult species have confirmed that prolonged cooling for 24 to 72 hours initiated within 6 hours of injury is associated with persistent behavioral and histological protection (21, 46, 54-56).

If some is good, is more better?

There appears to be a critical depth of cerebral hypothermia between 32 and 34°C required for effective neuronal rescue. In fetal sheep cooled from 90 minutes after ischemia, substantial neuroprotection was seen only in fetuses in whom there was a sustained decrease in the extradural temperature to less than 34°C (normal temperature in the fetal sheep is 39.5°C) (17). In the adult gerbil, cooling to a rectal temperature of 32°C was associated with greater behavioral and histological neuroprotection than 34°C (56). Although we do not know the optimal degree of cerebral cooling in newborns, the first controlled trials of hypothermia after cardiac arrest in adults strongly support this target range, with improved neurological outcome in patients cooled to between 32 and 34°C (57, 58).

There is a clear trade-off, however, between the adverse systemic effects of cooling, which increase markedly below a core temperature of approximately 34°C (59), and the potential cerebral benefit. For example, in the adult dog, deep hypothermia (15°C) after cardiac arrest was detrimental, whereas mild hypothermia (34 to 36°C), from 10 minutes until 12 hours after cardiac arrest was beneficial (60).

Is it possible to "selectively" cool the head?

In order to provide adequate neuroprotection with minimal risk of systemic adverse effects in sick, unstable neonates, ideally only the brain would be cooled. Although this has been demonstrated experimentally using cardiac bypass procedures (61), it is clearly impractical in routine practice. Pragmatically, partially selective cerebral cooling can be obtained using a cooling cap applied to the scalp, while the body is warmed by some method such as an overhead heater to limit the degree of systemic hypothermia (62-64). A mild (~34 to 35°C) degree of systemic hypothermia is still desirable during head cooling, firstly to reduce the steepness of the intracerebral gradient which develops during true selective head cooling (65), avoiding excessively cold cap temperatures which might cause scalp injury or exacerbate local scalp edema (64), and to provide at least some cooling of deep cerebral structures such as the brain stem. This approach has recently been demonstrated in studies in the piglet to be associated with a substantial (median, 5.3°C), sustained decrease in deep intracerebral temperature at the level of the basal ganglia compared with the rectal temperature (66, 67). In asphyxiated newborns, although direct temperature measurements are not feasible, head cooling has been shown to increase the gradient between nasopharyngeal and rectal temperature by approximately 1°C (62).

CLINICAL IMPLICATIONS

Caveats for clinical trials: will hypothermia always 'work'?

The experimental studies discussed above suggest that a prolonged duration of moderate hypothermia may be able to improve outcome if it is started within 6 hours of hypoxic-ischemic injury. These studies, however, used very carefully standardized insults, occurring at a precisely known time. In contrast, although the precipitating insult in neonatal encephalopathy may certainly be a well defined event such as placental abruption that is terminated at birth, in other cases it seems to evolve over hours during labor, and indeed the infant may be compromised even before labor starts (68).

Consistent with this, some infants with apparent hypoxic-ischemic encephalopathy do not show any initial recovery of cerebral oxidative metabolism, and have extremely poor outcomes (69). Such cases may reflect either a significant interval of evolution of injury before birth or more simply the most extreme insults. Both interpretations suggest that hypothermia is unlikely to be effective. If the former interpretation is correct, for example, then the latent phase is already over and there would no time available for treatment before the start of secondary deterioration (43, 70). Alternatively, if these cases represent the most severe insults, it is known experimentally that hypothermia seems to be less protective with the most severe cerebral injuries, even with very early initiation of cooling (21, 54, 70).

Nevertheless, many infants with moderate to severe hypoxic-ischemic encephalopathy do show initial, transient recovery of cerebral oxidative metabolism. In those cases, secondary cerebral energy failure does not occur until 6 to 15 hours after birth (14, 69). Even though the onset of energy failure likely represents the outer limit of the therapeutic window for hypothermia, this delay still suggests a reasonable potential window of opportunity for treatment for at least some infants.

Clinical trials of hypothermia

Small controlled trials of head cooling with mild hypothermia (62, 64, 71, 72) and of whole body cooling (73) in asphyxiated newborns have now been reported, in addition to several case series (74-76). Although none of these studies were powered to evaluate neurological outcome, there is a suggestion of improved short term (72,76,77) and long term outcomes (71, 77, 78).

For example, in a controlled study of head cooling among infants with early stage 2 or 3 encephalopathy, mild systemic hypothermia was associated with a trend to reduced cerebral palsy in survivors (odds ratio 0.46 [0.08, 2.56] vs normothermia) (71). A retrospective study of whole body cooling to between 32 and 34°C in 10 infants found a significant reduction of major neurologic abnormalities and abnormal MRI findings at follow-up compared with 11 historical controls (78). Finally, a larger randomized pilot study of head cooling with mild hypothermia compared to normothermia found a significant reduction in neuron specific enolase (NSE) levels in cerebral spinal fluid with cooling (26.2+/-10.8 vs 34.6+/-17.1 mg/L, P<0.05) but only a small increase in normal developmental outcome at 6 months of age in 18 of 23 cooled patients (78.3 %) compared with 19 of 27 (70.4 %) normothermic infants (77).

EXTRACEREBRAL EFFECTS OF HYPOTHERMIA

While the above studies have suggested that mild hypothermia is generally safe they have also highlighted the importance of understanding the extracerebral, physiologic effects of hypothermia (59).

Cardiovascular adaptation

Consistent with the known electrocardiographic effects, hypothermia slows the atrial pacemaker and intracardiac conduction. Consequently, hypothermia to less than approximately 35.5°C is associated with sustained sinus bradycardia in most infants (64, 73). Electrocardiograms done in infants with sustained heart rates of <90 bpm confirmed markedly prolonged QT duration above the 98th percentile corrected for age and heart rate, without arrhythmia. These changes resolve with rewarming (79). Although such prolonged QT in the absence of ventricular arrhythmia may be safe, close monitoring is clearly essential and other therapies which lengthen the QT interval (such as macrolide antibiotics) should be avoided.

During initiation of cooling there is a significant increase in blood pressure, both experimentally (42) and clinically (74). This response is mediated by rapid peripheral vasoconstriction, i.e. centralization of blood flow (80). Cooling resulted in a marked reduction in carotid blood flow compared with sham cooled fetuses, with prolongation of secondary hypoperfusion and abolition of hyperperfusion during delayed seizures. This relative reduction is mediated by reduced metabolism not by nonspecific peripheral vasoconstriction (17). Many studies, mostly in the piglet, have shown that cerebral blood flow and metabolism remain closely coupled, even during deep hypothermia (81).

Respiratory management

Persistent pulmonary hypertension is frequent associated with perinatal asphyxia. Experimentally, moderate hypothermia (31±0.4°C) increases pulmonary vascular resistance (82). One case series suggested that hypothermia is associated with a modest but consistent increase in FIO_2 (74). In contrast other controlled studies found no apparent change in the oxygen or ventilatory requirements of infants with persistent pulmonary hypertension of the newborn during induction of hypothermia or rewarming (64, 73). An important technical point is that the partial pressure of blood gases including oxygen and carbon dioxide are reduced by hypothermia. Thus measured levels will be artefactually increased if the blood gas is analyzed at 37°C. Similarly, measured pH values are reduced if not corrected for a reduction in the patient's temperature.

Nonshivering thermogenesis

Unlike adults, infants respond to cooling with intense nonshivering thermogenesis. Active cooling reveals underlying changes in this endogenous heat production system which are normally masked by the routine use of servo-controlled warming. For example, hypoxia or sedation, which potently inhibit thermogenesis, lead to a decrease in temperature (74). On the other hand, seizures can increase peripheral heat production and ventilation without warm gases can cause significant heat loss (74). It is important to anticipate the potential for these changes in order to avoid large swings in temperature. During head cooling with mild systemic hypothermia, keeping the overhead heater on maximum is one way to minimize the contribution of these changes in endogenous heat production and thus keep a more stable balance over time.

Metabolic effects

Hypokalemia and mild metabolic acidosis may occur in infants cooled to below 34°C. Hypokalemia occurs in animal models during deep hypothermia, but corrects spontaneously during rewarming suggesting that this change is due to intracellular redistribution (83). Consistent with this, a mild decrease in serum potassium was reported in a series of infants cooled to between 33 and 34°C (75), whereas no change was found in studies using milder systemic cooling (73). Thus maintenance potassium administration during cooling must be used cautiously, since 'correction' of the reversible hypokalemia during hypothermia may lead to rebound *hyper*kalemia on rewarming (84).

CONCLUSION

There is now good experimental evidence that moderate post-asphyxial cerebral cooling can be associated with long-term neuroprotection. The key requirements are that hypothermia is initiated as soon as possible in the latent phase, prior to secondary deterioration, and continued for a sufficient period in relation to the evolution of delayed encephalopathic processes, typically 48 hours or more. Although, experimentally, cooling can be partially effective if started up to 6 hours after relatively short insults, cooling started as soon as possible, within at most a few hours of birth, is most likely to be effective.

Preliminary studies of both whole body cooling and head cooling combined with mild systemic hypothermia support the general safety of selective hypothermia even in sick asphyxiated infants, but these data should not be over interpreted. These studies are too small, and were not designed to either test the efficacy of treatment or to detect uncommon adverse events. This is now being addressed by large multicenter trials of different cooling strategies with adequate power to assess longer-term outcome.

Acknowledgments

The authors' work reported in this review has been supported by National Institutes of Health grant RO-1 HD32752, and by grants from the Health Research Council of New Zealand, Lottery Health Board of New Zealand, and the Auckland Medical Research Foundation.

REFERENCES

1. Gunn AJ, Gunn TR. Changes in risk factors for hypoxic-ischaemic seizures in term infants. *Aust N Z J Obstet Gynaecol* 1997; 37:36-39.
2. Westin B, Miller JA, Jr., Boles A. Hypothermia induced during asphyxiation: its effects on survival rate, learning and maintenance of the conditioned response in rats. *Acta Paediatr* 1963; 52:49-60.
3. Westin B, Miller JA, Jr., Nyberg R, Wedenberg E. Neonatal asphyxia pallida treated with hypothermia alone or with hypothermia and transfusion of oxygenated blood. *Surgery* 1959; 45:868-879.
4. Miller JA, Jr., Miller FS, Westin B. Hypothermia in the treatment of asphyxia neonatorum. *Biol Neonat* 1964; 20:148-163.
5. Cordey R. Resuscitation of the newborn in white asphyxia by means of hypothermia alone or combined with intra-arterial transfusion of oxygenated blood. *Bull Fed Soc Gynecol Obstet Lang Fr* 1961; 13:507-509.
6. Cordey R. Hypothermia in resuscitating newborns in white asphyxia; a report of 14 cases. *Obstet Gynecol* 1964; 24:760-767.
7. Cordey R, Chiolero R, Miller JA, Jr. Resuscitation of neonates by hypothermia: report on 20 cases with acid-base determination on 10 cases and the long-term development of 33 cases. *Resuscitation* 1973; 2:169-181.
8. Silverman WA, Fertig JW, Berger AP. The influence of the thermal environment upon the survival of newly born premature infants. *Pediatrics* 1958; 22:876-886.
9. Nurse S, Corbett D. Direct measurement of brain temperature during and after intraischemic hypothermia: correlation with behavioral, physiological, and histological endpoints. *J Neurosci* 1994; 14:7726-7734.
10. Banasiak KJ, Xia Y, Haddad GG. Mechanisms underlying hypoxia-induced neuronal apoptosis. *Prog Neurobiol* 2000; 62:215-249.
11. Tan WK, Williams CE, During MJ, et al. Accumulation of cytotoxins during the development of seizures and edema after hypoxic-ischemic injury in late gestation fetal sheep. *Pediatr Res* 1996; 39:791-797.
12. Zipfel GJ, Babcock DJ, Lee JM, Choi DW. Neuronal apoptosis after CNS injury: the roles of glutamate and calcium. *J Neurotrauma* 2000; 17:857-869.
13. Williams CE, Gunn A, Gluckman PD. Time course of intracellular edema and epileptiform activity following prenatal cerebral ischemia in sheep. *Stroke* 1991; 22:516-521.
14. Roth SC, Edwards AD, Cady EB, et al. Relation between cerebral oxidative metabolism following birth asphyxia, and neurodevelopmental outcome and brain growth at one year. *Dev Med Child Neurol* 1992; 34:285-295.
15. Lorek A, Takei Y, Cady EB, et al. Delayed ("secondary") cerebral energy failure after acute hypoxia-ischemia in the newborn piglet: continuous 48-hour studies by phosphorus magnetic resonance spectroscopy. *Pediatr Res* 1994; 36:699-706.
16. Gunn AJ, Parer JT, Mallard EC, Williams CE, Gluckman PD. Cerebral histologic and electrocorticographic changes after asphyxia in fetal sheep. *Pediatr Res* 1992; 31:486-491.
17. Gunn AJ, Gunn TR, de Haan HH, Williams CE, Gluckman PD. Dramatic neuronal rescue with prolonged selective head cooling after ischemia in fetal lambs. *J Clin Invest* 1997; 99:248-256.
18. Beilharz EJ, Williams CE, Dragunow M, Sirimanne ES, Gluckman PD. Mechanisms of delayed cell death following hypoxic-ischemic injury in the immature rat: evidence for apoptosis during selective neuronal loss. *Mol Brain Res* 1995; 29:1-14.

19. Laptook AR, Corbett RJ, Sterett R, et al. Modest hypothermia provides partial neuroprotection when used for immediate resuscitation after brain ischemia. *Pediatr Res* 1997; 42:17-23.

20. Yager J, Towfighi J, Vannucci RC. Influence of mild hypothermia on hypoxic-ischemic brain damage in the immature rat. *Pediatr Res* 1993; 34:525-529.

21. Bona E, Hagberg H, Loberg EM, Bagenholm R, Thoresen M. Protective effects of moderate hypothermia after neonatal hypoxia- ischemia: short- and long-term outcome. *Pediatr Res* 1998; 43:738-745.

22. Sirimanne ES, Blumberg RM, Bossano D, et al. The effect of prolonged modification of cerebral temperature on outcome after hypoxic-ischemic brain injury in the infant rat. *Pediatr Res* 1996; 39:591-597.

23. Kuboyama K, Safar P, Oku K, et al. Mild hypothermia after cardiac arrest in dogs does not affect postarrest cerebral oxygen uptake/delivery mismatching. *Resuscitation* 1994; 27:231-244.

24. Laptook AR, Corbett RJ, Burns DK, Sterett R. A limited interval of delayed modest hypothermia for ischemic brain resuscitation is not beneficial in neonatal swine. *Pediatr Res* 1999; 46:383-389.

25. Kuboyama K, Safar P, Radovsky A, et al. Delay in cooling negates the beneficial effect of mild resuscitative cerebral hypothermia after cardiac arrest in dogs: a prospective, randomized study. *Crit Care Med* 1993; 21:1348-1358.

26. Shuaib A, Trulove D, Ijaz MS, Kanthan R, Kalra J. The effect of post-ischemic hypothermia following repetitive cerebral ischemia in gerbils. *Neurosci Lett* 1995; 186:165-168.

27. Busto R, Dietrich WD, Globus MY, Ginsberg MD. Postischemic moderate hypothermia inhibits CA1 hippocampal ischemic neuronal injury. *Neurosci Lett* 1989; 101:299-304.

28. Kil HY, Zhang J, Piantadosi CA. Brain temperature alters hydroxyl radical production during cerebral ischemia/reperfusion in rats. *J Cereb Blood Flow Metab* 1996; 16:100-106.

29. Kubota M, Nakane M, Narita K, et al. Mild hypothermia reduces the rate of metabolism of arachidonic acid following postischemic reperfusion. *Brain Res* 1998; 779:297-300.

30. Thoresen M, Satas S, Puka-Sundvall M, et al. Post-hypoxic hypothermia reduces cerebrocortical release of NO and excitotoxins. *Neuroreport* 1997; 8:3359-3362.

31. Thoresen M, Penrice J, Lorek A, et al. Mild hypothermia after severe transient hypoxia-ischemia ameliorates delayed cerebral energy failure in the newborn piglet. *Pediatr Res* 1995; 37:667-670.

32. Thoresen M, Bagenholm R, Loberg EM, Apricena F, Kjellmer I. Posthypoxic cooling of neonatal rats provides protection against brain injury. *Arch Dis Child Fetal Neonatal Ed* 1996; 74:F3-F9.

33. Edwards AD, Yue X, Squier MV, et al. Specific inhibition of apoptosis after cerebral hypoxia-ischaemia by moderate post-insult hypothermia. *Biochem Biophys Res Commun* 1995; 217:1193-1199.

34. Tooley JR, Satas S, Porter H, Silver IA, Thoresen M. Head cooling with mild systemic hypothermia in anesthetized piglets is neuroprotective. *Ann Neurol* 2003; 53:65-72.

35. Xu RX, Nakamura T, Nagao S, et al. Specific inhibition of apoptosis after cold-induced brain injury by moderate postinjury hypothermia. *Neurosurgery* 1998; 43:107-114.

36. Inamasu J, Suga S, Sato S, et al. Postischemic hypothermia attenuates apoptotic cell death in transient focal ischemia in rats. *Acta Neurochir Suppl* 2000; 76:525-527.

37. Samejima K, Villa P, Earnshaw WC. Role of factors downstream of caspases in nuclear disassembly during apoptotic execution. *Philos Trans R Soc Lond B Biol Sci* 1999; 354:1591-1598.

38. Gottron FJ, Ying HS, Choi DW. Caspase inhibition selectively reduces the apoptotic component of oxygen-glucose deprivation-induced cortical neuronal cell death. *Mol Cell Neurosci* 1997; 9:159-169.
39. Phanithi PB, Yoshida Y, Santana A, et al. Mild hypothermia mitigates post-ischemic neuronal death following focal cerebral ischemia in rat brain: immunohistochemical study of Fas, caspase-3 and TUNEL. *Neuropathology* 2000; 20:273-282.
40. Tomimatsu T, Fukuda H, Endo M, et al. Effects of hypothermia on neonatal hypoxic-ischemic brain injury in the rat: phosphorylation of Akt, activation of caspase-3-like protease. *Neurosci Lett* 2001; 312:21-24.
41. Fukuda H, Tomimatsu T, Watanabe N, et al. Post-ischemic hypothermia blocks caspase-3 activation in the newborn rat brain after hypoxia-ischemia. *Brain Res* 2001; 910:187-191.
42. Gunn AJ, Gunn TR, Gunning MI, Williams CE, Gluckman PD. Neuroprotection with prolonged head cooling started before postischemic seizures in fetal sheep. *Pediatrics* 1998; 102:1098-1106.
43. Gunn AJ, Bennet L, Gunning MI, Gluckman PD, Gunn TR. Cerebral hypothermia is not neuroprotective when started after postischemic seizures in fetal sheep. *Pediatr Res* 1999; 46:274-280.
44. Colbourne F, Corbett D. Delayed and prolonged post-ischemic hypothermia is neuroprotective in the gerbil. *Brain Res* 1994; 654:265-272.
45. Colbourne F, Corbett D. Delayed postischemic hypothermia: a six month survival study using behavioral and histological assessments of neuroprotection. *J Neurosci* 1995; 15:7250-7260.
46. Colbourne F, Li H, Buchan AM. Indefatigable CA1 sector neuroprotection with mild hypothermia induced 6 hours after severe forebrain ischemia in rats. *J Cereb Blood Flow Metab* 1999; 19:742-749.
47. Colbourne F, Corbett D, Zhao Z, Yang J, Buchan AM. Prolonged but delayed postischemic hypothermia: a long-term outcome study in the rat middle cerebral artery occlusion model. *J Cereb Blood Flow Metab* 2000; 20:1702-1708.
48. Dietrich WD, Busto R, Alonso O, Globus MY, Ginsberg MD. Intraischemic but not postischemic brain hypothermia protects chronically following global forebrain ischemia in rats. *J Cereb Blood Flow Metab* 1993; 13:541-549.
49. Nurse S, Corbett D. Neuroprotection after several days of mild, drug-induced hypothermia. *J Cereb Blood Flow Metab* 1996; 16:474-480.
50. Coimbra C, Drake M, Boris-Moller F, Wieloch T. Long-lasting neuroprotective effect of postischemic hypothermia and treatment with an anti-inflammatory/antipyretic drug. Evidence for chronic encephalopathic processes following ischemia. *Stroke* 1996; 27:1578-1585.
51. Trescher WH, Ishiwa S, Johnston MV. Brief post-hypoxic-ischemic hypothermia markedly delays neonatal brain injury. *Brain Dev* 1997; 19:326-338.
52. Baena RC, Busto R, Dietrich WD, Globus MY, Ginsberg MD. Hyperthermia delayed by 24 hours aggravates neuronal damage in rat hippocampus following global ischemia. *Neurology* 1997; 48:768-773.
53. Kim Y, Busto R, Dietrich WD, Kraydieh S, Ginsberg MD. Delayed postischemic hyperthermia in awake rats worsens the histopathological outcome of transient focal cerebral ischemia. *Stroke* 1996; 27:2274-2280.
54. Nedelcu J, Klein MA, Aguzzi A, Martin E. Resuscitative hypothermia protects the neonatal rat brain from hypoxic- ischemic injury. *Brain Pathol* 2000; 10:61-71.

55. Wagner BP, Nedelcu J, Martin E. Delayed postischemic hypothermia improves long-term behavioral outcome after cerebral hypoxia-ischemia in neonatal rats. *Pediatr Res* 2002; 51:354-360.

56. Colbourne F, Auer RN, Sutherland GR. Characterization of postischemic behavioral deficits in gerbils with and without hypothermic neuroprotection. *Brain Res* 1998; 803:69-78.

57. Bernard SA, Gray TW, Buist MD, et al. Treatment of comatose survivors of out-of-hospital cardiac arrest with induced hypothermia. *N Engl J Med* 2002; 346:557-563.

58. The Hypothermia after Cardiac Arrest Study Group. Mild therapeutic hypothermia to improve the neurologic outcome after cardiac arrest. *N Engl J Med* 2002; 346:549-556.

59. Schubert A. Side effects of mild hypothermia. *J Neurosurg Anesthesiol* 1995; 7:139-147.

60. Weinrauch V, Safar P, Tisherman S, Kuboyama K, Radovsky A. Beneficial effect of mild hypothermia and detrimental effect of deep hypothermia after cardiac arrest in dogs. *Stroke* 1992; 23:1454-1462.

61. Wass CT, Waggoner JR, Cable DG, et al. Selective convective brain cooling during normothermic cardiopulmonary bypass in dogs. *J Thorac Cardiovasc Surg* 1998; 115:1350-1357.

62. Gunn AJ, Gluckman PD, Gunn TR. Selective head cooling in newborn infants after perinatal asphyxia: a safety study. *Pediatrics* 1998; 102:885-892.

63. Simbruner G, Haberl C, Harrison V, Linley L, Willeitner AE. Induced brain hypothermia in asphyxiated human newborn infants: a retrospective chart analysis of physiological and adverse effects. *Intensive Care Med* 1999; 25:1111-1117.

64. Battin MR, Penrice J, Gunn TR, Gunn AJ. Treatment of term infants with head cooling and mild systemic hypothermia (35.0 degrees C and 34.5 degrees C) after perinatal asphyxia. *Pediatrics* 2003; 111:244-251.

65. Laptook AR, Shalak L, Corbett RJ. Differences in brain temperature and cerebral blood flow during selective head versus whole-body cooling. *Pediatrics* 2001; 108:1103-1110.

66. Thoresen M, Simmonds M, Satas S, Tooley J, Silver I. Effective selective head cooling during posthyoxic hypothermia in newborn piglets. *Pediatr Res* 2001; 49:594-599.

67. Tooley J, Satas S, Eagle R, Silver IA, Thoresen M. Significant selective head cooling can be maintained long-term after global hypoxia ischemia in newborn piglets. *Pediatrics* 2002; 109:643-649.

68. Westgate JA, Gunn AJ, Gunn TR. Antecedents of neonatal encephalopathy with fetal acidaemia at term. *Br J Obstet Gynaecol* 1999; 106:774-782.

69. Azzopardi D, Wyatt JS, Cady EB, et al. Prognosis of newborn infants with hypoxic-ischemic brain injury assessed by phosphorus magnetic resonance spectroscopy. *Pediatr Res* 1989; 25:445-451.

70. Haaland K, Loberg EM, Steen PA, Thoresen M. Posthypoxic hypothermia in newborn piglets. *Pediatr Res* 1997; 41:505-512.

71. Battin MR, Dezoete JA, Gunn TR, Gluckman PD, Gunn AJ. Neurodevelopmental outcome of infants treated with head cooling and mild hypothermia after perinatal asphyxia. *Pediatrics* 2001; 107:480-484.

72. Akisu M, Huseyinov A, Yalaz M, Cetin H, Kultursay N. Selective head cooling with hypothermia suppresses the generation of platelet-activating factor in cerebrospinal fluid of newborn infants with perinatal asphyxia. *Prostaglandins Leukot Essent Fatty Acids* 2003; 69:45-50.

73. Shankaran S, Laptook A, Wright LL, et al. Whole-body hypothermia for neonatal encephalopathy: animal observations as a basis for a randomized, controlled pilot study in term infants. *Pediatrics* 2002; 110:377-385.

74. Thoresen M, Whitelaw A. Cardiovascular changes during mild therapeutic hypothermia and rewarming in infants with hypoxic-ischaemic encephalopathy. *Pediatrics* 2000; 106:92-99.
75. Azzopardi D, Robertson NJ, Cowan FM, et al. Pilot study of treatment with whole body hypothermia for neonatal encephalopathy. *Pediatrics* 2000; 106:684-694.
76. Debillon T, Daoud P, Durand P, et al. Whole-body cooling after perinatal asphyxia: a pilot study in term neonates. *Dev Med Child Neurol* 2003; 45:17-23.
77. Zhou WH, Shao XM, Cao Y, Chen C, Zhang XD. Safety study of hypothermia for treatment of hypoxic-ischemic brain damage in term neonates. *Acta Pharmacol Sin* 2003; 23:64-68.
78. Compagnoni G, Pogliani L, Lista G, et al. Hypothermia reduces neurological damage in asphyxiated newborn infants. *Biol Neonate* 2002; 82:222-227.
79. Gunn TR, Wilson NJ, Aftimos S, Gunn AJ. Brain hypothermia and QT interval. *Pediatrics* 1999; 103:1079.
80. Gordon CJ, Heath JE. Integration and central processing in temperature regulation. *Annu Rev Physiol* 1986; 48:595-612.
81. Walter B, Bauer R, Kuhnen G, Fritz H, Zwiener U. Coupling of cerebral blood flow and oxygen metabolism in infant pigs during selective brain hypothermia. *J Cereb Blood Flow Metab* 2000; 20:1215-1224.
82. Benumof JL, Wahrenbrock EA. Dependency of hypoxic pulmonary vasoconstriction on temperature. *J Appl Physiol* 1977; 42:56-58.
83. Sprung J, Cheng EY, Gamulin S, Kampine JP, Bosnjak ZJ. The effect of acute hypothermia and serum potassium concentration on potassium cardiotoxicity in anesthetized rats. *Acta Anaesthesiol Scand* 1992; 36:825-830.
84. Zydlewski AW, Hasbargen JA. Hypothermia-induced hypokalemia. *Mil Med* 1998; 163:719-721.

Chapter 10

HEMORRHAGIC SHOCK AND EXSANGUINATION CARDIAC ARREST

Samuel A. Tisherman, MD
Safar Center for Resuscitation Research, University of Pittburgh, Pittsburgh, PA, USA

INTRODUCTION

The first example of hypothermia being used for therapeutic use dates back to the Edwin Smith papyrus, which described the use of cold applications to wounds of the head. Hypocrites advocated packing patients in snow and ice to reduce hemorrhage (1). Later, during the War of 1812, Napoleon's Surgeon-General, Baron Larrey, noted that soldiers who were closest to the fire died more rapidly than those who remained more hypothermic (2). The latter observations may have been related to beneficial physiologic effects of hypothermia or the detrimental effects of superficial warming leading to afterdrop. During the French-Indochina war in the 1950s, the French attempted to use hypothermia for their soldiers unable to tolerate anesthesia and surgery at normal body temperature (3).

When discussing therapeutic hypothermia, the level and timing of hypothermia always need to be clearly defined. For this review, the levels of hypothermia are defined as: *mild* (33-36°C), *moderate* (28-32°C), *deep* (11-20°C), *profound* (6-10°C), and *ultraprofound* (≤5°C). Unless otherwise specified, core temperature (esophageal, pulmonary artery, rectal) is used. Timing is defined in relation to the ischemic event.

A clear distinction must be made between accidental, exposure hypothermia and intentional, therapeutic hypothermia. Trauma patients are predisposed to hypothermia because of exposure by removal of clothing and opening of body cavities, and administration of cold intravenous (IV) fluids and blood products. In addition, they have a decreased ability to maintain normothermia because of hemorrhagic shock (HS), anesthetic agents, and alcohol or drug intoxication. Consequently, they are often already cool in the Emergency Department (ED) (4,5). The degree of uncontrolled hypothermia in trauma patients has been correlated with Injury Severity Score (ISS) (4) and Trauma Score (5). Shivering, which increases oxygen demands and increases acidosis, can occur. Therapeutic, controlled hypothermia, should optimally include the use of anesthetics to modulate natural homeostatic mechanisms, i.e., produce poikilothermia, to allow rapid, homogeneous cooling and prevent shivering. Thus, to consider the risks vs. benefits of hypothermia in trauma patients one must consider this difference between the uncontrolled, exposure hypothermia that occurs in most severely injured trauma patients and the controlled, therapeutic hypothermia that has never been systematically applied in this patient population.

The relationship between hypothermia and outcome from traumatic HS is less clear than it is for other insults discussed in this book. Mechanisms and outcome-oriented studies in animal models have documented benefits from therapeutic (controlled) mild hypothermia during HS and resuscitation (6-20). In contrast, clinical data suggests that spontaneous (uncontrolled) hypothermia is deleterious to trauma patients (21-24). In this review, laboratory data regarding hypothermia during HS is presented and the clinical data regarding hypothermic trauma patients is critically examined. Explanations for the disparity between these findings are discussed and ways to answer the questions regarding the deleterious vs. beneficial effects of hypothermia in future laboratory and clinical studies are proposed.

For the trauma victim with exsanguinating hemorrhage leading to cardiac arrest, current therapy is inadequate; survival remains <10% (25). This is despite aggressive fluid resuscitation and ED thoracotomy. A new approach for rapid hypothermic-pharmacologic preservation of the organism (suspended animation) is presented.

HYPOTHERMIA AND HEMORRHAGIC SHOCK

Laboratory Studies

Regarding *protection*, Schumer, et al (26), showed that pre-insult moderate hypothermia could decrease lactic acidosis and improve survival after HS. Clinically, pre-treatment is not possible. During and after HS, moderate hypothermia has also been shown to be beneficial to the heart (7), liver (27), and skeletal muscle (28,29).

Blalock (30) found that hemorrhagic shock caused a reduction in blood flow to the extremities that was greater than that to the vital organs. External rewarming may result in peripheral vasodilatation and resultant detrimental effects. Thus, he found that *hyper*thermia shortened survival, whereas *hypo*thermia increased survival time.

Tanaka, et al (31), showed that deep hypothermia improved survival from hemorrhagic shock in rats. This level of hypothermia in humans would cause cardiac arrest, necessitating extracorporeal circulatory support, which could not currently be initiated rapidly enough.

After prolonged, pressure-controlled HS (to the point of 80% reuptake of shed blood) in awake rats, Sori, et al (6), found that, compared to active warming to maintain rectal temperature (Tr) of 34-36°C, allowing rats to cool spontaneously during HS to 29°C improved survival (50% vs. 0%). This is in spite of the fact that duration of shock, based on reuptake of shed blood, was longer in the cooler group. Meyer and Horton (7-9) examined the role of mild hypothermia (33°C), induced and reversed by peritoneal lavage, with and without correction of metabolic acidosis, in the treatment of HS in dogs. Hypothermic dogs had a lower heart rate, respiratory rate, coronary sinus lactate levels, total body and myocardial oxygen consumption, and left ventricular developed pressure (+dp/dt) compared to the normothermic dogs. Subendocardial ischemia was found in the normothermic group only. Most importantly, hypothermia improved survival (9).

The group at the Safar Center for Resuscitation Research of the University of Pittsburgh began to explore the use of hypothermia for HS resuscitation in 1991. Using a model of volume controlled HS (3.25 ml/100 gm blood withdrawn over 20 min) in awake rats without resuscitation, the effects on survival time of several treatments that could be initiated by medics in the field were examined (10). Hypothermia by surface cooling to 30°C or FiO_2 1.0 breathing increased MAP and prolonged survival ($p < 0.05$). In a follow-up study with fluid resuscitation in awake rats, the combination of FiO_2 1.0 breathing and hypothermia allowed 100% long-term survival compared to 0% survival with room air breathing and normothermia (11).

The pressure and volume-controlled HS models cited above do not adequately duplicate the physiologic changes that occur in the trauma patient with ongoing bleeding. Consequently, a 3-phased model of uncontrolled HS (UHS) via tail cut in rats was developed, including UHS phase I, resuscitation phase II, and observation phase III to 72 h (32,33). Both moderate hypothermia (30°C) and limited fluid resuscitation (to maintain MAP 40 mmHg) improved long-term survival (12). The best outcome was with the combination of limited fluid resuscitation and hypothermia. In a model of lethal UHS in rats, using only Phase I of the 3-phased model, simulating battlefield conditions of the casualty with temporarily uncontrolled bleeding waiting for evacuation, moderate hypothermia doubled survival time, whereas breathing 100% oxygen had no effect (13). Using the same model, the effect of mild hypothermia was compared to normothermia and moderate hypothermia at three levels of inhaled oxygen (FiO$_2$ 0.25, 0.5, 1.0). Survival time was significantly improved with both mild and moderate hypothermia (14). Oxygen inhalation had no effect. In a long-term study with fluid resuscitation, both mild and moderate hypothermia increased blood pressure and improved long-term survival time and rate, compared to normothermia (p<0.05) (15). Oxygen inhalation again had no benefit.

In these studies both mild and moderate hypothermia increase blood pressure during HS. This finding was pursued further, since the beneficial effect of hypothermia during UHS may in part be secondary to the blood pressure effect and not the metabolic effects of hypothermia. Using a pressure controlled HS rat model, mild hypothermia was still beneficial (16).

Therapeutic hypothermia may be a double-edged sword; complications, such as coagulopathy, arrhythmias, acidosis, and infection are possible. There is evidence that ischemia and reperfusion of the viscera is one of the driving forces behind the systemic inflammatory response syndrome. Consequently, better preservation of the viscera with regional cooling alone could improve outcome without undesired side effects of systemic hypothermia. This hypothesis was tested during HS in rats with laparotomy and temporary evisceration of the intestines to allow differential cooling of the gut vs. the organism (17). As in other studies, systemic cooling significantly improved survival, but regional cooling of the gut had no effect.

In most of these studies, hypothermia was initiated during HS, which may not be possible clinically. Delaying cooling until the beginning of fluid resuscitation can still improve survival time (18). In addition, if spontaneous cooling occurs during HS, as it frequently does in patients, continuing hypothermia can improve survival time after severe HS compared to early rewarming (19).

In military and rural trauma situations, the time from injury to surgical hemostasis may be several hours. After such prolonged (6 h) HS, mild hypothermia improves survival in rats (20).

These studies have generally been performed in small animals without significant tissue trauma and without intensive care life support. Prior to considering clinical trials, a large animal study in a clinically-relevant model was needed. Wu, et al (34), developed a pig model with trauma (laparotomy and spleen injury followed by splenectomy) and 24 h intensive care. This study tested the hypothesis that mild hypothermia (34°C) during HS would increase survival. In addition, they tested the hypothesis that infusion of ice-cold saline, rather than room-temperature saline, would increase the rate of cooling and further increase survival. Fluids were administered for hypotensive (limited) fluid resuscitation during HS simulating field resuscitation. Six of eight animals survived in the mild hypothermia group with room temperature fluid administration, which was significantly better than the normothermic group with only 2 of 8 surviving. The infusion of ice-cold fluid seemed to result in increased vasoconstriction and less fluid requirement during HS. Only 4 of 8 survived, which was not different than the other groups.

Clinical Studies

Luna, et al (21), retrospectively found that, compared to normothermic patients, hypothermic patients had higher ISS. Survival correlated with temperature: 78% who remained normothermic survived, compared to 59% with mild hypothermia (34-36°C), and 41% with severe hypothermia (<34°C). In a similar retrospective review, Jurkovich, et al, (22) found that higher ISS, presence of shock, and large transfusion requirements were risk factors for becoming hypothermic. Controlling for these factors, it appeared that hypothermia remained a risk factor for mortality. Even though they concluded that hypothermia is associated with increased mortality in trauma patients, they questioned, "whether it is the hypothermia per se or the severity of the injury producing the hypothermia that is responsible for the subsequent mortality." Both of these studies included small numbers of patients and used the ISS (35), an anatomic, not physiologic, system for stratification.

To test the hypothesis that using physiologic, in addition to anatomic, measures of injury severity would more appropriately predict outcome in hypothermic trauma patients, Steinemann, et al (36), retrospectively, compared outcomes of trauma patients with a core temperature of less than 35°C to those of patients who remained normothermic. Hypothermia correlated with higher ISS, lower (worse) trauma score and systolic blood pressure, and greater fluid requirements and base deficit. Hypothermic patients were less likely to survive when stratified by ISS. However, when the patients were stratified by their probability of survival using the TRISS methodology (37) there was no significant difference in survival and length of stay in the ICU between the hypothermic and normothermic groups. This suggests that development of hypothermia in trauma patients is more of an epiphenomenon, not a primary factor that leads to mortality.

The only prospective study related to hypothermia in trauma patients was that conducted by Gentilello, et al, (23,24). In hypothermic (≤34.5°C) trauma patients in the intensive care unit, they randomly compared standard rewarming vs. rapid rewarming, using a novel continuous arterio-venous rewarming (CAVR) technique with a heparin-bonded, counter-current heat exchanger (Level I Technologies, Rockland, MA) and large catheters placed into the femoral artery and vein. Total fluid requirement over the first 24 hours and time required to achieve normothermia were significantly lower in the CAVR group compared to the control group. The frequencies of organ system failures were not different and there was no difference in survival to discharge from the hospital between the two groups (66% with CAVR, 50% with standard rewarming). Five complications occurred directly secondary to CAVR. These authors found no evidence of coagulation differences between groups. These results are difficult to interpret for several reasons. First, the two groups were not equivalent at the beginning of the study. The CAVR group had twice as many patients who had undergone a laparotomy as the control group. Perhaps the hypothermia was from exposure in the operating room, instead of shock. Second, the treatment (rewarming) was not initiated until the patients were in the intensive care unit. Third, the study was unblinded, leading to potential bias. It is important to recognize that this study did not involve controlled, therapeutic hypothermia with induction of poikilothermia.

Laboratory vs. Clinical Data

There are several differences between the laboratory and the clinical setting which need to be discussed to help explain the disparities in outcome. Laboratory models do not mimic the clinical setting because of: a lack of tissue trauma and coagulation abnormalities; the use of fresh, autologous (not banked donor) blood transfusions (38); and the need for anesthesia prior to, and during, HS. The latter may profoundly affect physiologic responses to hemorrhage (39,40). Clinical studies are difficult to interpret because of a lack of a prospective, randomized trial of therapeutic, controlled hypothermia, or even a large, prospective observational study; inadequate assessment of physiologic status; lack of temperature control; inability to control for underlying disease states; and poorly defined outcome measures.

The effect of hypothermia on the coagulation system of trauma patients may be critical to the potential detrimental effect of hypothermia that is suspected clinically. Hypothermia has been shown to increase blood loss intra-operatively during trauma laparotomies (41). In general, however, no consistent changes in specific coagulation factors have been found (42,43). Decreased platelet counts and platelet function seem to be the most consistent findings. The hypothermia-induced platelet trapping in capillaries seems reversible. Increased fibrinolytic activity during hypothermia has also been suggested. Clinical data on coagulation in hypothermic patients may be confounded because standard measurements are performed with warming of the blood to 37°C. Gubler, et al (44), cooled and/or diluted the blood of healthy volunteers and ICU patients *ex vivo* to measure the effects of these two interventions on standard blood coagulation tests (prothrombin time, activated partial thromboplastin time, and platelet function). Cooling had similar effects on undiluted and diluted blood. Although there were statistically significant changes at 35°C, these changes did not reach clinical significance until the temperature was decreased to 33 or 31°C. Similarly, Reed, et al (45), found that consistent and significant coagulation changes didn't occur unless body temperature was 33°C or less. Gentillello, et al (24), did not find significant coagulation differences between their standard rewarming and CAVR groups. In clinical trials of hypothermia after severe traumatic brain injury, Resnick, et al (46), found no increase in bleeding in the hypothermia group. These findings suggest that mild hypothermia (33-36°C) in patients does not have significant effects on the coagulation system. In critically ill trauma victims with hypothermia, metabolic acidosis, and hemodilution, the independent effects of each of these factors are difficult to determine.

The animal studies above have been performed with minimal tissue trauma. Any clinically-significant coagulation abnormalities secondary to hypothermia would not have been demonstrated. To examine the effects of mild hypothermia (34°C) on bleeding during HS, a pig model of pressure-controlled HS (MAP 40 mmHg for 60 min) with hemodilution during HS (to decrease the pig's natural hypercoagulabilty) was developed (47). A laparotomy was performed; a small slice of the liver edge was excised and allowed to bleed freely. There was no significant difference in early blood loss between the normothermic and hypothermia groups, although there was a suggestion of increased bleeding after 1 hour with hypothermia. There were also no differences in coagulation studies, platelet counts, or thromboelastograms. Systemic anticoagulation with heparin in this model resulted in massive bleeding and rapid death.

Clinical Trial of Mild Hypothermia for Hemorrhagic Shock

Retrospective studies and poorly controlled prospective studies will never be able to answer the question of whether or not therapeutic, controlled hypothermia has a beneficial effect on outcome after traumatic HS. A prospective, randomized, controlled trial is needed. Such a trial should be performed at multiple centers with well-integrated trauma systems. The patient population, i.e., trauma victims with evidence of HS, needs to be clearly defined. Mild cooling should be initiated as quickly as possible during resuscitation (i.e., in the field or Emergency Department), yet in a controlled manner, preventing over-shoot. Since many trauma patients become hypothermic anyway, the hypothermic group may just need to be kept cool while the normothermic control group undergoes active rewarming. To prevent shivering, patients in both groups need to be sedated, paralyzed, and intubated until all are rewarmed to normothermia. All physiologic parameters need to be as well controlled, by protocol, as possible. The primary outcome variable should be long-term survival. Secondary endpoints could include fluid requirements, clotting studies, morbidity (cardiac, infectious), and development of organ system failure.

The appropriate level of hypothermia to be tested in clinical trials seems to be mild hypothermia (34°C) since this level has had as much benefit in animal models as moderate hypothermia, and should have fewer complications. The ideal duration for mild therapeutic hypothermia during HS and resuscitation remains unanswered. Most laboratory studies have examined only 1-2 hours of cooling. Would more prolonged hypothermia improve outcome? Recent recommendations regarding mild, therapeutic hypothermia following resuscitation from cardiac arrest suggest continuing hypothermia for 12-24 h (48). It may be that 12 h of hypothermia would be the appropriate duration following HS.

SUSPENDED ANIMATION

When cardiac arrest is caused by trauma-induced internal truncal hemorrhage, with the bleeding site not immediately controllable, there has been near 100% mortality in military and civilian casualties, in spite of emergency thoracotomy in trauma centers.

In 1984, U.S. Army surgeon Ronald Bellamy and anesthesiologist Peter Safar met and discussed the pathophysiology of rapid death in combat casualties killed in action (48). Similar patterns have been observed in civilian victims of penetrating truncal injuries (25). Until the 1980s, it had been considered impossible to resuscitate victims of truncal internal exsanguination to cardiac arrest, which occurs over a few minutes, because the surgery required for stopping the hemorrhage cannot be performed rapidly enough in the field. Bellamy and Safar recommended research into a new approach: "suspended animation" for preservation of the organism until hemostasis, followed by delayed resuscitation. Pharmacologic and hypothermic preservation potentials seemed worth exploring (49).

Laboratory Studies of Suspended Animation

In the late 1980s the Pittsburgh group first embarked on a systematic study of suspended animation in a newly developed dog model of normothermic HS followed by exsanguination cardiac arrest, with deep and profound hypothermia induced and reversed with cardiopulmonary bypass (CPB) (50-55). In the first suspended animation studies, after 60 min pressure-controlled HS at normothermia, rapid cooling was induced via closed-chest CPB. Circulation was then stopped (no flow) for up to 120 min. CPB was also used for resuscitation-rewarming. For cardiac arrest of 120 min, deep hypothermia (about 15°C, tympanic membrane temperature [Tty]) (50) was less preservative than profound hypothermia (10°C) (51). Cardiovascular resuscitability from cardiac arrest of 120 min at 10°C was remarkable, but was followed by brain damage. Using 10°C, the University of Wisconsin organ preservation solution (52) was not beneficial. The studies above were conducted with a standard CPB system and systemic anti-coagulation, which would be deleterious in the traumatized patient. Fortunately, the elimination of systemic heparinization with the use of heparin-bonded equipment (53) did not reduce the cerebral outcome benefit of profound hypothermia. A "first" was study #6 (55): after a preceding normothermic HS of 60 min, an exsanguination cardiac arrest period of 60 min at 10°C allowed complete functional recovery with histologically normal brains.

For elective brain surgery, Taylor, et al (56,57), extended profound hypothermic exsanguination to 3 h in dogs, not with no-flow, but rather with low-flow or trickle-flow by cold asanguinous perfusion, using CPB with special stasis (intracellular) and purge (extracellular) solutions ("Hypothermosol"). Their goal was to develop a technique for brain preservation during otherwise infeasible neurosurgical procedures.

Rhee, et al (58,59), have also explored suspended animation in a clinically relevant exsanguination model in pigs. Using readily-available equipment, they induced profound hypothermia by aortic flush, both proximally and distally, via a thoracotomy and direct aortic cannulation. Repair of the aortotomy was accomplished during no flow. After total circulatory arrest of up to 40 min, normal neurologic recovery could be achieved (58). The same group under Alam, et al (59), found normal cognitive function after exsanguinating hemorrhage from a vessel injury and prolonged asanguinous low flow (by CPB) at 10°C.

CPB with blood cooling cannot be initiated rapidly in the field by paramedics. Therefore, since 1998, the Pittsburgh group have studied, in dogs, an aortic flush of cold isotonic saline solution, without CPB, to rapidly induce preservation. CPB remains needed for reversal of suspended animation (resuscitation). Outcome evaluation was to 72 h. For cardiac arrest 15 min, at Tty 36°C after flush, 72 h outcome was overall performance category (OPC) 1 (normal), but with some histologic brain damage (60). For cardiac arrest 20 min (61), Tty 36°C achieved by saline flush at 24°C, did not achieve OPC 1. This model was therefore used for determining whether the addition of one or more drugs would achieve OPC 1 and histologically normal brains. Of 14 single drugs that were explored by aortic flush, thiopental with phenytoin achieved OPC 1 (in just three dogs). The only drug that achieved statistically significant benefit, but not histologic normality, was the antioxidant tempol (62). It therefore seemed that the effects of hypothermia were much greater than that of pharmacologic strategies.

For cardiac arrest longer than 20 min, cold flush had to include the spinal cord to prevent hind leg weakness and viscera to prevent organ system failure. Very large volumes of cold saline flushed into the abdominal aorta was needed to achieve survival with OPC 1 and histologically normal brains after cardiac arrest 30 min with Tty 28°C (63), after cardiac arrest 60 min with Tty 15°C, and after cardiac arrest 90 min with Tty 10°C (64). Exsanguination cardiac arrest periods of 120 min can be reversed, but OPC 1 is difficult to achieve and significant brain damage is found at necropsy (64).

While aortic flush initiated at cardiac arrest 2 min or 5 min proved highly preservative, delaying the flush initiation to normothermic cardiac arrest 8 min failed to preserve the brain during cardiac arrest 30 min no-flow (65).

To achieve preservation for cardiac arrest 90-120 min, with field-feasible fluid volumes, novel solutions and novel drug combinations should be explored. Methods for rapid vessel access and portable devices for fluid cooling-pumping need to be developed.

Suspended Animation and Trauma

The studies described above did not include significant tissue trauma. Clinically, however, patients who exsanguinate will usually have massive trauma. When a laparotomy, splenic injury, and thoracotomy were added to the model of 90 min exsanguination cardiac arrest, the animals died of extracerebral organ system failure. Consequently, the period of arrest was decreased to 60 min and outcome was compared to the same insult without trauma (66). Animals without trauma survived with good neurologic outcome. Some of the animals with trauma had normal recovery, but others suffered extracerebral organ system dysfunction. The encouraging finding was that all of these animals had normal brain histopathology, suggesting that long-term outcome with intensive care could be normal. In a follow-up study, plasma exchange could improve the multiple organ system dysfunction and possibly improve neurologic outcome (67).

SUMMARY

Laboratory studies have consistently found benefit of mild, therapeutic hypothermia during prolonged HS. In contrast, retrospective clinical studies suggest that hypothermia may be directly detrimental. Only a controlled clinical trial can determine if therapeutic mild hypothermia can be beneficial in trauma victims. Safety and feasibility trials may be appropriate prior to initiating a randomized clinical trial.

For victims of exsanguinating hemorrhage, a novel approach, suspended animation induced via aortic flush to achieve profound cerebral hypothermia, may allow survival from otherwise lethal injuries. Clinical trials suspended animation for exsanguination cardiac arrest should be considered using currently available equipment.

REFERENCES

1. Adams F. *The genuine works of Hippocrates*. New York: William Wood; 1886, pp. 238-239.
2. Larrey IJ. *Memoirs of military service and campaigns of the French armies* (Translated by RW Hall), Baltimore, J Cushing, 1814, pp 156-164.
3. Chippaux C. Application of artificial hibernation to war surgery in Indochina. *Internat Rec Med Gen Pract Clinics* 1954; 167:328.
4. Gregory JS, Flancbaum L, Townsend C, et al. Incidence and timing of hypothermia in trauma patients undergoing operations. *J Trauma* 1991; 31:795-798.
5. Little RA, Stoner HB. Body temperature after accidental injury. *Br J Surg* 1981; 68:221-224.
6. Sori AJ, El-Assuooty A, Rush BF, Engler P. The effect of temperature on survival in hemorrhagic shock. *Am Surg* 1987; 53:706-710.
7. Meyer DM, Horton JW. Effect of different degrees of hypothermia on myocardium in treatment of hemorrhagic shock. *Journal of surgical research* 1990; 48:61-67.
8. Meyer DM, Horton JW. Effect of moderate hypothermia in the treatment of canine hemorrhagic shock. *Annals of Surgery* 1988; 207:462-9.
9. Meyer DM, Horton JW. Prolonged survival times with induction of hypothermia after severe hemorrhagic shock. *Curr Surg* 1988; 45:295-8.
10. Crippen D, Safar P, Porter L, et al. Improved survival of hemorrhagic shock with oxygen and hypothermia in rats. *Resuscitation* 1991; 21:271-281.
11. Leonov Y, Safar P, Sterz F, Stezoski SW. Extending the golden hour of hemorrhagic shock tolerance with oxygen plus hypothermia in awake rats. An exploratory study. Resuscitation 2002; 52:193-202.
12. Kim S, Stezoski W, Safar P, et al. Hypothermia and minimal fluid resuscitation increase survival after uncontrolled hemorrhagic shock in rats. *J Trauma* 1997; 42:213-222.
13. Kim S, Stezoski SW, Safar P, et al. Hypothermia, but not 100% oxygen breathing, prolongs survival during uncontrolled hemorrhagic shock in rats. *J Trauma* 1998; 44:485-491.
14. Takasu A, Carrillo P, Stezoski SW, et al. Mild or moderate hypothermia, but not increased oxygen breathing, prolongs survival during lethal uncontrolled hemorrhagic shock in rats, with measurement of visceral dysoxia. *Crit Care Med* 1999; 27:1557-1564.
15. Takasu A, Stezoski SW, Stezoski J, et al. Mild or moderate hypothermia, but not increased oxygen breathing, increases long term survival after uncontrolled hemorrhagic shock in rats. *Crit Care Med* 2000; 28:2465-2474.
16. Prueckner S, Safar P, Kentner R, et al. Mild hypothermia increases survival from severe pressure controlled hemorrhagic shock in rats. *J Trauma* 2001; 50:253-262.
17. Wu X, Stezoski J, Safar P, et al. Systemic hypothermia, but not regional gut hypothermia, improves survival from prolonged hemorrhagic shock in rats. *J Trauma* 2002; 53:654-662.
18. Wu X, Safar P, Stezoski J, et al. Delayed mild hypothermia prolongs survival following severe hemorrhagic shock (HS) in rats. *Shock* 2001; 15 (suppl):49 (abstract).
19. Wu X, Stezoski J, Safar P, et al. After spontaneous hypothermia during hemorrhagic shock, continuing mild hypothermia (34°C) improves early, but not late, survival in rats. *J Trauma* 2003; 55:308-316.
20. Wu X, Safar P, Stezoski J, et al. Early or delayed mild hypothermia (34°C) during prolonged (6 h) hemorrhagic shock (HS) improves survival in rats. *Shock* 2003; 19:59.

21. Luna GK, Maier MV, Palvin EG, et al. Incidence and effect of hypothermia in seriously injured patients. *J Trauma* 1987; 27:1014-1018.

22. Jurkovich GJ, Greiser WB, Luterman A, et al. Hypothermia in trauma victims: an ominous predictor of survival. *J Trauma* 1987; 27:1019-1024.

23. Gentilello LM, Cobean RA, Offner PJ, et al. Continuous arteriovenous rewarming: rapid reversal of hypothermia in critically ill patients. *J Trauma* 1992; 32:316.

24. Gentilello LM, Jurkovich GJ, Stark MS, et al. Is hypothermia in the victim of major trauma protective or harmful? *Ann Surg* 1997; 226:439.

25. Rhee PM, Acosta J, Bridgeman A, et al. Survival after emergency department thoracotomy: review of published data from the past 25 years. *J Am Coll Surg* 2000; 190:288-98.

26. Schumer W. Moderate hypothermia in controlled hemorrhage in dogs. Physiochemical response of the microcirculation. *Amer Surg* 1966; 32:347-354.

27. Johannigman JA, Johnson DJ, Roettger R. The effect of hypothermia on liver adenosine triphosphate (ATP) recovery following combined shock and ischemia. *J Trauma* 1992; 32:190-195.

28. Hagberg S, Haljamae H, Rockert H. Shock reactions in skeletal muscle. IV. The effect of hypothermic treatment on cellular electrolyte responses to hemorrhagic shock. *Acta Chir Scand* 1970; 136:23-28.

29. Haljamae H. Effects of hemorrhagic shock and treatment with hypothermia on the potassium content and transport of single mammalian skeletal muscle cells. *Acta Physiol Scand* 1970; 78:189-200.

30. Blalock A, Alfred X, Mason MF. A comparison of the effects of heat and cold in the prevention and treatment of shock. *Arch Surg* 1941; 42:1054.

31. Tanaka J, Sato T, Berezesky IK, et al. Effect of hypothermia on survival time and ECG in rats with acute blood loss. *Adv Shock Res* 1983; 9:219-232.

32. Capone A, Safar P, Stezoski SW, et al. Uncontrolled hemorrhagic shock outcome model in rats. *Resuscitation* 1995; 29:143-152.

33. Capone AC, Safar P, Stezoski W, et al. Improved outcome with fluid restriction in treatment of uncontrolled hemorrhagic shock. *J Am Coll Surg* 1995; 180:49-56.

34. Wu X, Kochanek P, Stezoski SW, Tisherman SA. Mild hypothermia improves survival after prolonged, traumatic hemorrhagic shock in pigs. J Trauma 2004; 57:445 (abstract).

35. Baker SP, Oneill B. The Injury Severity Score: An update. *J Trauma* 1976; 16:882 -885.

36. Steinemann S, Shackford SR, Davis JW. Implications of admission hypothermia in trauma patients. *J Trauma* 1990; 30:200-202.

37. Champion HR, Sacco WL, Copes WS. Trauma scoring. In: Feliciano D, Moore EE, Mattox KL (eds): *Trauma*. Norwalk, Appleton & Lange, 1996, p 53-67

38. Collins JA. Problems associated with the massive transfusion of stored blood. *Surgery*, 1974; 75: 274.

39. Adamicza A, Tarnoky K, Nagy A, Nagy S. The effect of anaesthesia on the haemodynamic and sympathoadrenal responses of the dog in experimental haemorrhagic shock. *Acta Physiologica Hungarica* 1985; 65:239-254.

40. Longnecker DE, Sturgill BC. Influence of anesthetic agent on survival following hemorrhage. *Anesthesiology* 1976; 45:516-521.

41. Bernabei AF, Levison MA, Bender JS. The effects of hypothermia and injury severity on blood loss during trauma laparotomy. *J Trauma* 1992; 33:835-839.

42. Patt A, McCroskey BL, Moore EE. Hypothermia-induced coagulopathies in trauma. *Surg Clin NA* 1988; 69:775-785.

43. Rohrer MJ, Natale AM. Effect of hypothermia on the coagulation cascade. *Crit Care Med* 1992; 20:1402-5.

44. Gubler KD, Gentilello LM, Hassantish SA, Miaer RV. The impact of hypothermia on dilutional coagulopathy. *J Trauma* 1994; 36:847-851.

45. Reed RL, Johnston TD, Hudson JD, Fischer RP. The disparity between hypothermic coagulopathy and clotting studies. *J Trauma* 1992; 33:465-470.

46. Resnick DK, Marion DW, Darby JM. The effect of hypothermia on the incidence of delayed traumatic intracerebral hemorrhage. *Neurosurgery* 1994; 34:252-255.

47. Wu X, Safar P, Subramanian M, et al. Mild hypothermia (34°C) does not increase initial bleeding from the injured liver after hemorrhagic shock (HS) in pigs. *Crit Care Med* 2001; 29 (Suppl.):A188.

48. Nolan JP, Morley PT, Vanden Hoek TL, et al. Therapeutic hypothermia after cardiac arrest: an advisory statement by the advanced life support task force of the International Liaison Committee on Resuscitation. *Circulation* 2003; 108:118-121.

49. Bellamy RF. The causes of death in conventional land warfare: implications for combat casualty care research. Mil Med. 1984; 149(2):55-62.

50. Bellamy R, Safar P, Tisherman SA, et al. Suspend animation for delayed resuscitation. *Crit Care Med* 1996; 24 (Suppl):S24-S47.

51. Tisherman SA, Safar P, Radovsky A, et al. Therapeutic deep hypothermic circulatory arrest in dogs: A resuscitation modality for hemorrhagic shock with 'irreparable' injury. *J Trauma* 1990; 30:836-847.

52. Tisherman SA, Safar P, Radovsky A, et al. Profound hypothermia (<10°C) compared with deep hypothermia (15°C) improves neurologic outcome in dogs after two hours' circulatory arrest induced to enable resuscitative surgery. *J Trauma* 1991; 31:1051-1062.

53. Tisherman SA, Safar P, Radovsky A, et al. Profound hypothermia does, and an organ preservation solution does not, improve neurologic outcome after therapeutic circulatory arrest of 2 h in dogs. *Crit Care Med* 1991; 19:S89.

54. Tisherman S, Safar P, Radovsky A, et al. Cardiopulmonary bypass without systemic anticoagulation for therapeutic hypothermic circulatory arrest during hemorrhagic shock in dogs. *Crit Care Med* 1992; 20:S41.

55. Tisherman S, Safar P, Radovsky A. "Suspended animation" research for otherwise infeasible resuscitative traumatologic surgery. *Prehosp Disaster Med* 1993; 8:S131.

56. Capone A, Safar P, Radovsky A, et al. Complete recovery after normothermic hemorrhagic shock and profound hypothermic circulatory arrest of 60 minutes in dogs. J Trauma 1996; 40:388-394.

57. Taylor MJ, Bailes JE, Elrifai AM, et al. A new solution for life without blood: asanguinous low-flow perfusion of a whole-body perfusate during 3 hours of cardiac arrest and profound hypothermia. *Circulation* 1995; 91:431-444.

58. Bailes JE, Alrifai AM, Taylor MJ, et al. Ultraprofound hypothermia combined with blood substitution: a new protocol for extending the safe limits of cardiac arrest for up to three hours. *Neurologic Surg* 1993; XLIV:564-567.

59. Rhee P, Talon E, Eifert S, et al. Induced hypothermia during emergency department thorac60otomy: an animal model. *J Trauma* 2000; 48:439-447.

60. Alam HB, Bowyer MW, Koustova E, et al. Learning and memory is preserved following induced asanguinous hyperkalemic hypothermic arrest in a swine model of traumatic exsanguination. *Surgery* 2002; 132:278-288.

61. Woods RJ, Prueckner S, Safar P, et al. Hypothermic aortic arch flush for preservation during exsanguination cardiac arrest of 15 minutes in dogs. *J Trauma* 1999; 47:1028-1038.

62. Behringer W, Prueckner S, Safar P, et al. Rapid induction of mild cerebral hypothermia by cold aortic flush achieves normal recovery in a dog outcome model with 20-minute exsanguination cardiac arrest. *Acad Emerg Med* 2000; 7:1341-1348.

63. Behringer W, Safar P, Kentner R, et al. Antioxidant Tempol enhances hypothermic cerebral preservation during prolonged cardiac arrest in dogs. *J Cereb Blood Flow Metab* 2002; 22:105-117.

64. Behringer W, Prueckner S, Kentner R, et al. Rapid hypothermic aortic flush can achieve survival without brain damage after 30 min cardiac arrest in dogs. *Anesthesiology* 2000; 93:1491-1499.

65. Behringer W, Safar P, Wu X, et al. Survival without brain damage after clinical death of 60-120 mins in dogs using suspended animation by profound hypothermia. *Crit Care Med* 2003; 31:1523-1531.

66. Behringer W, Safar P, Wu X, et al. Delayed intra-ischemic aortic cold flush for preservation during prolonged cardiac arrest in dogs. *Crit Care Med* 2001; 29 (12, Suppl.): A17.

67. Nozari A, Safar P, Wu X, et al. Suspended animation can allow survival without brain damage after traumatic exsanguination cardiac arrest of 60 min in dogs. *J Trauma*, in press.

68. Nozari A, Safar P, Tisherman S, et al. Suspended animation and plasma exchange (SAPEX) enables full neurologic recovery from lethal traumatic exsanguinations, even after 2 h period of no flow. *Crit Care Med* 2003; 31 (12, suppl):A9.

Chapter 11

ADULT RESPIRATORY DISTRESS SYNDROME AND SEPSIS

Jesús Villar, MD, PhD, Elena Espinosa, MD, PhD
Hospital Universitario NS de Candelaria, Santa Cruz de Tenerife, Canary Islands, Spain

INTRODUCTION

Critical illness in adults is often followed by acute lung injury (ALI). The most severe form of ALI, termed Acute Respiratory Distress Syndrome (ARDS), has a mortality rate of about 50% in most series and higher than 90% when it is associated with severe sepsis and multiple system organ failure (1). Among the clinical conditions associated with the development of ARDS, sepsis is the most common and lethal. Despite recent advances in critical care medicine, the current therapeutic approach for ALI and ARDS is just supportive, not curative. Significant improvements in supportive treatment in the intensive care unit (e.g., more specific antibiotic treatment, improved mechanical ventilation, improved monitoring of circulation, better nursing care, etc.) are mainly responsible for improvements in survival in ARDS and sepsis. However, the incidence of sepsis is rising while a third of septic patients will succumb to this devastating syndrome (2). The septic insult results in a complex cascade of inflammatory mediators, such as cytokines, that is initiated by the organisms themselves or by their soluble products. Although cytokine production is not unique to systemic infection, measurement of circulating inflammatory mediators can confirm the presence of host inflammation, but may not distinguish crucial pathways involved in disease progression and outcome (3).

The exact cause of death in patients with ARDS and sepsis remains elusive. An analysis of studies in recent years has demonstrated that the risk of severe morbidity and death from sepsis is significantly correlated with a hyper-inflammatory state and the effectiveness of anti-inflammatory treatment (4). In this chapter, we will review the use of hypothermia in patients with sepsis and acute lung injury as an alternative approach to reduce the associated unacceptably high mortality, including its pathophysiological rationale and relevant experimental and clinical data. In addition, we will include some thoughts on the possible use of hypothermia in the future.

HYPOTHERMIA IN DISEASE STATES: FRIEND OR FOE?

There is a vast body of literature concerning the physiologic effects of hypothermia. Mice and rats usually respond to infections by becoming hypothermic. For nearly one hundred years, scientists have observed that experimental animals injected with Gram-negative bacteria and kept at an elevated ambient temperature had higher mortality rates than normothermic controls (5). The fundamental rationale for the application of hypothermia has been the reduction of oxygen requirements in the face of reduced blood flow to the tissues. Hypothermia decreases the metabolic rate of an organism. Hypothermia could potentially affect the transport and utilization of O_2 by its effect on at least 7 mechanisms (6): (a) metabolic rate, (b) O_2 solubility, (c) acid-base status, (d) oxygen-hemoglobin dissociation, (e) cardiac output or regional blood flow, (f) concentration of hemoglobin, and (g) critical level of PO_2. The main justification for its use in clinical medicine is to depress the metabolic rate and thus the vulnerability of tissue to ischemic damage. As the temperature decreases, more O_2 will be dissolved in the blood at a given partial pressure. However, hemoglobin concentrations can also affect the solubility of O_2, independently of temperature (7). At lower temperatures, the PO_2 at 50% hemoglobin saturation with oxygen (P_{50}) decreases, thereby leading to low mixed venous oxygen tension and thus low tissue PO_2 values. Although the mechanism is not completely clear, tissues seem to be able to tolerate lower oxygen tensions during periods of decreased temperature. It has been reported that, in the intact animal, the cardiac output decreases by about one-half for every 10°C decrease in temperature (8).

Induced hypothermia, as adjunctive therapy, has been the subject of considerable research interest. It is crucial to distinguish between spontaneous hypothermia (as an adaptive response or accidental) and induced (therapeutic) hypothermia (9, 10). Induced hypothermia (to normothermia or below) involves surface and other cooling methods, sedation and muscle relaxation, each of which reduces oxygen demand. In most experimental and clinical studies, hypothermia (33-35°C) has been induced by surface cooling using cooling blankets, skin washing with alcohol, and ice bags. Techniques involving the use of an endovascular heat exchange catheter (11) or by continuous veno-venous haemofiltration (12) have been recently reported to be superior for rapid and more stable induction of hypothermia.

Induced hypothermia is physiologically very different from spontaneous hypothermia as analyzed by Clemmer et al (13), Brun-Buisson et al (14) and Pittet et al (15), where inadequate rather than excessive metabolism is the problem. These studies demonstrated that septic patients who become hypothermic spontaneously have a significantly worse prognosis than those who are normothermic or febrile. However, other reports have indicated that accidental hypothermia in patients found outdoors with alcohol intoxication or drug overdoses appeared to have exerted a strongly protective effect by reducing the incidence and severity of organ damage (16, 17).

Hypoxia causes body temperature to decrease in a number of different animal models (18). Hypoxia-induced hypothermia has been shown to be beneficial, primarily because it lowers metabolic rate, and thus O_2 need, when O_2 availability is limited.

Lethal response to endotoxin could be altered markedly by small changes in body temperature. In penicillin-treated pneumococcal sepsis in rabbits, suppression of fever is effective in preventing deaths not prevented by antibiotics alone (5). It is possible that hypothermia enhances the immune system by attenuating the violent host inflammatory response that endotoxin initiates, and therefore augments clearance of endotoxin by the reticuloendothelial system. Hypothermia prolonged the mean survival time of mice challenged with an LD_{100} of pneumococci and improved survival after sublethal inocula (19).

The capability of hypothermia to allow organ system recovery from otherwise lethal periods of ischemia has been attributed to its capacity to reduce tissue oxygen utilization (20). In an experimental model of partial hind limb ischemia in skeletal muscle, it was postulated that induced hypothermia markedly attenuated subsequent and further reperfusion-associated oxidative injury due to a down-regulation of the neutrophil chemotactic response (21).

INDUCED HYPOTHERMIA IN SEVERE SEPSIS AND ACUTE LUNG INJURY

Laboratory studies

All experimental studies of oxygen uptake and distribution during induced hypothermia (6, 22-24), with one exception (24), have been limited to healthy animals with normal lungs. Johnston et al (24) reported the effects of systemic hypothermia to 32°C in dogs with oleic acid-induced acute lung injury. Although systemic cooling failed to improve arterial oxygenation and tissue delivery, it decreased systemic oxygen demands, thereby improving the oxygen supply-demand balance. However, these data must be analysed with caution since the model of oleic acid-induced lung injury and the short duration of the experiment (<7 hours) make their results quite difficult to interpret. Theoretical and experimental studies have shown that a left-shifted oxyhemoglobin dissociation curve, as would occur during hypothermia, may increase tissue O_2 utilization under conditions of severe hypoxemia (6, 25). Wetterberg et al (26) found that the application of hypothermia markedly improved survival in an experimental model of hypercapnic hypoxemia. These investigators reported that hypothermia increased alveolar PO_2 by lowering both CO_2 production and the saturated water vapour pressure in the alveoli. Since hypothermia is able to lower the metabolic production of CO_2 and consumption of O_2, a corollary is that hypothermia could be induced to attenuate or reduce ventilator-induced lung injury in patients with severe acute lung injury by producing lower levels of hypercapnia or normal levels of $PaCO_2$. This in turn would allow a further reduction of the tidal volume without the side-effects of hypercapnia (27).

On the other hand, prolonged periods of ischemia are associated with organ injury and distant organ dysfunction in experimental models. Patel et al (28) tested the effects of local hepatic hypothermia in a rat model of hepatic ischemia and reperfusion injury and found that peak serum tumor necrosis factor (TNF)-alpha levels, hepatic neutrophil infiltration and liver necrosis was significantly reduced by more than 50% in hypothermic rats compared to normothermic. In addition, measurements of myeloperoxidase activity and Evans blue extravasation (as indicators of acute lung injury) were reduced by 40% with the application of local hepatic hypothermia compared with animals undergoing normothermic ischemia and reperfusion (28).

Clinical studies

Induced hypothermia could preserve organ function and enhance survival in critically ill patients, but this only has been directly tested and clinically documented in patients with anoxic cerebral injury after cardiac arrest (29, 30) and in patients with traumatic brain injury (31). Besides the use of hypothermia as a means for preventing brain damage, the application of therapeutic hypothermia in humans for respiratory failure or sepsis has been mostly limited to uncontrolled, sporadic reports in patients with several acute and critical conditions (12, 32-39) (Table 11-1). Haeger (32) treated 18 moribund patients with various infections and non-infectious conditions by cooling patients to 32°C. Twelve patients survived. Blair et al (33) reported 17 deaths from a large series of 33 patients with sepsis and shock treated with mild hypothermia when other forms of therapy were considered to have failed. Cockett and Goodwin (34) induced hypothermia in 12 patients with bacteremia and shock following urological surgery. Only one death was observed, a mortality rate much lower than expected. The uncontrolled nature of these early studies, however, prevents us from drawing any definitive conclusions.

Table 11-1. Published reports on therapeutic hypothermia in critically ill patients with acute respiratory failure and sepsis or septic shock.

Year	Indication for hypothermia	Type of study	No. patients	Survival	Authors (*Ref.*)
1957	Moribund patients	Uncontrolled	18	66.6%	Haeger *(32)*
1961	Septic shock	Uncontrolled	33	48.5%	Blair *(33)*
1961	Septic shock	Uncontrolled	12	91.7%	Cockett *(34)*
1983	Paediatric ARDS	Case report	1	100%	Gilston *(35)*
1985	Adult ARDS	Case Report	1	100%	Hurst *(36)*
1992	Acute severe asthma	Case Report	1	100%	Browning *(37)*
1992	Pneumonia, ARDS	Case Report	1	100%	Wetterberg *(38)*
1993	Septic ARDS	Concurrent-controlled	9 hypothermia 10 normothermia	33% 0%	Villar *(39)*
1995	ARDS & Sepsis	Uncontrolled	27	48.1%	Pernerstorfer *(12)*

ARDS = acute respiratory distress syndrome.

The first published use of therapeutic hypothermia in the management of severe respiratory failure was in 1983 by Gilston (35). He induced mild hypothermia (33-34°C) for 3 days in a 16-month old child suffering severe pulmonary edema. A marked improvement in the PaO_2 at the lower temperature was noted and the child recovered. The use of therapeutic hypothermia in adult ARDS was first reported by Hurst, et al, in 1985 (36). They cooled a 32-year old woman with severe ARDS to 33°C for 10 days. They reported decreased white cell and platelet counts, but the patient fully recovered. Browning and Goodrum (37) treated a 20-year old woman in status asthmaticus who failed to respond to conventional therapy with hypothermia at 30°C for almost 5 days. Reducing CO_2 production as a direct effect of induced hypothermia allowed lower minute ventilation and lower airway pressures. Wetterberg and Steen (38) cooled a 20-year old male with post-traumatic ARDS complicated with pneumonia from 40 to 33°C for 11 days. The patient was successfully weaned from the ventilator and recovered without complications.

Villar and Slutsky (39) were the first to systematically study and document the therapeutic efficacy of hypothermia (as opposed to normothermia) in improving oxygenation and survival in humans with septic ARDS. Research into ARDS has revealed many complex biochemical and physiological derangements, aggravated and even precipitated by sepsis (1). There is an increasing recognition that changes in lung structure and function during acute lung injury and ARDS are merely some of the early and obvious manifestations of a syndrome caused by the overwhelming sepsis-induced host response, which attacks all tissues and vital organs (40). Mortality rate for gram-negative sepsis is still high, despite adequate antimicrobial therapy. Villar and Slutsky performed a non-randomized, concurrent-controlled study. Nineteen consecutive moribund septic ARDS patients (mean age 40±14 years old) with an expected mortality of 100% were studied. The expected mortality was based on an historical control group of patients admitted into the same ICU with a $P(A-a)O_2 > 500$ mmHg during mechanical ventilation using ≥ 10 cm H_2O of positive end-expiratory pressure (PEEP) for more than 36 hours. Currently, hypoxia is not the dominant or even a major factor in the high mortality of these patients (1), although 15-20% of non-survivors from ARDS die as a result of refractory hypoxemia. At a PaO_2 of 50 mmHg, arterial oxygen saturation is 85%, which is normally sufficient to prevent acidosis (41). Inadequate cardiac output is a far more common cause of inadequate oxygen delivery. In the Villar and Slutsky study, prior to the application of hypothermia, PaO_2 ranged between 47 and 101 mmHg at FiO_2 of 100%. Ten patients were assigned to receive conventional treatment and 9 patients to conventional treatment plus mild hypothermia (33.7±0.6°C) instituted as a last resort. In this study, hypothermia was used when all other forms of available therapy were considered to have failed. All patients, whether or not they were treated with hypothermia, received a combination of neuromuscular blockade and sedation to abolish muscle activity and reduce metabolic activity, both major components of resting oxygen consumption. The mean duration of hypothermia was 70±15 hours. Total body cooling was associated with a 20% reduction in heart rate and cardiac index, and with a significant reduction in $P(A-a)O_2$ and intrapulmonary shunt. Despite the fact that the cardiac index decreased, there were no significant differences in oxygen transport and oxygen consumption before and during treatment with hypothermia, although the O_2 extraction rate increased by 15% during hypothermia, despite the fact that it remained within normal values (between 22 and 32%). Inappropriately low O_2 extraction rate during septic shock may be as much due to tissue edema and blood flow distribution as to increased O_2 demand (9). These inappropriately low O_2 extraction values could account for the unchanged oxygen consumption since O_2 balance is difficult to determine due to maldistribution of tissue blood flow, as occurs during severe sepsis. An increase in blood pressure during hypothermia in most patients in the Villar and Slutsky's report allowed for the decrease in vasopressor requirements. Peripheral factors that determine regional oxygen delivery are of major importance in determining organ viability. These factors may also be important for predicting survival during sepsis. The improved ability to extract O_2 during hypothermia could be the result of improvements in tissue O_2 diffusion mediated primarily by regional blood flow redistribution (42). There is currently no way of determining how the extra oxygen is distributed among vital organs and non-vital tissues.

The most surprising finding of the study by Villar and Slutsky was that hypothermia improved survival, even though oxygen consumption did not decrease. Three out of nine patients survived in the hypothermic group, while none of the control patients survived (Table 11-1). The number of patients in each group was too small to evaluate other differences between survivors and non-survivors under hypothermia.

One report on induced hypothermia in patients with sepsis and ARDS (12) aimed to test whether mild hypothermia, established by continuous veno-venous hemofiltration, could optimize values for oxygen delivery. Oxygen transport and oxygen consumption decreased and the decreases were more pronounced in non-survivors. The mechanism for this improved survival is unknown. In most patients in this study, hypothermia improved arterial oxygenation, making it possible to reduce the inspired concentration of oxygen within the first 24 hours of treatment.

It could be argued that suppression or attenuation of the cellular inflammatory response in sepsis by hypothermia should be beneficial and might expect to improve outcome. There is some evidence suggesting that the decrease in temperature diminishes the uncontrolled, self-destructive inflammatory response. *In vitro* experiments have found that the cooling of stimulated peripheral mononuclear cells delayed the nuclear factor (NF)-κB activation and the release of interleukin-1β, interleukin-6, and tumor necrosis factor, compared with cells kept normothermic after stimulation (43). Interleukin-1 and interleukin-6 are key mediators of the cellular inflammatory response and are critical in the perpetuation of lung damage during the systemic inflammatory response induced by sepsis. Endothelial damage is not only a feature of severe sepsis, but one of the manifestations of widespread tissue injury and a crucial factor in the pathogenesis and fatal outcome of septic shock (44). A recent experimental study (45), evaluating the protective effect of moderate hypothermia (27°C) in a model of endotoxin-induced lung injury, found that pre-treatment with hypothermia was associated with a decreased sequestration of neutrophils in the lung, leading to a favourable balance between pro and anti-inflammatory cytokines and attenuated lung injury. These results need to be verified when hypothermia is instituted after the onset of endotoxin-induced lung inflammation.

CONCLUSIONS

Induced hypothermia has long been employed in medicine to preserve tissue integrity. Several experimental and clinical reports have documented the therapeutic potential of systemic hypothermia in brain injury, sepsis and lung injury. The mechanism for this efficacy may be due to a number of factors including: (a) better regional blood flow redistribution, (b) a leftward shift of the oxygen dissociation curve and improved tissue oxygenation during severe hypoxemia, and (c) enhancement of the immune system by delaying the violent host inflammatory response initiated by endotoxin. Further research on the clinical use of therapeutic hypothermia in ARDS and sepsis is warranted. Specifically, there is a need for high-quality, carefully controlled studies on the clinical efficacy of hypothermia in sepsis. An evaluation of mild hypothermia as an adjunct to specific therapy in sepsis, independently of the presence of ARDS, deserves a randomized controlled study focusing on the role of pro-inflammatory and anti-inflammatory cytokines, and suppression of the production of free radical and multiple other compounds directly implicated in organ injury. It is plausible that mild hypothermia might also prove to be useful in the treatment of less severe stages of sepsis, with or without ARDS.

REFERENCES

1. Villar J, Petty TL, Slutsky AS. ARDS in its middle age: what have we learned? *Appl Cardiopulm Pathophysiol* 1998; 7:167-172.
2. Riedermann NC, Guo RF, Ward PA. The enigma of sepsis. *J Clin Invest* 2003; 112:460-467.
3. Dinarello CA. Proinflammatory and anti-inflammatory cytokines as mediators in the pathogenesis of septic shock. *Chest* 1997; 112(Suppl):321S-329S.
4. Eichacker PQ, Parent C, Kalil A, et al. Risk and the efficacy of anti-inflammatory agents: retrospective and confirmatory studies of sepsis. *Am J Respir Crit Care Med* 2002; 166:1197-1205.
5. Klastersky J, Kass EH. Is suppression of fever or hypothermia useful in experimental and clinical infectious diseases? *J Infect Dis* 1970; 121:81-86.
6. Willford DC, Hill EP, Moores WY. Theoretical analysis of oxygen transport during hypothermia. *J Clin Monit* 1986; 2:30-43.
7. Christoforides C, Hedley-Whyte J. Effect of temperature and haemoglobin concentration on solubility of O_2 in blood. *J Appl Physiol* 1969; 27:592-596.
8. Hegnauer AH, D'Amato H. Oxygen consumption and cardiac output in the hypothermic dog. *Am J Physiol* 1954; 173:138-142.
9. Gilston A. Oxygen dynamics and induced hypothermia in sepsis. *Resuscitation* 1994; 28:65-70.
10. Bernard S. Induced hypothermia in intensive care medicine. *Anaesth Intens Care* 1996; 24:382-388.
11. Keller E, Imhof HG, Gasser S, et al. Endovascular cooling with heat exchange catheters: a new method to induce and maintain hypothermia. *Intensive Care Med* 2003; 29:939-943.
12. Pernerstorfer T, Krafft P, Fitzgerald R, et al. Optimal values for oxygen transport during hypothermia in sepsis and ARDS. *Acta Anaesthesiol Scand* 1995; 107 (Suppl):223-227.
13. Clemmer TP, Fisher CJ Jr, Bone RC, et al. Hypothermia in the sepsis syndrome and clinical outcome. The Methylprednisolone Severe Sepsis Study Group. *Crit Care Med* 1992; 20:1395-1401.
14. Brun-Buisson C, Doyon F, Carlet J, et al. Incidence, risk factors, and outcome of severe sepsis and septic shock in adults. A multicenter prospective study in intensive care units. French ICU Group for Severe Sepsis. *JAMA* 1995; 274:968-974.
15. Pittet D, Thievent B, Wenzel RP, et al. Bedside prediction of mortality from bacteremic sepsis. A dynamic analysis of ICU patients. *Am J Respir Crit Care Med* 1996; 153:684-693.
16. Block R, Jankowski JAZ, Lacoux P, Pennington CR. Does hypothermia protect against the development of hepatitis in paracetamol overdose? *Anaesthesia* 1992; 47:789-791.
17. Megarbane B, Axler O, Chary I, et al. Hypothermia with indoor occurrence is associated with a worse outcome. *Intensive Care Med* 2000; 26:1843-1849.
18. Wood SC. Interactions between hypoxia and hypothermia. *Annu Rev Physiol* 1991; 53:71-85.
19. Eiseman B, Wotkyns RS, Hirose H. Hypothermia and infection: three mechanisms of host protection in type III pneumococcal peritonitis. *Ann Surg* 1964; 160:994-1006.
20. Bigelow WG, Lindsay WK, Harrison RC, et al. Oxygen transport and utilization in dogs at low body temperatures. *Am J Physiol* 1950; 160:125-137.
21. Yoshioka T, Shires GT, Fantini GA. Hypothermia relieves oxidative stress in reperfused skeletal muscle following partial ischemia. J Surg Res 1992; 53:408-416.

22. Kuhn LA, Turner JK. Alterations in pulmonary and peripheral vascular resistance in immersion hypothermia. *Circ Res* 1959; 7:366-374.

23. Gutierrez G, Warley AR, Dantzker DR. Oxygen delivery and utilization in hypothermic dogs. *J Appl Physiol* 1986; 60:751-757.

24. Johnston WE, Vinten-Johansen J, Strickland RA, et al. Hypothermia with and without end-expiratory pressure in canine oleic acid pulmonary edema. *Am Rev Respir Dis* 1989; 140:110-117.

25. Eaton JW, Skelton TD, Berger E. Survival at extreme altitude: protective effect of increased haemoglobin-oxygen affinity. *Science* 1974; 183:743-744.

26. Wetterberg T, Sjoberg T, Steen S. Effects of hypothermia in hypercapnia and hypercapnic hypoxemia. Acta Anaesthesiol Scand 1993; 37:296-302.

27. Faenza S. Hypothermia: an adverse effect or a missing partner? *Intensive Care Med* 1997; 23:1015-1017.

28. Patel S, Pachter HL, Yee H, et al. Topical hepatic hypothermia attenuates pulmonary injury after hepatic ischemia and reperfusion. *J Am Coll Surg* 2000; 191:650-656.

29. The Hypothermia after Cardiac Arrest Study Group. Mild therapeutic hypothermia to improve the neurologic outcome after cardiac arrest. *N Engl J Med* 2002; 346:549-556.

30. Bernard SA, Gray TW, Buist MD, et al. Treatment of comatose survivors of out-of-hospital cardiac arrest with induced hypothermia. *N Engl J Med* 2002; 346:557-563.

31. Henderson WR, Dhingra VK, Chittock DR, et al. Hypothermia in the management of traumatic brain injury. Intensive Care Med 2003; 29:1637-1644.

32. Haeger VHM. Hypothermia in therapy of hyperpyrexia and poor general condition. *Nord Med* 1957; 57:246-249.

33. Blair E, Buxton RW, Cowley RA, Mansberger AR Jr. The use of hypothermia in septic shock. *JAMA* 1961; 178:916-919.

34. Cockett ATK, Goodwin WE. Hypothermia as a therapeutic adjunct in management of bacteremic shock after urological surgery. *J Urol* 1961; 85:358-364.

35. Gilston A. A hypothermic regime for acute respiratory failure. *Intensive Care Med 1983; 9:37-39.*

36. Hurst JM, DeHaven CB, Branson R, Solomkin JS. Combined use of high-frequency jet ventilation and induced hypothermia in the treatment of refractory respiratory failure. *Crit Care Med* 1985; 13:771-772.

37. Browning D, Goodrum DT. Treatment of acute severe asthma assisted by hypothermia. *Anaesthesia* 1992; 47:223-225.

38. Wetterberg T, Steen S. Combined use of hypothermia and buffering in the treatment of critical respiratory failure. *Acta Anaesthesiol Scand* 1992; 36:490-492.

39. Villar J, Slutsky AS. Effects of induced hypothermia in patients with septic adult respiratory distress syndrome. *Resuscitation* 1993; 26:183-192.

40. Gilston A. Oxygen balance in acute respiratory failure. *Appl Cardiopulm Pathophysiol* 1987; 2:211-214.

41. Finch CA, Lenfant C. Oxygen transport in man. *N Engl J Med* 1972; 286:407-415.

42. Dantzker DR, Foresman B, Gutierrez G. Oxygen supply and utilization relationship. A reevaluation. *Am Rev Respir Dis* 1991; 143:675-679.

43. Kimura A, Sakurada S, Ohkuni H, et al. Moderate hypothermia delays pro-inflammatory cytokine production of human peripheral blood mononuclear cells. *Crit Care Med* 2002; 30:1499-1502.

44. Gerlach H, Esposito C, Stern DM. Modulation of endothelial hemostatic properties: an active role in the host response. *Annu Rev Med* 1990; 41:15-24.

45. Lim CM, Kim MS, Ahn JJ, et al. Hypothermia protects against endotoxin-induced acute lung injury in rats. *Intensive Care Med* 2003; 29:453-459.

Chapter 12

LIVER FAILURE AND INTRACEREBRAL HYPERTENSION

Rajiv Jalan MBBS, MD[1], Christopher Rose, PhD[2]
[1] Institute of Hepatology, University College London Medical School, London, U.K
[2] Fundacion Valenciana de Investigaciones Biomedicas, Valencia, Spain

INTRODUCTION

Brain edema and encephalopathy are severe central nervous system complications of acute liver failure (ALF). Brain edema frequently results in an increase in intracranial pressure (ICP) which consequently leads to brain stem herniation: the major cause of mortality in patients with ALF. ICP is a critical measure which defines the prognosis in patients with ALF (1-5). Orthotopic liver transplantation (OLT) results in survival rates in excess of 70%, however 30-40% of patients with ALF die (primarily due to the deadly effects of raised ICP) while on the liver transplantation list waiting for a donor organ to become available. When uncontrolled intracranial hypertension develops, death occurs in over 90% of patients with ALF. Therefore, there is an urgent need for new therapeutic approaches to the prevention of brain edema and increased ICP in ALF. The potential targets for therapy and the currently used agents to treat increased ICP in ALF are illustrated in Figure 12-1.

HYPOTHERMIA

Induced hypothermia was first tested clinically to treat severe traumatic brain injury and later to improve neurological outcome due to cardiac arrest.

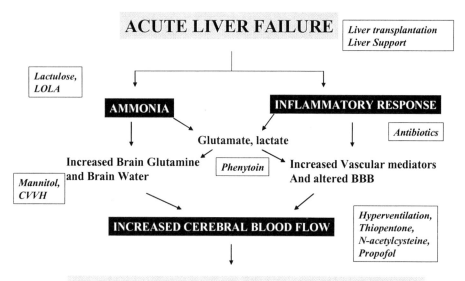

Figure 12-1. Factors involved in the development of increased ICP in patients with ALF and the currently used therapeutic interventions to target these pathophysiological factors. Ammonia related neurotoxicity and brain edema are possibly the first events and are therefore important targets for therapy. CBF autoregulation is lost in patients with ALF resulting in cerebral hyperemia and in the advanced stages there is an associated loss of oxygen and glucose extraction by the brain. There is also an increasing body of literature suggesting that the systemic inflammatory response may play an important modulating role and also contribute to the altered CBF and cellular bioenergetics. The alterations in ammonia metabolism and its effects upon Krebs cycle results in increased brain lactate and alterations in the reuptake mechanisms result in an increase in extracellular glutamate which initiate further brain swelling. Targets for therapy include (1) ammonia and brain swelling (2) CBF and metabolism (3) inflammatory response and (4) treatments that affect multiple pathways (Figure 12-3). Data obtained from experimental models and also from humans suggest that hypothermia may affect most of these pathophysiological factors. LOLA: L-ornithine L-aspartate, CVVH: Continuous veno-venous hemofiltration. (Figure modified from reference 39).

The success of mild hypothermia has led to a broadening of its application to many other neurological emergencies. For liver failure, hypothermia was first tested experimentally in rodents, for which hypothermia prevented the central nervous system consequences of pure hyperammonemia (6) and of hepatectomy (7). Traber, et al, (8) first demonstrated a beneficial effect of moderate hypothermia (<32°C) in rats with ALF (hepatic devascularization). Here, hypothermia extended the survival time and prevented an increase in brain water content in rats with ALF compared to normothermia. However, moderate hypothermia has potential detrimental consequences such as cardiac arrhythmias and coagulation defects (9). Fortunately, mild hypothermia (33-35°C), which should be safer, has demonstrated beneficial effects by prolonging the time of onset of hepatic encephalopathy and preventing brain edema in rats with liver devascularization (10). Lowering the core temperature by 2-4°C also delayed ammonia-induced brain edema and increased ICP in rats with portacaval anastomosis (11).

Effect on ammonia

The pathophysiological mechanisms responsible for the development of brain edema and increased ICP in ALF are not fully understood. However, a large body of evidence suggests that ammonia plays a major role. Hyperammonemia and increased brain ammonia are consistent findings observed in patients with fulminant hepatic failure as well as in different experimental animal models of ALF which lead to brain edema and increased ICP. Also, to emphasize the importance of ammonia, a positive correlation has been reported between arterial ammonia concentrations and the appearance of brain stem herniation in patients with ALF (12).

The mechanisms by which hypothermia protects rats with ALF from the onset of brain edema remains to be determined. However, the beneficial effects of hypothermia are not mediated by an effect on blood ammonia, but on cerebral spinal fluid (CSF) ammonia. Blood ammonia levels in hypothermic rats with ALF were similar to those in normothermic rats; but CSF ammonia concentrations were significantly less (10). These findings suggest that one of the beneficial mechanisms of action of mild hypothermia in ALF may be attenuating the transfer of ammonia across the blood-brain barrier.

Effect on cerebral blood flow (CBF)

An increase in CBF causing cerebral hyperemia and consequently a higher delivery of ammonia to the brain has been strongly suggested to be implicated in the development of brain edema and increased ICP in ALF. The attenuation of raised ICP demonstrated with mild hypothermia in ammonia-infused rats with portacaval anastomosis was accompanied by a reduction in CBF (11). These findings support the importance of increased ICP and CBF in ALF. However, the mechanisms responsible for increased CBF in ALF are elusive. There is some evidence showing that the vasodilator nitric oxide (NO) plays a stimulating role. The source of NO remains unknown, but clinical studies suggest that NO production arises as a result of inflammation and increased cytokine production. Furthermore, increased activation of N-methyl-D-aspartate (NMDA) receptors due to ammonia toxicity in the brain results in increased NO synthase activity and NO production (13).

Effect on brain glutamine

The only possible way to remove ammonia in the brain is through the production of glutamine from glutamate. This is achieved with the enzyme glutamine synthetase, found solely in astrocytes. It is believed that glutamine accumulation in the astrocyte results in increased cellular osmolarity which leads to cell swelling and subsequently to brain edema in ALF (14). This is supported by studies both *in vitro* and *in vivo* where the administration of methionine sulfoximine, a glutamine synthetase inhibitor, reduced ammonia-induced cell swelling (15-17). However, we found that rats with ALF that protection against brain edema by hypothermia was not accompanied by a reduction in microdialysate (extracellular) brain glutamine (10). Furthermore, in the same model, using nuclear magnetic resonance (NMR) techniques, Chatauret, et al (18), also found that hypothermia-induced reductions in brain water content in rats with ALF were not associated with significant reductions in brain glutamine (18) at time points associated with brain edema in normothermic ALF rats. This suggests that mild hypothermia's major protective effect on brain edema is not mediated via an effect on brain glutamine synthesis.

Recently it has been suggested that alterations of brain osmolytes are responsible for astrocyte swelling. This is supported by findings that significant reductions in severity of brain edema and encephalopathy in ALF by hypothermia occur concomitantly with significant attenuation of decreases of myo-inositol and taurine (19).

Effect on brain glutamate

Using *in vivo* microdialysis techniques, increased extracellular brain glutamate has been a consistent finding in different experimental animal models of ALF (20-23). Increased extracellular brain glutamate leads to increased glutamatergic neurotransmission; a pathway believed to be implicated in the pathogenesis of encephalopathy and brain edema in ALF (24). This is supported with studies demonstrating that memantine, a noncompetitive antagonist of the glutamate receptor (NMDA), reduces the severity of neurological signs of hepatic encephalopathy in rats with ALF (25). Mild hypothermia led to a significant lowering of extracellular brain glutamate concentrations in rats with ALF, concomitant with the delay in the onset of severe encephalopathy and brain edema, as well as a reduction in CSF ammonia (10). It is therefore strongly suggested that increased extracellular brain glutamate is important in the pathogenesis of hepatic encephalopathy and the onset of brain edema in ALF. An increase in extracellular brain glutamate occurs as a result of increased glutamate release and/or decreased glutamate uptake (clearance) from the extracellular space (26). Knecht, et al (27), measured a loss in expression of the astrocytic glutamate transporter, EAAT-2 (GLT-1) in rats with ALF; this downregulation could explain the increase in extracellular brain glutamate. This is supported *in vitro*, in which cultured astrocytes treated with ammonia had decreased glutamate transporter expression (28). These findings suggest that hypothermia possibly prevents a decrease in glutamate uptake by removing the ammonia inhibition on glutamate transporters.

Effect on energy metabolism

It is commonly known that ammonia inhibits the enzyme α-ketoglutarate dehydrogenase in the tricarboxylic acid cycle (29), which may explain new data suggesting ammonia has an effect on cerebral energy metabolism (30). When applied to cultured astrocytes, ammonia stimulates an increase in lactate dehydrogenase activity and, subsequently, an increase in lactate production (31). This observation was found *in vivo* where an increase in CSF lactate was measured during severe encephalopathy and brain edema in rats with ALF (32). Similarly, extracellular brain lactate concentrations were increased in relation to increased ICP in patients with ALF (33). An increase in lactate production indirectly suggests that anaerobic pathways (increased glycolytic activity) may be stimulated to compensate for a decreased pyruvate oxidation to maintain adenosine triphosphate production. Increased alanine production is also another indirect metabolite suggesting stimulation of anaerobic pathways. It has also been demonstrated that brain alanine is elevated in the hyperammonemic brain (23, 34, 35) and more recently in rats with ALF using NMR spectroscopy (18). Furthermore, decreased concentrations of the neuronal marker molecule N-acetylaspartate (NAA) have been demonstrated in frontal cortex of rats in coma stages of HE as a result of ALF, reflecting neuronal mitochondrial dysfunction (18). However mild hypothermia has demonstrated to prevent the increase in brain lactate, alanine and decrease in NAA in frontal cortex concomitant with the prevention of encephalopathy and brain edema (18). Therefore, one possible mechanism of action of hypothermia in ALF is the facilitation of pyruvate oxidation as a consequence of decreased ammonia in the brain. Hypothermia, therefore removes the ammonia inhibition in the TCA cycle, decreases brain lactate, alanine, and increases NAA production, restoring proper energy metabolism within the brain.

CLINICAL IMPLICATIONS OF MILD HYPOTHERMIA

Hypothermia has been extensively practiced and studied in head injured patients; however, little data is known on patients with ALF treated with hypothermia. As discussed above, animal studies provided the rationale for the evaluation of the role of hypothermia in patients with ALF. In our unit, we have demonstrated a beneficial effect of mild hypothermia in 3 separate studies.

Study 1

The first study was performed to investigate whether hypothermia could be used as a bridge to liver transplantation in patients with acute liver failure who had uncontrolled intracranial hypertension (defined as persistently elevated ICP to levels of 25 mmHg or more despite treatment with 2 boluses of mannitol and removal of 500 ml of fluid with haemofiltration). Twenty patients fulfilling this criteria were cooled to 32°C. Six of these patients were eventually not suitable candidates for OLT and died following rewarming (Figure 12-2). Thirteen of the 14 transplant candidates were successfully bridged to transplantation, undergoing approximately 32 hrs of cooling. The longest period without occurrence of increased ICP was 118 hours, at which time the patient was successfully transplanted. On average, upon cooling, ICP was high (36.5 (SD 2.7) mmHg) but was reduced following 4 hours of cooling (17.1 (0.9) mmHg) and was sustained for 24 hours (16.3 (1.3) mmHg) ($p < 0.001$). Recurrence of episodes of increased ICP to above 20 mmHg responded to additional treatment with mannitol.

Hypothermia had a significant impact on many important pathophysiological mechanisms. Arterial ammonia concentration was reduced by approximately 30% and ammonia delivery to the brain by 66%. This was coupled with a reduction in ammonia extraction across the brain from about 11% to values close to zero (36). Production of glutamine across the brain was reduced following cooling, suggesting that hypothermia reduces the activity of the major ammonia metabolizing enzyme, glutamine synthetase. However this reduction in glutamine production could also be due to a reduction of ammonia levels in the brain. CBF was also significantly reduced following 4 hours of cooling and was sustained for 24 hours ($p < 0.001$). In a previous report, mild hypothermia restored CBF autoregulation (37). Furthermore, in this selected group of patients, peripheral cytokine production was very high; hypothermia reduced the pro-inflammatory cytokines TNFα, IL-1β and IL-6 significantly [unpublished data]. These effects on ICP and CBF were associated with significant improvement in cardiovascular hemodynamics manifested by increased mean arterial pressure and systemic vascular resistance and reduced noradrenaline requirements.

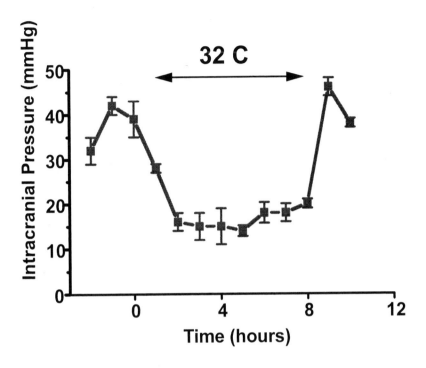

Figure 12-2. This figure shows the effect of hypothermia on ICP in patients with ALF who have intracranial hypertension that is uncontrolled with currently available therapies. The changes in ICP during the cooling and the rewarming suggests that the effects are likely to be mediated by hypothermia (data from reference 36).

Study 2

The second study was performed to investigate whether mild hypothermia could prevent the occurrence of surges of increased ICP (starting ICP<20 mmHg) in patients with ALF and severe hepatic encephalopathy. Five patients were studied and cooled to 35°C from the time of the need for mechanical ventilation until OLT, spontaneous recovery or death. Three of the 5 patients were successfully bridged to OLT with a mean cooling period of 54 hours. The longest period that a patient was cooled was 120 hours. One of the patients recovered without need for OLT and 1 patient died 120 hours after inclusion into the study from sepsis and multiorgan failure. Prior to cooling, the ICP was elevated at a mean of 17.6 (2.7) mmHg and this was reduced to 15.2 (0.9) mmHg at 4 hours, which was sustained at

24 hours (15.9 (1.3) mmHg) (p<0.05). With this group of patients the starting CBF was not significantly high and there were no significant changes in CBF during the cooling period [unpublished data].

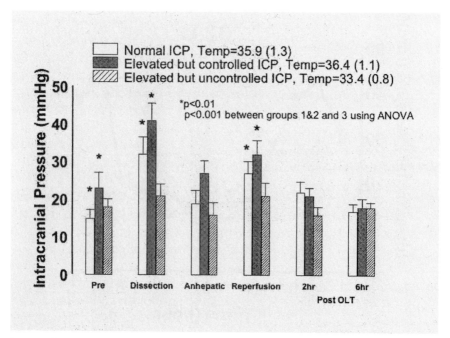

Figure 12-3. This figure shows the changes in ICP in patients undergoing liver transplantation. □ represents a group of patients that were normothermic during transplantation, prior to the transplant they did not require any specific therapy for increased ICP. ■ represents a group of patients that were normothermic during transplantation, prior to the transplant they required specific therapy for increased ICP. ▨ represents a group of patients that were transplanted hypothermic. The data show that during transplantation, there is a marked and significant increase in ICP in the patients during the dissection and the reperfusion phases that are transplanted normothermic. In those patients that are transplanted with their core temperatures at 32-33°C, such increases in ICP are prevented. (data from reference 38).

Study 3

The third study was performed to ask whether hypothermia could prevent the occurrence of episodes of increased ICP during the dissection and reperfusion phases of liver transplantation where increases in ICP are inevitable and current therapies are limited to the use of barbiturates with their attendant complications. In this study we compared the changes in ICP between a group that was hypothermic and another group that was normothermic during liver transplantation. There were significant increases in ICP in the normothermic group during the dissection and reperfusion phases of the operation, which was not observed in the hypothermic group (Figure 12-3). The rise in the ICP in the normothermic group was associated with significant increase in CBF, which was not observed in the hypothermic patients (38).

CONCLUSIONS

To date, studies using hypothermia as a treatment for patients with ALF provide convincing evidence of efficacy and safety in patients with uncontrolled ICP and those who are undergoing liver transplantation. In patients who have severe hepatic encephalopathy but do not have increased ICP, mild hypothermia reduces the risk of developing increases in ICP. However, a randomized controlled study is clearly warranted to confirm hypothermia as an effective, safe, easy-to-use and inexpensive method to treat intracranial hypertension in ALF as a bridge to OLT or recovery of liver function. Overall, the mechanisms in which hypothermia is beneficial are multi-factorial as hypothermia acts non-specifically both peripherally and centrally. Hypothermia is a useful therapeutic tool to help explore and understand the pathophysiology of ALF. Hypothermia displays many beneficial effects on brain water and ICP which seem to be related to reductions of blood-brain ammonia transfer (decreased brain ammonia concentrations), normalization of extracellular brain glutamate, restoration of cerebral blood flow, decrease in mediators of inflammation and improvement in brain energy metabolism which together are thought to underlie the pathophysiology of severe increases in ICP in patients with ALF.

REFERENCES

1. Trey C, Davidson CS. The management of fulminant hepatic failure. In: Popper (H. Schaffner F, ed.) Progress in liver disease, Grune and Stratton, New York, volume III, pp. 282-298.
2. O'Grady JG, Alexander GJM, Hayllar KM, Williams R. Early indicators of prognosis in fulminant hepatic failure. *Gastroenterology* 1989; 97:439-445.
3. Ascher NL, Lake JR, Emond JC and Roberts JP. Liver transplantation for fulminant hepatic failure. *Arch Surg* 1993; 128:677-682.
4. Makin AJ, Wendon J, Williams R. A 7-year experience of severe acetaminophen-induced hepatotoxicity (1987-1993). *Gastroenterology* 1995; 109:1907-16.
5. Hoofnagle JH, Carithers RL, Chapiro C, Ascher NL. Fulminant hepatic failure: Summary of a Workshop. *Hepatology* 1995; 21:240-252.
6. Schenker S, Warren KS. Effect of temperature variation on toxicity and metabolism of ammonia in mice. *J Lab Clin Med* 1962; 60:291-301.
7. Peignoux M, Bernuau J, Benhamou JP. Total hepatectomy and vascular exclusion in the rat. A comparison, with special reference to the influence of body temperature. *Clin Sci* 1982; 62:273-277.
8. Traber P, Canto M, Ganger D, Blei AT. Effect of body temperature on brain edema and encephalopathy in the rat after hepatic devascularization. *Gastroenterology* 1989; 96:885-91.
9. Shubert A. Side effects of mild hypothermia. *J Neurosurg Anesthesiol* 1995; 7:139-147.
10. Rose, C., Michalak, A., Rambaldi, A., et al. Mild hypothermia delays the onset of coma and prevents brain edema and extracellular brain glutamate accumulation in rats with acute liver failure. *Hepatology* 2000; 31:872-877.
11. Cordoba J, Crespin J, Gottstein J., Blei AT. Mild hypothermia modifies ammonia-induced brain edema in rats after portacaval anastomosis. *Gastroenterology* 1999; 116:686-693.
12. Clemmensen JO, Larsen FS, Kondrup J, et al. Cerebral herniation in patients with acute liver failure is correlated with arterial ammonia concentration. *Hepatology* 1999; 29:648-653.
13. Hermenegildo C, Monfort P, Felipo V. Activation of NMDA receptors in rat brain in vivo following acute ammonia intoxication. Characterization by in vivo microdialysis. *Hepatology* 2000; 31:709-715.
14. Cordoba J, Gottstein J, and Blei AT. Glutamine, myoinositol, and organic osmolytes after portacaval anastomosis in the rat: Implications for ammonia-induced brain edema. *Hepatology* 1996; 27:919-923.
15. Norenberg MD, Bender AS. Astrocyte swelling in liver failure: role of glutamine and benzodiazepines. *Acta Neurochir Suppl (Wien)* 1994; 60:24-27.
16. Takahashi H, Koehler RC, Brusilow SW, Traysman RJ. Inhibition of brain glutamine accumulation prevents cerebral edemain hyperammonemic rats. *Am J Physiol* 1991; 261:H825-H829.
17. Chodobski A, Szmydynger-Chodobska J, Urbanska A, Szczepnaska-Sadowska E. Intracranial pressure, cerebral blood flow, and cerebrospinal fluid formation during hyperammonemia in the cat. *J Neurosurg* 1986; 65:86-91.

18. Chatauret N, Zwingmann C, Rose C, et al. Effects of hypothermia on brain glucose metabolism in acute liver failure: A 1H/13C-nuclear magnetic resonance study. *Gastroenterology* 2003; 125:815-824.

19. Zwingmann C, Chatauret N, Rose C, et al. Selective alterations of brain osmolytes in acute liver failure: protective effect of mild hypothermia. *Brain Res* 2004; 999:113-118.

20. Michalak A, Rose C, Butterworth J, Butterworth RF. Neuroactive amino acides and glutamate (NMDA) receptors in frontal cortex of rats with experimental acute liver failure. *Hepatology* 1996; 24:908-914.

21. Bosman DK, Deutz NEP, Maas MAW, et al. Amino acid release from cerebral cortex in experimental acute liver failure, studied by in vivo cerebral cortex microdialysis. *J Neurochem* 1992; 59:591-599.

22. de Knegt RJ, Schalm SW, van der Rijt CCD, et al. Extracellular brain glutamate during acute liver failure and during acute hyperammonemia simulating acute liver failure: an experimental study based on in vivo brain dialysis. *J Hepatol* 1994; 20:19-26.

23. Hilgier W, Zielinska M, Borkowska HD, et al.. Changes in the extracellular profiles of neuroactive amino acids in the rat striatum at the symptomatic stage of hepatic failure. *J Neurosci Res* 1999; 56:76-84.

24. Butterworth RF. Hepatic encephalopathy and brain edema in acute hepatic failure: does glutamate play a role? *Hepatology* 1997; 25:1032-1035.

25. Vogels BAP, Maas MAW, Daalhuisen J, et al.. Memantine, a non-competitive NMDA-receptor antagonist improves hyperammonemia-induced encephalopathy and acute hepatic encephalopathy in rats. *Hepatology* 1997; 25:820-827.

26. Rose C.. Increased extracellular brain glutamate in acute liver failure: Decreased uptake or increased released? *Metab Brain Dis* 2002; 17:251-261.

27. Knecht K, Michalak A, Rose C, et al. Decreased glutamate transporter (GLT-1) expression in frontal cortex of rats with acute liver failure. *Neurosci Lett* 1997; 229:201-203.

28. Chan H, Hazell AS, Desjardins P, Butterworth RF. Effects of ammonia on glutamate transporter (GLAST) protein and mRNA in cultured rat cortical astrocytes. *Neurochem Int* 2000; 37:243-248.

29. Lai JCK, Cooper AJL. Brain α-ketoglutarate dehydrogenase complex: kinetic properties, regional distribution and effects of inhibitors. *J Neurochem* 1986; 47:1376-1386.

30. Rao KV, Norenberg MD. Cerebral energy metabolism in hepatic encephalopathy and hyperammonemia. *Metab Brain Dis* 2001; 16:67-78.

31. Bélanger M, Chan H, Hazell AS, Butterworth RF. Increased lactate dehydrogenase (LDH) expression and activity in cultured astrocytes exposed to ammonia. *J Neurochem* 2001; 78:25.

32. Chatauret N, Rose C, Therrien G, Butterworth RF. Mild hypothermia prevents cerebral edema and CSF lactate accumulation in acute liver failure. *Metab Brain Dis* 2001; 16:95-102.

33. Tofteng F, Jorgensen L, Hansen BA et al. Cerebral microdialysis in patients with fulminant hepatic failure. *Hepatology* 2002; 36:1333-1340.

34. Swain M, Butterworth RF, Blei AT. Ammonia and related amino acids in the pathogenesis of brain edema in acute liver failure in rats. *Hepatology* 1992; 15:449-453.

35. Mans AM, De Joseph MR, Hawkins RA. Metabolic abnormalities and grade of encephalopathy in acute hepatic failure. *J Neurochem* 1994; 63:1829-1838.

36. Jalan R, Olde Damink SWM, Deutz NEP et al. Treatment of uncontrolled intracranial hypertension in acute liver failure with moderate hypothermia. *Lancet* 1999; 354:1164-68.

37. Jalan R, Olde Damink SW, Deutz NE, et al. Restoration of cerebral blood flow autoregulation and reactivity to carbon dioxide in acute liver failure by moderate hypothermia. *Hepatology* 2001; 34:50-54.
38. Jalan R, Olde Damink SWM, Deutz NEP et al. Moderate hypothermia prevents cerebral hyperemia and increase in intracranial pressure in patients undergoing liver transplantation for acute liver failure. *Transplantation* 2003; 75:2034-39.

Chapter 13

MYOCARDIAL ISCHEMIA AND INFARCTION

Sharon L. Hale, BS[1], Robert A. Kloner, MD, PhD[1], Shoichi Katada, MD[2], Toshihiko Obayashi, MD[2], Takeshi Ishii, MD[2], Susumu Nakajima, MD[2], Naoki Yahagi, MD, MSc[2]

[1]*University of Southern California, Los Angeles, CA, USA*
[2]*University of Tokyo, Tokyo, Japan*

INTRODUCTION

Atherosclerotic heart disease is the leading cause of death in developed nations. Manifestations include myocardial ischemia or infarction. In addition, some patients develop cardiovascular insufficiency, with the additional risk of systemic ischemia. Hypothermia has been shown to protect tissues during ischemia and thus may have clinical benefit in patients with cardiovascular disorders. This chapter will explore the potential therapeutic role for hypothermia in regional and global myocardial ischemia, as well as systemic ischemia secondary to heart failure.

ACUTE CORONARY OCCLUSION AND MYOCARDIAL ISCHEMIA

A long standing focus of research in cardiology has been preservation of ischemic myocardium. In the early phase of myocardial ischemia due to coronary artery occlusion, all compromised cells remain viable, but, over time, cells begin to die if blood flow is not restored. What has been described as a "wavefront" of necrosis occurs (1). First identified in a canine model of coronary artery occlusion, this phenomenon relates to the fact that necrosis begins in the sub-endocardium, where coronary collateral flow is the least, and spreads to the sub-epicardium where collateral flow is greater. In this model, the process may last for hours. The extent of cell death depends on the duration of ischemia, the degree of reduction in blood flow and the amount of collateral flow present in the jeopardized region. Many strategies have been tested in an attempt to protect the ischemic heart. Currently, the treatment of choice by cardiologists is reperfusion therapy. If timely reflow can be established, either by thrombolytic therapy or angioplasty and stenting, tissue will be salvaged; however reperfusion therapy for acute myocardial infarction cannot be performed in all patients. Even in patients who receive this therapy, the time needed for the blockage to be removed or bypassed may be hours after the onset of chest pain. If reperfusion takes place after the cells are irreversibly injured by ischemia, the cells die. Cells that are reperfused while still reversibly injured may be salvaged.

Despite aggressive therapy, many patients develop complications, such as congestive heart failure, and even die, as a result of arrhythmias or extensive myocardial damage. In addition, a significant number of patients show persistent ST- segment elevation even after successful restoration of epicardial flow, a phenomenon consistent with microvascular injury. Indeed, the fact that infarct size is one of the most important predictors of early and late survival after acute myocardial infarction indicates the clear need for new approaches to improve myocyte preservation before and during reperfusion therapy.

Another factor related to ischemia/reperfusion that cardiologists are paying increasing attention to is the so-called "no-reflow phenomenon": even when the infarct-related coronary artery is successfully opened, restoration of blood flow at the microvascular level may be sub-optimal.

Thus, continuing challenges in treating acute myocardial infarction are the issues that many patients do not receive reperfusion therapy, time to reperfusion may be lengthy and complete reflow may not occur on a microvascular level. Methods to protect ischemic myocardium and to delay cell necrosis after acute myocardial infarction are still needed. Treatments to reduce no-reflow and enhance microvascular perfusion are important, as such therapy may improve healing and reduce deleterious infarct expansion and ventricular remodeling.

In addition to myocardial ischemia and infarction from coronary occlusion, another setting in which protecting myocardium is critically important is during cardiac surgery, particularly minimally invasive cardiac bypass procedures during which bypass is performed on the beating heart without extracorporeal circulation. Areas of the heart may become ischemic during surgery. Thus there is a need to develop methods to protect potentially ischemic myocytes during this procedure.

Hypothermia and Global Myocardial Ischemia

For at least half a century, cardiac surgeons have used hypothermia to protect the non-working heart (2). Successful organ preservation depends heavily on hypothermia. Cold cardioplegia and localized cooling are used by thoracic surgeons to preserve the heart during traditional coronary artery bypass and other intra-cardiac procedures. Moderate to deep hypothermia protects the donor heart during global ischemia prior to transplantation. The application of whole-body and global cardiac hypothermia are well-established procedures. Hypothermia is thought to protect against hypoxia due to its ability to slow cellular metabolism, reduce myocardial oxygen demand, slow the rate of adenosine triphosphate (ATP) depletion, and increase tolerance to the accumulation of metabolic wastes. The use and effects of hypothermia in the nonworking heart have been well explored. However the feasibility of using this concept of cardioprotection in the working heart, subjected to regional ischemia, has only been explored in the last several decades.

POTENTIAL MECHANISMS OF PROTECTION

The mechanisms for the protective effect of hypothermia in the ischemic, beating heart have yet to be conclusively determined. In general, tissue metabolic rate decreases as body temperature decreases. One potential mechanism is a reduction in high-energy phosphate depletion. In the absence of ischemia, a reduction in temperature elevates myocardial creatine phosphate levels and has no effect on ATP (3). In the presence of ischemia, cooling may help prevent the decrease of ATP. In the liver of rabbits, topical hypothermia of 30°C significantly maintains ATP levels after 15 and 30 minutes of ischemia (4). In isolated, perfused, working rabbit hearts hypothermic perfusion (31°C) initiated before 2 hours of global ischemia resulted in increased myocardial ATP preservation during ischemia and reperfusion compared with a normothermic control group (5).

Another potential mechanism could be the induction of heat shock proteins by hypothermia. Heat shock proteins have been shown to confer protection to the myocardium in the setting of ischemia and reperfusion. These proteins are expressed in response to cold stress in addition to that of hyperthermia. One study showed that levels of heat shock protein (Hsp-70) messenger ribonucleic acid (mRNA) was three times higher in hearts exposed to hypothermic perfusion before ischemia (5). It is, however, unlikely that these proteins can explain the acute protection observed with cooling, since their expression takes several hours.

Cell death after ischemia and reperfusion may be due in part to apoptosis. A study of transient global cerebral ischemia showed that hypothermic treatment applied for 3 hours after ischemia promoted expression of BCL-2, an anti-apoptotic protein, and reduced cellular apoptosis compared with normothermia (6). Other studies have shown a similar reduction in the number of apoptotic cells with hypothermic treatment for focal cerebral ischemia (7, 8). Ning and coworkers (9) noted that hypothermic perfusion in isolated rabbit hearts subjected to ischemic cardioplegic arrest altered the expression of 6 genes related to apoptosis, including increasing expression of anti-apoptotic BCL-2. These investigators concluded that hypothermia-induced myocardial protection might be due to a beneficial modification to signaling pathways for apoptosis.

Hypothermia may protect microvasculature and promote reflow by reducing post-ischemic endothelial injury due to free-radical release at reperfusion. In an isolated rat liver model of ischemia and reperfusion, mild hypothermic perfusion (34°C) decreased the formation of reactive oxygen species at reperfusion and reduced post ischemic vascular resistance (10). Another study showed improved reflow to previously ischemic myocardium in rabbits treated with regional hypothermia during acute coronary artery occlusion and reperfusion (11).

EFFECTS OF MILD HYPOTHERMIA ON THE ISCHEMIC WORKING HEART

Left ventricular function

If cardiac function is depressed by hypothermia, this intervention may not be beneficial in the setting of acute myocardial infarction, where ventricular function may already be compromised. Deep hypothermia has been associated with deterioration in cardiac function. Indices of left ventricular (LV) function including LV pressure, LV dP/dt $_{max}$ (maximum rate of LV pressure rise) and cardiac output have been reported to decrease dramatically in dogs cooled to 25°C (3). In rats cooled to ~15°C the same decrease in LV function was observed. In addition, when the rats were rewarmed to baseline temperature, these parameters remained significantly depressed (12).

In contrast, mild hypothermia ($\geq$31°C) appears to have little effect on, or may improve, LV function. Weisser and colleagues found that mild hypothermia in non-ischemic pig hearts resulted in an increase in myocardial contractility. Although heart rate decreased, cardiac output, stroke volume and LV dP/dt $_{max}$ increased (13). Other investigators showed that in ischemic pig hearts cardiac output was maintained under hypothermia because of an increase in stroke volume, despite a decrease in heart rate (14). In a dog model, cardiac output increased until a body temperature of 33°C was reached. However, after that, as temperature was lowered to 25°C cardiac output decreased. Also dP/dt$_{max}$ increased during cooling to 33°C but returned to baseline as the temperature decreased (15). Data from these few studies suggest that mild hypothermia does not cause a significant decline in left ventricular function and may improve it.

Myocardial contractility depends on temperature. In an animal study using pigs, a depression of systolic function occurred during cooling at a constant atrial-paced heart rate of 150 beats/min (normal, resting heart rate being around 100 beats/min in human-sized pigs) (16). However, when heart rate is allowed to vary, the opposite effect is observed. For example, in anesthetized, unpaced dogs subjected to veno-venous cooling, Goldberg showed that systolic function, as measured using a strain gauge to assess contractile force, was augmented as temperature decreased (17). This result has been confirmed by others using load-independent techniques (18-20). These apparently contradictory results may be reconciled if alterations in heart rate modulate the changes in cellular activity induced by hypothermia. Weisser et al recently investigated the influence of mild hypothermia (37 to 31°C) on isometric twitch force, sarcoplasmic reticulum (SR) calcium (Ca^{2+}) content, and intracellular Ca^{2+} transients in ventricular muscle strips from human and porcine myocardium, as well as on *in vivo* hemodynamic parameters in unpaced pigs (21). In their *in vitro* experiments, they used muscle strips from 5 nonfailing human and 8 pig hearts, while in their *in vivo* experiments 8 pigs were monitored using Millar-tip (left ventricle) and Swan-Ganz (pulmonary artery) catheters. Hemodynamic parameters were assessed under baseline conditions (37°C), and after stepwise cooling (during cardiopulmonary bypass) to 35, 33, and 31°C. Hypothermia increased isometric twitch force significantly (by 91±16% in human and by 50±9% in pig myocardium). Rapid cooling did not change contractions or aequorin light emission significantly. In the anesthetized pigs, mild hypothermia resulted in an increase in hemodynamic parameters related to myocardial contractility. While heart rate decreased from 111±3 to 73±1 beats/min, cardiac output increased from 2.4±0.1 to 3.1±0.3 l/min, and stroke volume from 21±1 to 41±3 ml. Neither systemic nor pulmonary vascular resistance changed significantly during cooling. Thus, mild hypothermia exerted significant positive inotropic effects on the unpaced human and porcine myocardium, but it did not increase intracellular Ca^{2+} transients or the SR Ca^{2+} content.

Lewis et al, using a validated load-independent method, demonstrated that during hypothermia, left ventricular contractility was reduced at a maintained higher heart rate in cardiac surgical patients (22). At 37°C, increasing the heart rate increased contractility (at 80 beats/min, 100%; at 120 beats/min, 205.9%; P=0.0021), but, at 33°C contractility fell as heart rate increased at (80 beats/min, 100%; at 120 beats/min, 53.7%; P=0.0014).

The mechanisms for the effects of hypothermia on contractility are unclear. Myocardial contractility is dependent on myosin/actin crossbridge formation, and is sensitive to the concentration of calcium ($[Ca^{2+}]$) prevailing within the cell. The $[Ca^{2+}]$ is dependent both on the duration of the action potential and on the activity of the ATP-dependent ion-exchange pumps situated within the cell wall and in the SR (22). Since enzymatic activity is directly related to temperature, the effect of cooling is dependent on the relative thermal sensitivity of each enzymatic reaction step. As a consequence, the effects of hypothermia on systolic function cannot easily be predicted. If the inhibitory effects of a decrease in temperature are greater on myosin/actin crossbridge formation, contractility will decrease, but if they are greater on $[Ca^{2+}]$, contractility may increase. In fact, Henderson, et al, showed more than 25 years ago that in rat myofibrils the force of contraction increased with decreases in temperature down to 29°C, suggesting that Ca^{2+} handling is the more temperature-sensitive of the two processes (23). Indeed, variations in Ca^{2+} handling with temperature, causing an increase in the intracellular Ca^{2+} concentration, have been demonstrated *in vitro* at the level of the Ca^{2+} channel in animals, the Ca^{2+}/Na^+ exchange pump in humans, and the SR Ca^{2+} pump, Ca^{2+}/Na^+ exchanger, sarcolemmal Ca^{2+} pump, and mitochondrial Ca^{2+} uniporter in small mammals (21, 24).

Regional myocardial blood flow

Cooling of the heart might cause a decrease in myocardial blood flow due to vasoconstriction. This could be harmful in the setting of regional ischemia. At a body temperature of 25°C myocardial blood flow was reduced to an average of 34% of baseline in non-ischemic canine hearts (3). However mild hypothermia (~32-34°C) appears not to adversely affect myocardial blood flow in either dogs (25, 26) or rabbits (27) during coronary artery occlusion or reperfusion. In fact, hypothermia administered during coronary artery occlusion may improve reflow to the jeopardized ischemic region during reperfusion. Hale and Kloner (11) showed that rabbit hearts made hypothermic late in the ischemic period had smaller than predicted anatomic regions of "no-reflow" (an anatomic area of hypoperfusion and decreased regional myocardial blood flow observed in animal models and humans after transient coronary artery occlusion and reperfusion). In addition, return of absolute myocardial blood flow to the risk region during reperfusion was higher in hearts treated with hypothermia.

EFFECTS OF HYPOTHERMIA ON EXPERIMENTAL INFARCT SIZE

The concept of using hypothermia for protection in the beating, regionally ischemic heart evolved in the late 1970's beginning with experimental studies by Abendschein and coworkers (28). One of the first studies to test the hypothesis that hypothermia could reduce myocardial infarct size examined the effects of whole-body hypothermia in dogs subjected to 5 or 10 hours of coronary artery occlusion without reperfusion. Beginning 30 minutes after occlusion, body temperature was reduced by covering the dogs with bags of ice and by circulating ice water in a rubber mat under the animals. Approximately two hours of cooling were required to reduce body temperature to 26°C. Hypothermia was maintained for the duration of the protocol. Even though hypothermia was not begun until 30 minutes after the onset of coronary artery occlusion, infarct size, measured after five hours of coronary artery occlusion, was reduced 40% compared to that in normothermic hearts. In addition they noted that sham-operated hearts from dogs subjected to hypothermia had no evidence of necrosis; thus hypothermia per se was not damaging. A later study using a similar method to induce hypothermia was that by Voorhees and coworkers (25). Their study confirmed that a reduction in body temperature reduced infarct size in an experimental canine model. In addition, this study showed that blood flow to ischemic myocardium was not reduced by hypothermia and that hypothermia did not interact with myocardial infarction to produce or exacerbate cardiogenic shock, again suggesting the safety of this technique.

An alternative approach tested to reduce myocardial temperature was hypothermic synchronized coronary venous retroperfusion. This technique was investigated in several studies for its potential to protect jeopardized myocardium after coronary artery occlusion using a canine model of myocardial ischemia (29-31). Briefly, a cuffed catheter was inserted into the great cardiac vein serving the ischemic area. Cooled, shunted arterial blood was pulsed during diastole (with the cuff inflated) for ischemic zone retroperfusion; during systole the cuff was deflated to permit venous drainage. Using this technique, a temperature decrease in the myocardium of 5°C was achieved after approximately 15 minutes of retroperfusion. In one study in which blood was perfused at 20°C, infarct size was reduced from 72% of the ischemic zone in control hearts to 29% in cooled hearts after 6 hours of coronary occlusion (29). In another study (30), infarct size, measured after two hours, was reduced from 65% of the area at risk in control hearts to 24% in hearts perfused at 32°C and to 6% in hearts perfused at 15°C.

These initial studies showed the feasibility of using temperature reduction during ischemia, and the potential of hypothermia to limit infarct size, at least in the setting of myocardial ischemia without reperfusion.

Relationship between temperature and the development of necrosis

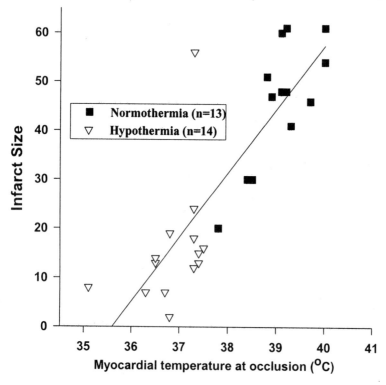

Figure 13-1. Relationship between myocardial temperature before coronary artery occlusion and eventual infarct size (as a percentage of the risk zone). Note that infarct size is closely correlated with temperature.

The importance of temperature on the development of necrosis after myocardial ischemia and reperfusion was shown by studies conducted in many animal models including rabbits (27, 32), pigs (33, 34), dogs (26) and rats (35). These studies have shown that there is a strong correlation between body, blood and pericardial temperatures and eventual myocardial infarct size. For example, Hale and Kloner (27) found a close relationship between the amount of the ischemic risk region that became necrotic and the temperature of the heart (Figure 13-1).

Chien and coworkers studied the effects of body temperature in the relatively normothermic to hyperthermic range (35 to 42°C) on myocardial infarct size development in rabbits. They found that infarct size was closely correlated with body temperature in both paced and unpaced hearts (32).

A correlation between temperature and infarct size was noted by Schwartz and colleagues in the open-chest dog model of coronary artery occlusion (26). They placed a thermister in the pericardial space under the heart. Using multivariate analysis, they determined that not only was collateral blood flow (a known determinate of infarct size development in dogs) a major predictor of infarct size, but pericardial temperature was as well. The effect of decreased temperature was greatest in dogs with little collateral blood flow during occlusion.

Another study investigated the effect of temperature on infarct size in pigs (33). Again, a strong correlation was noted between body core temperature and the proportion of the ischemic risk zone that became necrotic. These investigators emphasized the importance of controlling for temperature in studies testing interventions aimed at reducing infarct size.

Hypothermia in experimental models of ischemia and reperfusion

Mild hypothermia initiated before the onset of ischemia

Hale and Kloner tested the potential use of mild hypothermia as a therapeutic maneuver to protect ischemic myocardium in an anesthetized open-chest rabbit model of ischemia and reperfusion. Using topical regional hypothermia produced by placing a bag filled with ice and water on the heart, the temperature in hearts in treated animals was reduced from about 39°C to 35°C before coronary artery occlusion (27). Cooling was maintained for the 30 minutes of coronary artery occlusion and for 15 minutes into a total of 3 hours of reperfusion. Infarct size was closely correlated to myocardial temperature at the start of coronary occlusion. A reduction of only about 4°C in the region that would become ischemic reduced infarct size by 65%. Regional hypothermia reduces heart rate in this model. However, the protection was independent of the reduction in heart rate.

When hearts were paced to 230 beats/minute (above control heart rate), a profound decrease in infarct size was still observed. This study confirmed the important role of myocardial temperature level in the progression of necrosis and also showed the therapeutic potential of topical regional hypothermia to reduce infarct size (Figure 13-2).

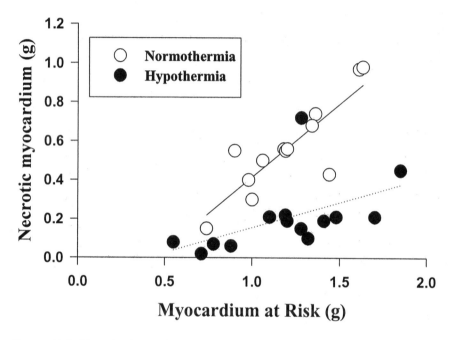

Figure 13-2. Necrotic tissue plotted as a function of risk region in normothermic and hypothermic hearts. On average, for any given size of risk region, a smaller infarct developed in hypothermic hearts.

Hypothermia initiated after ischemia

For hypothermia to be used as a therapeutic modality in the clinical setting of acute myocardial infarction, the question of whether it is of benefit when initiated after ischemia is of utmost importance. Studies performed in animal models have addressed this question and in general data shows a positive benefit of cooling in reducing infarct size even when started well after coronary occlusion. In the rabbit model, cooling initiated at 10 or 20 minutes after a coronary artery occlusion of 30 minutes total duration still resulted in a pronounced reduction in myocardial infarct size (36, 37).

Another study confirmed this finding using a pig model (14). Cooling was begun at 20 minutes into a 60-minute coronary artery occlusion and continued for 15 minutes of reperfusion. An 80% reduction in infarct size was found in the hearts of pigs receiving hypothermic treatment.

It is important however that cooling be initiated as quickly as possible after the onset of ischemia. For example, Hale and colleagues found that if cooling was initiated at 10 minutes of coronary artery occlusion (total duration of ischemia 30 minutes) infarct size was reduced by about 50%, but when cooling was not begun until 25 minutes of ischemia it failed to reduce infarct size (36). In general, if cooling is begun right at reperfusion or after reperfusion, but is not present during the phase of ischemia, hypothermia is not protective.

Myocardial cooling can be achieved within minutes in small animals, but humans have a much greater thermal mass and cooling would be expected to be slower. The extent and timing of mild hypothermia instituted after the onset of ischemia was addressed by Dae and coworkers (14) using human-sized pigs as a model. The method they used to reduce temperature in treated animals was endovascular cooling using a heat-exchange balloon catheter (SetPoint Endovascular Temperature Management System; Radiant Medical Inc., Redwood City, CA) introduced into the inferior vena cava. The investigators found that core temperature could be reduced by 4°C after 40 minutes, suggesting that this technique could be applied in humans, and that it might be practical to use therapeutic hypothermia as a clinical treatment for acute myocardial infarction.

CLINICAL APPLICATION OF HYPOTHERMIA FOR ACUTE MYOCARDIAL INFARCTION

Induction of hypothermia in humans

Methods used to induce cooling in experimental models include venous retroperfusion (29-31), surface cooling (25, 28), topical organ cooling (27), heat exchange devices (14) and various other techniques. For use in humans, the method used to induce cooling must be safe and effective, i.e. a reduction in body temperature must be achieved as quickly as possible in order to provide maximum protection for ischemic tissue. To date, the method of choice used to reduce temperature in patients with acute myocardial infarction, who are participating in clinical studies, is catheter-based, endovascular cooling. A catheter is inserted via the femoral vein into the inferior vena cava and inflated. A closed-circuit pumping system is then used to move a cooled solution through the catheter, reducing temperature systemically. This technique has been shown to be safe (38) and relatively rapid in reducing body temperature. In this study, the target core body temperature was 33°C, with cooling being maintained for 3h after reperfusion. Re-warming to 36.5°C was then performed over a 1 to 2h period. Shivering was suppressed using skin warming with the aid of a forced-air blanket, together with oral buspirone (30-60 mg), and intravenous meperidine (75-100 mg loading dose over 15 min, followed by an intravenous infusion at 25-35 mg/h). The results of such endovascular cooling suggest that: 1) mild systemic hypothermia can be induced in awake patients with acute myocardial infarction using an endovascular heat-exchange catheter: 2) endovascular cooling is safe and well tolerated during acute myocardial infarction; and 3) shivering can be suppressed successfully in awake patients during endovascular cooling through skin warming and pharmacologic intervention.

Preliminary clinical trials

So far, results have been published from one study by Dixon and colleagues showing the safety and efficacy of mild hypothermia used in patients receiving percutaneous coronary intervention for acute myocardial infarction (38). Although this study was not powered to show a reduction in myocardial infarct size (total patient population was 42), the median infarct size was lower in the treated group, and adverse cardiac events were reduced to 0% compared with 10% in normothermic patients. Currently studies such as "Hypothermia as an Adjunctive Therapy to Percutaneous Intervention in Patients with Acute Myocardial Infarction: COOL-MI" and "ICE-IT" are assessing the effects of mild hypothermia on myocardial infarct size. It will be crucial that cooling is instituted as soon as possible in these clinical trials. If cooling is instituted only at the time of, or after, reperfusion, it is unlikely to have a protective effect. The therapeutic window appears to be short in animal studies.

CARDIOVASCULAR INSUFFICIENCY

Hypothermia is known to suppress cellular automaticity (39). On the basis of this effect, the application of moderate hypothermia to infants with postoperative junctional tachycardia has been reported (40-43). Recently, hypothermia has been shown to have beneficial effects on the treatment of severe circulatory insufficiency of various etiologies including myocardial ischemia (44-47). This section will address the use of therapeutic systemic hypothermia as an adjunct to the treatment of low cardiac output states of various etiologies, including myocardial ischemia.

Mild hypothermia should theoretically decrease tissue oxygen demand and increase cardiac function, without increasing cardiac oxygen consumption. In addition, reducing metabolic demand by means of hypothermia has been reported to protect various organs during surgery (44-46). Indeed, mild hypothermia of between 33 and 35.5°C may improve oxygenation and survival in patients with lung failure. Moreover, a recent study in critically ill patients by Manthous and colleagues showed significant decreases in oxygen (VO_2) and carbon dioxide (VCO_2) consumption with cooling (48).

Sun et al, who studied the effects of coronary artery bypass during mild versus moderate hypothermia, noted a significantly lower incidence of postoperative atrial fibrillation in the mild hypothermia group (34°C) than in the moderate hypothermia group (28°C) (49). Use of moderate, but not mild, hypothermic cardiopulmonary bypass evoked a significant sympathetic response, with increases in plasma norepinephrine and neuropeptide Y concentrations. They also reported that increasing age is a significant determinant of postoperative atrial fibrillation (50).

Sympathetic activation, which is believed to be a normal defense mechanism against cold stress in humans, occurs at a core temperature of 34°C during general anesthesia (51). This sympathetic activation may lead to an increase in cardiac output and/or to spontaneous shivering and thermoregulatory peripheral vasoconstriction. Since deeper hypothermia has a negative chronotropic effect on the heart, one would expect cardiac output and heart rate to be reduced when core temperature is depressed further (52, 53). To prevent the development of such an undesirable situation, core temperature should be kept above 34°C.

Such mild hypothermia tends slightly to reduce VO_2, the actual decrease being related almost linearly to the decrease in temperature. The physiologic coupling between oxygen delivery (DO_2) and VO_2 seems to remain intact in survivors of the acute respiratory distress syndrome, according to one study (54). During cooling an increase in DO_2 occurred without an increase in VO_2. This markedly improved the O_2 extraction ratio, which decrease from a mean of 44.8% to 34.5%. This finding may be important, since a lower O_2 extraction ratio is associated with a reduced mortality rate in critically ill patients (55, 56). In the above patients, an optimal DO_2 could be maintained regardless of the temperature, and the authors could find no evidence of altered pulmonary function, inasmuch as there was no reduction in either PaO_2 or inspired O_2 consumption.

Mild hypothermia, with appropriate sedation, is a simple and useful procedure for improving the circulation in postcardiac surgical patients who develop severe heart failure despite the use of intra-aortic balloon pump, thus potentially relieving or preventing tissue hypoxia or subsequent organ failure.

Urine output may increase significantly by the hypothermia (45). One explanation is reduced reabsorption in the distal tubule of the kidney, which has been reported during hypothermia at 28°C (57). This enhanced urine flow could facilitate management of fluid balance, decreasing risk of pulmonary edema; but may also lead to inappropriate intravascular volume depletion.

Activated coagulation time (ACT), platelet count, and volume of chest-tube blood loss did not change as a result of the hypothermia in the above study (45). In trauma patients, hypothermia to below 34°C, especially in combination with acidosis, is associated with clinically significant bleeding, despite adequate blood, plasma, and platelet replacement (58). In another study, there was a negative correlation between local tissue temperature and bleeding time, although use of a systemic body temperature of 32°C together with local warming of the arm skin to 34°C restored the bleeding time to normal (59). The reason why mildly hypothermic patients did not show an increased blood loss (45) could be related to the use of adequate, but not excessive, sedation. Sedation or light anesthesia may produce sufficient vasodilation to maintain local tissue perfusion, thus keeping the tissue temperature and pH high enough to avoid the increase in bleeding time seen by other researchers (58).

It has been suggested that the extent of myocardial depression or decreased inotropy in the presence of hypothermia in normal hearts depends on the level of sedation and use of a vasodilator to prevent sympathetic adverse effects such as shivering or muscle rigidity and to maintain homeostasis (59). Some have recommended that the difference between the core body temperature and the peripheral body temperature (monitored on the palm of the hand) during cooling should ideally be less than 2°C (45). From experience of handling cardiopulmonary bypass, arrhythmia does not occur until a core body temperature of 30°C is reached, even at a maximal cooling rate. One advantage that postcardiac surgery patients have during hypothermia is that they already have temporary pacing wires placed on the surface of the heart, which could be used to control arrhythmias that might occur. In fact, in the study by Yahagi, et al (45), none of the patients had intractable arrhythmias during hypothermia.

Finally, it should be pointed out that care is needed in setting the optimal heart rate during mild hypothermia, since a pronounced prolongation of contraction and relaxation times limits the beneficial effects of cooling due to diastolic dysfunction (21, 22).

POTENTIAL NEGATIVE CONSEQUENCES OF HYPOTHERMIC THERAPY

Deep hypothermia is associated with adverse consequences such as decreased myocardial blood flow (3), deterioration in ventricular function (3, 12) and conduction disturbances including ventricular fibrillation (60, 61), but mild hypothermia has not been associated with these complications. Shivering is an adverse effect related to temperature reduction. To reduce shivering in humans, a combination of surface warming and pharmaceutical intervention with combined meperidine and buspirone (38, 62) have been used with success.

The issue of whether hypothermia slows thrombolysis must also be addressed before cooling can be used in patients receiving this intervention as treatment for coronary blockage. At least one *in vitro* study has suggested that the thrombolytic action of tissue plasminogen activator (tPA) is temperature dependent (63) and that its efficacy is reduced with even mild hypothermia.

SUMMARY

Data from many studies in various animal models have shown the importance of temperature on the progression of necrosis after acute myocardial infarction. Although cooling has long been used clinically for cardioprotection in the non-working heart, the use of hypothermia as therapy for acute myocardial infarction is only now being tested. Experimentally, cooling has been produced by various means including whole-body hypothermia, synchronized hypothermic coronary venous retro-perfusion, heat exchangers and regional hypothermia targeting the heart alone. It has been shown that cooling significantly reduces infarct size when initiated before or soon after the onset of ischemia. The reduction in temperature required to induce cardioprotection is mild (32-34°C), which appears to have no detrimental effects on left ventricular function or regional myocardial blood flow. In fact mild hypothermia may improve microvascular reflow to previously ischemic heart tissue. Clinical trials will determine the safety and efficacy of this intervention in humans suffering from acute myocardial infarction.

Mild hypothermia may also have benefit during cardiac insufficiency. Many questions remain, including understanding the mechanisms of the effects seen, the optimal combination of cooling and heart rate control, optimal speed of cooling and rewarming, and duration of hypothermia. Additional clinical studies are needed.

REFERENCES

1. Reimer KA, Jennings RB. The "wavefront phenomenon" of myocardial cell death. II. Transmural progression of necrosis with the framework of ischemic bed size (myocardium at risk) and collateral flow. *Lab Invest* 1979; 40:633-644.

2. Bigelow WG, Lindsay WK, Greenwood WF. Hypothermia. Its possible role in cardiac surgery: An investigation of factors governing survival in dogs at low body temperature. *Ann Surg* 1950; 132:849-866.

3. Tveita T, Mortensen E, Hevrøy O, et al. Experimental hypothermia: effects of core cooling and rewarming on hemodynamics, coronary blood flow, and myocardial metabolism in dogs. *Anesth Analg* 1994; 79:212-218.

4. Eidelman Y, Glat PM, Pachter HL, et al. The effects of topical hypothermia and steroids and ATP levels in an in vivo liver ischemia model. *J Trauma* 1994; 37:677-681.

5. Ning X-H, Xu C-S, Song YC, et al. Hypothermia preserves function and signaling for mitochondrial biogenesis during subsequent ischemia. *Am J Physiol* 1998; 274:H786-H793.

6. Zhang Z, Sobel RA, Cheng D, et al. Mild hypothermia increases Bcl-2 protein expression following global cerebral ischemia. *Brain Res Mol Brain Res* 2001; 95:75-85.

7. Edwards AD, Yue X, Squier MV, et al. Specific inhibition of apoptosis after cerebral hypoxia-ischaemia by moderate post-insult hypothermia. *Biochem Biophys Res Commun* 1995; 217:1193-1199.

8. Phanithi PB, Yoshida Y, Santana A, et al. Mild hypothermia mitigates post-ischemic neuronal death following focal cerebral ischemia in rat brain: immunohistochemical study of Fas, caspace-3 and TUNEL. *Neuropathology* 2001; 20:273-282.

9. Ning XH, Chen SH, Xu CS, et al. Hypothermic protection of the ischemic heart via alterations in apoptotic pathways as assessed by gene array analysis. *J Appl Physiol* 2002; 92:2200-2207.

10. Zar HA, Tanigawa K, Kim YM, et al. Mild therapeutic hypothermia for postischemic vasoconstriction in the perfused rat liver. *Anesthesiology* 1999; 90:1103-1111.

11. Hale SL, Dae M, Kloner RA. Hypothermia during reperfusion limits "no-reflow" injury in a rabbit model of acute myocardial infarction. *Cardiovasc Res* 2003; in press.

12. Tveita T, Skandfer M, Refsum H, et al. Experimental hypothermia and rewarming: changes in mechanical function and metabolism of rat heart. *J Appl Physiol* 1996; 80:291-297.

13. Weisser J, Martin J, Bisping E, et al. Influence of mild hypothermia on myocardial contractility and circulatory function. *Basic Res Cardiol* 2001; 96:198-205.

14. Dae MW, Gao DW, Sessler DI, et al. Effect of endovascular cooling on myocardial temperature, infarct size and cardiac output in human-sized pigs. *Am J Physiol* 2001; 282:H1584-H1591.

15. Lauri T, Leskinen M, Timisjarvi J. Effects of surface-induced hypothermia and rewarming on canine cardiac contraction-relaxation cycle. *Int J Circumpolar Hearth* 1997; 56:40-48.

16. Green PS, Cameron DE, Mohlala ML, et al. Systolic and diastolic left ventricular dysfunction due to mild hypothermia. *Circulation* 1989; 80: III44-48.

17. Goldberg LI. Effects of hypothermia on contractility of the intact dog heart. *Am J Physiol* 1958; 194:92-98.

18. Suga H, Sagawa K. Instantaneous pressure-volume relationships and their ratio in the excised, supported canine left ventricle. *Circ Res* 1974; 35:117-126.

19. Suga H, Goto Y, Igarashi Y, et al. Cardiac cooling increases Emax without affecting relation between O2 consumption and systolic pressure-volume area in left ventricle. *Circ Res* 1988; 63:61-71.

20. Mikane T, Araki J, Suzuki S, et al. O2 cost of contractility but not of mechanical energy increases with temperature in canine left ventricle. *Am J Physiol* 1999;277: H65-73.

21. Weisser J, Martin J, Bisping E, et al. Influence of mild hypothermia on myocardial contractility and circulatory function. *Basic Res Cardiol* 2001; 96:198-205.

22. Lewis ME, Al-Khalidi AH, Townend JN, et al. The effects of hypothermia on human left ventricular contractile function during cardiac surgery. *J Am Coll Cardiol* 2002; 39:102-108.

23. Henderson AH, Cattel MR. Length-induced changes in activation during contraction. *Circ Res* 1976; 38:289-296.

24. Mattheussen M, Mubagwa K, Van Aken H, et al. Interaction of heart rate and hypothermia on global myocardial contraction of the isolated rabbit heart. *Anesth Analg* 1996; 82:975-981.

25. Voorhees WD III, Abendchein DR, Tacker WA Jr. Effect of whole-body hypothermia on myocardial blood flow and infarct salvage during coronary artery occlusion in dogs. *Am Heart J* 1984; 107:945-949.

26. Schwartz LM, Verbinski SG, Vander Heide RS, Reimer KA. Epicardial temperature is a major predictor of infarct size in dogs. *J Mol Cell Cardiol* 1997; 29:1577-1583.

27. Hale SL, Kloner RA. Myocardial temperature in acute myocardial infarction: protecting ischemic myocardium with mild regional hypothermia in rabbits. *Am J Physiol* 1997; 273:H220-H227.

28. Abendschein, DR, Tacker WA Jr, Babbs CF. Protection of ischemic myocardium by whole-body hypothermia after coronary artery occlusion in dogs. *Am Heart J* 1978; 96:7722-780.

29. Meerbaum SM , Haendchen RV, Corday E, et al. Hypothermic coronary venous phased retroperfusion: A closed-chest treatment of acute regional myocardial ischemia. *Circulation* 1982; 65:1435-1445.

30. Wakida Y, Haendchen RV, Kobayashi S, et al. Percutaneous cooling of ischemic myocardium by hypothermic retroperfusion of autologous arterial blood: effects on regional myocardial temperature distribution and infarct size. *J Am Coll Cardiol* 1991; 18:293-300.

31. Haendchen RV, Corday E, Meerbaum S, et al. Prevention of ischemic injury and early reperfusion derangements by hypothermia retroperfusion. *J Am Coll Cardiol* 1983; 1:1067-1080.

32. Chien GL, Wolff RA, Davis RF, et al. "Normothermic range" temperature affects myocardial infarct size. *Cardiovasc Res* 1994; 28:1014-1017.

33. Duncker DJ, Klassen CL, Ishibashi Y, et al. Effect of temperature on myocardial infarction in swine. *Am J Physiol* 1996; 270:H1189-H1199.

34. McClanahan TB, Mertz TE, Martin BJ, et al. Pentostatin reduces infarct size in pigs only when combined with mild hypothermia (abstract). *Circulation* 1994; 90:I-478.

35. Van den Doel MA, Gho BCG, Duval SY, et al. Hypothermia extends the cardoprotection by ischaemic preconditioning to coronary artery occlusions of longer duration. *Cardiovasc Res* 1998; 37:76-81.

36. Hale SL, Dave RH, Kloner RA Regional hypothermia reduces myocardial necrosis even when instituted after the onset of ischemia. *Basic Res Cardiol* 1997; 92:351-357.

37. Miki R, Liu GS, Downey JM. Mild hypothermia reduces infarct size in the beating rabbit heart: a practical intervention for acute myocardial infarction? *Basic Res Cardiol* 1998; 93:372-383.

38. Dixon SR, Whitbourn RJ, Dae MW et al. Induction of mild systemic hypothermia with endovascular cooling during primary percutaneous coronary intervention for acute myocardial infarction. *J Am Coll Cardiol* 2002; 40:1928-1934.
39. Hoffmann BF. Temperature effects on cardiac transmembrane potentials. In: Dripps RD (ed). Physiology of induced hypothermia. Washington, DC: National Academy of Science, 1956: 302-326.
40. Bash SE, Shah JJ, Albers WH, et al. Hypothermia for the treatment of postsurgical greatly accelerated junctional ectopic tachycardia. *J Am Coll Cardiol* 1987; 10:1095-1099.
41. Balaji S, Sullivan J, Deanfield J, et al. Moderate hypothermia in the management of resistant automatic tachycardias in children. Br Heart J 1991; 66:221-224.
42. Till JA, Rowland E. Atrial pacing as an adjunct to the management of postsurgical His bundle tachycardia. *Br Heart J* 1991; 66:225-229.
43. Pfammatter JP, Paul T, Ziemer G, Kallfelz HC. Successful management of junctional tachycardia by hypothermia after cardiac operations in infants. *Ann Thorac Surg* 1995; 60:556-560.
44. Moriyama Y, Iguro Y, Shimokawa S, et al. Successful application of hypothermia combined with intra-aortic balloon pump support to low-cardiac-output state after open heart surgery. *Angiology* 1996; 47:595-599.
45. Yahagi N, Kumon K, Watanabe Y, et al. Value of mild hypothermia in patients who have severe circulatory insufficiency even after intra-aortic balloon pump. *J Clin Anesth* 1998; 10:120-125.
46. Moat NE, Lamb RK, Edwards JC, et al. Induced hypothermia in the management of refractory low cardiac output states following cardiac surgery in infants and children. Eur J Cardiothorac Surg 1992; 6:579-584.
47. Tisherman SA, Rodriguez A, Safar P. Therapeutic hypothermia in traumatology. *Surg Clin North Am* 1999; 79:1269-1289.
48. Manthous CA, Hall JB, Olson D, et al. Effect of cooling on oxygen consumption in febrile critically ill patients. *Am J Respir Crit Care Med* 1995; 151:10-14.
49. Sun LS, Adams DC, Delphin E, et al. Sympathetic response during cardiopulmonary bypass: mild versus moderate hypothermia. *Crit Care Med* 1997; 25:1990-1993.
50. Adams DC, Heyer EJ, Simon AE, et al. Incidence of atrial fibrillation after mild or moderate hypothermic cardiopulmonary bypass. Crit Care Med 2000; 28:309-311.
51. StØen R, Sessler DI. The thermoregulatory threshold is inversely proportional to isoflurane concentration. *Anesthesiology* 1990; 72:822-827.
52. Lauri T, Leskinen M, Timisjarivi J, et al. Cardiac function in hypothermia. *Arct Med Res* 1991; 50:63-66.
53. Gribbe P, Hirvonen L, Lind J, et al. Cineangiographic observations in hypothermic dogs. *Cardiologia* 1961; 39:341-362.
54. Pernerstorfer T, Kraff P, Fitzgerald R, et al. Optimal values for oxygen transport during hypothermia in sepsis and ARDS. *Acta Anaesth Scand* 1995; 107:223-227.
55. Shoemaker WC, Appel P, Bland R. Use of physiologic monitoring to predict outcome and to assist in clinical decisions in critically ill postoperative patients. *Am J Surg* 1983; 146:43-50.
56. Gilbert EM, Haupt MT, Mandanas RY, et al. The effect of fluid loading, blood transfusion, and catecholamine infusion on oxygen delivery and consumption in patients with sepsis. *Am Rev Respir Dis* 1986; 134:873-878.
57. Broman M, Kallskog O. The effects of hypothermia on renal function and haemodynamics in the rat. *Acta Physiol Scand* 1995; 153:179-184.

58. Ferrara A, MacArthur JD, Wright HK, et al. Hypothermia and acidosis worsen coagulopathy in the patient requiring massive transfusion. *Am J Surg* 1990; 160:515-518.

59. Wong KC. Physiology and pharmacology of hypothermia. *West J Med* 1983; 138:227-232.

60. Pattison CW, Dimitri WR, Williams BT. Persistent conduction disturbances following coronary artery bypass surgery: cold cardioplegia vs. intermittent ischaemic arrest (32 degrees C). *Scand J Thorac Cardiovasc Surg* 2001; 25:151-154.

61. Mouritzen, CV, Andersen MN. Mechanisms of ventricular fibrillation during hypothermia. *J Thorac Cardiovasc Surg* 1966; 5:585-589.

62. Mokhtarani M, Mahgoub A, Morioka N, et al. Buspirone and meperidine synergistically reduce the shivering threshold. *Anesth Analg* 2001; 93:1233-1239.

63. Shaw GJ, Dhamija A, Holland CK et al. Temperature dependence of tPA thrombolysis in an in-vitro clot model. *Acad Emerg Med* 2003; 10:438-439.

Chapter 14

COOLING METHODS

Gernot Kuhnen, PhD[1], Niels Einer-Jensen, DVM[2], Samuel A. Tisherman, MD[3]

[1]*Büro für Thermophysiologie, Pohlheim, Germany*
[2]*Institute of Medical Biology, University of Southern Denmark, Odense, Denmark*
[3]*Safar Center for Resuscitation Research, University of Pittsburgh, Pittsburgh, PA*

INTRODUCTION

Laboratory studies of therapeutic hypothermia have utilized animals that are much smaller than the average-sized human, making rapid cooling feasible. Cooling techniques can be very invasive without concern about the long-term risks. In addition, cooling is often started either before or early during the insult. For therapeutic hypothermia to be taken to clinical trials and, further, to become part of standard clinical practice, novel cooling techniques will be needed. The optimal technique for total body cooling should be easily applied, should cool the entire organism rapidly, and should carry little risk. Ideally, the technique should be applicable by lay people or physician extenders, preferably even in the field. In addition, techniques for selective brain cooling may provide the same benefits without the possible systemic side effects.

This chapter will describe several novel techniques for cooling that are currently being explored.

EXTERNAL COOLING

Cooling cap

Since the brain is the most vulnerable organ to ischemia and trauma and systemic hypothermia has potentially detrimental side effects, differential cooling of the brain while maintaining systemic normothermia is appealing. The simplest method to accomplish this would be to place an external cooling device on the head. In small animals (1-6), it is possible to differentially cool the brain, particularly if heating is applied to the rest of the body. In adults, however, with much larger brains and skulls, heat transfer from the brain through the scalp is much slower. Unfortunately, the high flow of warm blood through the cerebral circulation limits the effectiveness of this technique. Dennis, et al (7), utilized an anatomically realistic 3-D model of the head and neck to see if external cooling by ice packs or a head-cooling helmet could result in decreasing brain temperature to 33°C within 30 min. Neither technique was effective. The main limitation was the uncooled carotid artery supply, which would have to be decreased by a factor of 10 to allow adequate cooling. In contrast, Diao, et al (8), found that if the model included decreased brain perfusion at 20% normal, cooling of gray matter by 3°C would be feasible within 26 min in adults.

In patients with multiple sclerosis, Ku, et al (9), tested a portable cooling system and liquid cooling helmet. The helmet fits snugly on the subjects' head and neck. A solution of propylene glycol and water at <10°C is circulated through the helmet. Over 30 min, this device lead to a decrease in ear temperature of about 1°C and a decrease in oral temperature of 0.2-0.6°C. Intracranial blood flow decreased by about 33%.

Wang, et al (10), applied a cooling helmet designed from National Aeronautics and Space Administration technology to patients with severe stroke or head injury. The helmet has a conformal liquid cooling heat exchanger layer and a pressurized air bladder layer to improve the contact with the skin. Brain temperature 0.8 cm beneath the cortical surface was monitored. Within 1 h of helmet application, brain temperature decreased by 0.9-2.4°C. Brain temperature decreased to 34°C at 2-6 h. Systemic temperature decreased below 36°C slowly. A control group without the helmet had a slight increase in brain temperature.

Mellergard (11) applied various cooling techniques to patients with severe subarachnoid hemorrhage or traumatic brain injury. Application of blocks of frozen liquid to the scalp decreased epidural temperature by only 1°C. Intraventricular temperature did not change. Use of a cooling helmet circulating cold fluid only decreased epidural temperature by about 0.5-

0.6°C. Nasopharyngeal cooling with cold oxygen had almost no effect on brain temperature. In febrile patients, administration of paracetamol decreased rectal temperature by 0.6-1.2°C and brain temperature by 2°C. Interestingly, administration of a barbiturate for control of intracranial hypertension sometimes led to an increase in brain temperature associated with a decreased in systemic temperature. The only method that successfully decreased brain temperature was total body cooling using a combination of head cooling, paracetamol, fanning the body, washing with 70% alcohol, and ice packs placed in the axillary and inguinal regions.

Convection cooling

Convection cooling was used for cooling patients after cardiac arrest by the Hypothermia after Cardiac Arrest Study Group (12). A mattress (TheraKool, Kinetic Concepts, Wareham, United Kingdom) with a cover that delivers cold air was placed over the subject's body. Although the goal was to decrease core temperature to 32-34°C within 4 h after restoration of spontaneous circulation, the goal temperature was not reached for a median of 8 h. Application of ice packs increased the rate of cooling (13).

INTRAVENOUS FLUIDS

As a follow up to the successful randomized clinical trials that demonstrated improved outcome after cardiac arrest with induction of mild hypothermia after restoration of spontaneous circulation, Bernard, et al (14), performed a small feasibility study of bolus infusion of 30 ml/kg of ice-cold lactated Ringer's solution after restoration of spontaneous circulation. This resulted in a decrease in temperature from 35.5 to 33.8°C. Interestingly, the bolus also increased blood pressure. There was no comparison group, but it appears that this technique is safe to apply. Further study is needed to determine efficacy.

INTRAVASCULAR CATHETERS

Specialized central venous catheters

Cooling blood with an intra-corporeal device has gained interest because of its simplicity, safety, and potential for long-term use. The Cool Line™ (Alsius Corporation, Irvine, CA, USA) central venous catheter has 2 standard lumens, plus 2 balloons on the external surface of the catheter. It is inserted just like a standard central venous catheter. Cold or warm water is circulated through the balloons via the CoolGard 3000® system which regulates the temperature of this fluid to maintain the patient's temperature at the desired level. Blood that flows by the catheter is then warmed or cooled as needed. Schmutzhard, et al (15), demonstrated that this system can accurately maintain normothermia in a population of patients with severe neurologic diseases in a neurologic intensive care unit. The catheters were easily inserted, were well tolerated by patients, and had few complications. Similarly, Radiant Medical, Inc. (Redwood City, CA) has developed the Setpoint® endovascular temperature management system. The catheter utilized in this system has a helically-wound balloon mounted on the distal portion of the catheter. Doufas, et al (16), tested the ability of this system to cool neurosurgical patients to 34-34.5°C in the operating room. The core-cooling rate was 3.9±1.6°C/h. The rewarming rate was 2.0±0.5°C/h. No complications secondary to placement of the catheter occurred.

Intravascular venous heat exchangers (IVHE)

An alternative to the specialized central venous catheters is the use of IVHE, which combines a relatively high cooling rate with a minor surgical intervention. This approach could provide rapid core cooling, without selective brain cooling. This has developed and used in thermoregulatory studies in conscious goats (17).

Under sterile conditions and general anesthesia, one or more thin U-shaped polyethylene tubes were introduced into the venous vascular system with the U-turn-point advanced first. The tubes were covered by very thin silicone tubes to prevent blood from clotting around the tubes. From the point of entry into one jugular vein, the IVHE was guided into the superior vena cava, through the right atrium of the heart into the inferior vena cava, and advanced as far as the iliac bifurcation. The inlet and outlet of the U-shaped tube stayed extracorporeally and were connected to a cooling or heating device. The temperature and the flow of the fluid pumped through the U-shaped tubes determine the level of heat exchange.

In goats, about 5 W/kg could be extracted with the IVHE (about 200 W) (18). By using an increased pressure gradient of about 4 bar between inlet and outlet of the IVHE, the flow rate through the heat exchanger and the heat extraction could be increased to 9 W/kg (about 270 W) (17). In rabbits a heat subtraction of 5-6 W/kg was reached (19).

The use of an IVHE combines a high cooling capacity with technically simple surgical implantation of the tubes. However, this method does not allow selective brain hypothermia during core normothermia. This method seems to be more suitable for clinical usage than the method described below, however. The point of entry and length of the intravascular heat exchangers can be different from the example shown above. A similar set-up was used in a prospective pilot study in intensive care patients (15). However, due to low flow rate and a small heat exchange area, the set-up used in that study did not reach the same cooling capacity as that presented above.

EXTRACORPOREAL COOLING

Veno-venous cooling

Extracorporeal heat exchange with blood could provide even more efficient heat transfer than the catheter system above. Using 2 large-bore venous catheters or a double-lumen catheter, blood can readily be withdrawn from patients, cooled via an extra-corporeal circuit, and pumped back into the venous system.

Behringer, et al (20), tested a very simple veno-venous cooling system in anesthetized dogs. Two venous catheters were used. Blood was pumped by a small roller pump at 200 ml/min through intravenous fluid administration tubing that was immersed in ice water. Tympanic membrane temperature (Tty) decreased from 37.5°C to 34°C in approximately 5 min. In contrast, surface cooling with alcohol, a fan, and ice packs cooled Tty from 37.5°C to 34°C in 20 min.

In a cardiac arrest outcome study, Nozari, et al (21), examined the effects of mild hypothermia induction during cardiac arrest. Cooling was initiated with bolus infusion of ice-cold saline, which decreased Tty from 37.5°C to 36°C. Veno-venous cooling using the technique tested by Behringer, et al (20), then decreased Tty to 34°C within another 2 min. When the veno-venous cooling was continued during prolonged (40 min) cardiopulmonary resuscitation, Tty decreased to 27°C.

This system was designed to be as simple as possible, utilizing ice-cold water and just one pump, so that it could be feasible in the prehospital setting. In the hospital, a heat exchanger could be added along with a pump for counter-current flow of water. In addition, the technique could be simplified by using a large, double-lumen catheter for inflow and outflow instead of two separate peripheral venous catheters.

Extracorporeal carotid heat exchangers (ECHE) for independent control of brain and core temperatures

An extracorporeal heat exchanger (ECHE) could allow independent control of brain and core temperatures at predetermined levels. This was developed and used in thermoregulatory studies in conscious goats (22-24), and was recently modified and adapted to pigs to be used in basic studies of hypothermia (25, 26).

Because the brain is the most sensitive organ to ischemia and anoxia, there has been tremendous interest in improving cerebral outcome following a number of insults, including cardiac arrest, head trauma, and stroke. Given that induction of systemic hypothermia does carry some risk, selective brain cooling would be appealing. Unfortunately, simple methods, such as an ice cap (1-6), work well in small animals with a short distance from the scalp to deep brain, but would be ineffective in adult humans.

The brain is supplied mainly by the right and left carotid arteries (and to a small degree by the vertebral arteries). The hypothesis was that by placing extracorporeal heat exchangers in line with the carotid circulation, with one perfusing the brain and one returning blood to the systemic circulation, brain and core temperatures could be controlled independently.

The technique of ECHE is as follows:

Under sterile conditions and general anesthesia both carotid arteries were divided and exteriorized. After heparinization of the animal (500 IU/kg), one proximal end of the carotid artery was connected by silicone tubes (the silicone tubes were fitted to the vessels via Teflon connectors) and by a Y-piece to both distal carotid arteries (forming the head line). A heat exchanger inserted in this line controls the temperature of the blood supplying the brain and allows control of brain temperature (Figure 14-1). The second proximal carotid artery was connected to an external jugular vein to create an arteriovenous shunt (forming the core line). A heat exchanger in this line controls core temperature via the temperature of the blood flowing to the trunk (Figure 14-1). Flow measurements in conscious goats have shown that the 'Y-piece configuration' and the division of one jugular vein do not reduce the blood flow through the head (27). Measurements of temperature, heart rate, cardiac output, and arterial pressure have shown that this set-up allows isolated brain cooling without side-effects on core temperature or on the cardiovascular system (25).

By perfusing the heat exchanger with cold or warm water, heat could be subtracted from, or added to, the blood to keep the controlled temperature at a predetermined level. The heat exchange capacity depends on blood flow through the heat exchanger and the temperature difference between blood and temperature-controlled water passing through the heat exchanger. In general, in goats (body weights 35-55 kg) approximately 300 W could be subtracted from, and 140 W added to, the core while the values for the head line were about 100 W and 50 W, respectively. The basic requirement of this temperature controlling system is the low flow resistance of the heat exchanger and the good heat transfer inside the heat exchanger between blood and water flow.

During the experiments, when the full heat exchange capacity was not needed, the blood flow through the core line (arteriovenous shunt) was controlled to avoid chronic volume load of the heart. The development of clotting of blood in the tubes and the heat exchangers was hindered by a daily dose of an anticoagulant. Generally, the animals could be maintained in good condition for 3 to 9 months.

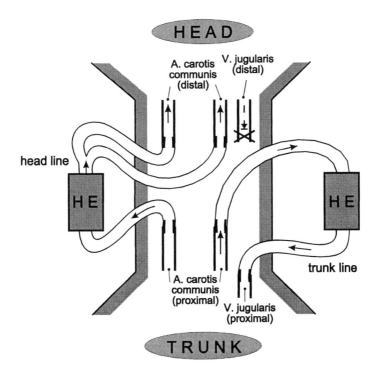

Figure 14-1. Schematic presentation of the set-up for the independent manipulation of head/brain and trunk temperatures. To control the heat exchange by the heat exchangers (HE), the blood flow through the HE and the blood temperatures before and after it, should be measured.

The presented technique allows the generation of brain hypothermia with maintenance of core normothermia at predetermined temperature levels. This avoids numerous unintentional physiological side effects which may accompany whole body hypothermia (28), e.g., decreased cardiac output, increased vascular resistance and cardiac arrhythmias (29, 30), myocardial ischemia (31), and impaired immune function (32).

Previous experimental approaches to selectively induced brain hypothermia have used two methods: The first is conductive cooling of the brain, which uses the cooling of the surface of the head (1-6). The second method is convective cooling, which uses an intravascular device (15), hemodilution with cold Ringer's lactate solution (33), or cooling blood from the femoral artery (34) or carotid artery (35). These methods have been unable to prevent a concomitant decrease in core temperature. As a result, core temperature could not be well controlled and brain temperature could be reduced, but not clamped at a precise predetermined level. Additionally, the conductive cooling of the head (e.g., cooling cap) causes large temperature differences within the brain.

The cooling capacity of the ECHE is high, and a predetermined cooling level could be reached quickly. For instance the brain temperature of young anesthetized pigs (25) could be lowered from 38 to 25°C within 3 minutes with a mean cooling rate of 4.3°C/min (up to 150 W were subtracted from the arterial blood). In this way, a steady state of deep brain hypothermia could be reached within a proposed 'therapeutic time window'. Even the cooling of a whole conscious adult goat (body weight 48 kg) can be accomplished with a cooling rate of 0.3°C/min (36). A constant level of temperature could be kept exactly. In most cases the temporal temperature dispersion is smaller than 0.1°C, even in conscious animals, which may attempt to autoregulate against a predetermined temperature level. Small brains may be cooled by conductive heat transfer, but the only effective way to cool large brains is convective cooling by means of their blood supply (11, 37).

Using the natural blood supply for temperature control results in a homogeneous temperature field. By using the carotid blood flow to control brain temperature by convective heat transfer, the temperature at all brain sites supplied predominantly by the carotid blood can be controlled. The temperature control is incomplete at brain sites, e.g., cerebellum, which receive (depending on the species) a considerable portion of their blood supply via the vertebral arteries (25). This disadvantage can be avoided by occluding the vertebral arteries (23).

A possible disadvantage of the present method may arise from the heparinization procedure. This would require surgical procedures, which could be accompanied by major bleeding, to be performed before the heparinization. However, in a recent study, delayed bleeding from surgical wounds nor macroscopically visible bleeding in the brain were observed at necropsy (25). Thus, the anticoagulation therapy did not restrict the experimental procedure used. Heparin-bonded catheters and heat exchangers could be used to avoid such complications of the procedure.

At this point it seems necessary to point out that the method was designed for basic experiments in animals; it may not be a practical method for use in patients. Additionally, the surgical procedure may limit the practical use. These problems may be reduced by percutaneous cannulation of the carotid artery which reduces the surgical intervention (but the cooling capacity, too, due to smaller diameter of the connectors) or by the use of the method described below.

LOCAL TRANSFER OF HEAT AND SUBSTANCES BETWEEN VESSELS

Counter current heat transfer takes place between two closely connected tubes where the flows have opposite directions (counter flow). The principle is used in mechanical engineering, e.g., to transfer heat from one fluid to the other without mixing the fluids.

The principle of local counter current transfer of substances has physiologic similarity to both traditional blood distribution of hormones and paracrine effects. Countercurrent transfer of heat will result in cooling or heating of an organ (testis) or part of an organ (maturating follicles). Countercurrent transfer of substances may be regarded as an intermittent feed back action between the two mentioned above, as the transfer may result in a semi-specific redistribution to organs like the ovary of substances (e.g. progesterone) produced by the organ. The blood and lymph vessels to an organ are often running closely together for a distance, therefore creating the possibility of counter current transfer. Transfer of heat has been described between vessels to several organ systems by Schmidt Nielsen (38). The present section will mainly review research in the area of counter current transfer in the reproductive organs and the brain. The review will speculate on possible therapeutic aspects of local heat transfer. In addition, heat transfer will be discussed as a tool for investigating transfer of substances and therefore also as a tool for development of local treatment.

Cooling of the testis and epididymis

The testis has a temperature 2-4°C below body temperature. The low temperature is thought to be essential for normal spermatogenesis or storage of the sperm in the caput of the epididymis (39). The low testicular temperature is induced by heat loss through the scrotal wall and maintained by a close to 100% effective cooling of the testicular arterial blood by the local venous outflow in the pampiniform plexus. The efficiency of the heat transfer was shown during *in vitro* experiments with bull testes kept at 35°C. The testicular veins and artery were perfused under controlled conditions: the flows, as well as the temperatures, of the fluids going in and out were measured (40). Since the heat transfer is extremely effective, only a limited amount of heat loss through the scrotum is needed, thus an expensive loss of energy is avoided.

Increased testicular temperature has created some interest in connection with infertility of men. Prolonged bathing in hot water is said to decrease both the sperm quality and numbers. Men may have impaired heat transfer, e.g., due to a varicocele in the pampiniform plexus. Long-term use of cooling devices covering the scrotum may improve sperm quality. In addition, cooling of the testes during systemic chemotherapy may protect the process of spermatogenesis.

Transfer of testosterone from the testicular vein blood to the testicular arterial blood creates a zone (the testis and the caput of epididymis) where the endogenous level of testosterone is higher than that in the rest of the body (41). It could seem logical to treat testosterone deficiency and impaired spermatogenesis with testicular implants of long acting testosterone preparations, but negative psychological reactions may be expected. Since there is a local, high, blood-carried testosterone concentration, the importance of the androgen binding protein for transport of testosterone from the testis to the caput should be re-evaluated.

Temperature differences within the ovary

The ovary and its blood vessels are localized in the middle of the pelvis, thus the organ should not be expected to be capable of inducing temperatures different from that of the rest of the body. However, there are strong suggestions of temperature differences within the ovary. Using a thermo camera to simultaneously register the difference between follicular and stromal temperatures immediately after the abdomen was opened and the ovary exposed, the temperature of large follicles was found to be 0.5 to 1.0°C below that of the ovarian stroma in rabbits (42) and pigs (43). Similar temperature differences were observed when the thermo camera was connected to an endoscope and the ovary photographed *in situ*. The decrease in follicular temperature seems to be based on two mechanisms: a heat consuming process during the rapid growth period of large follicles (44) and a very localized transfer of heat between the follicular vessels. The latter has not been measured, but is supported by anatomical studies of the vessels (45). The reason for the low follicular temperature is not clear, though it is interesting that both the male and female gamete seem to need a "below body temperature" environment.

Heat transfer between the main ovarian veins and artery has not been documented, since the idea has not been investigated. However, counter current transfer of substances including inert gases, steroids, peptides, and prostaglandins has been found in several animal species (46) and in women (47). In mono-ovulatory species, including man, one must expect a difference in hormonal levels between the two sides. Ovarian arterial blood does have a higher content of endogenous estradiol and progesterone than peripheral arterial blood; thus an ipsilateral communication takes place between the different ovarian structures. In ruminants, the luteolytic effects of prostaglandin $F_{2\alpha}$ of uterine origin are based on local transfer from the utero-ovarian veins to the ovarian artery. The Fallopian tube and the tubal part of the uterus (see below) are supplied by the ovarian artery and are therefore part of the local environment.

Transfer of heat from vagina to uterus and urethra

Local transfer of heat is a good indicator of a potential transfer of substances. There appears to be a correlation between transfer of heat and transfer of substances in experimental models where both types have been investigated. Documentation of heat transfer can therefore be taken as a strong indicator of substance transfer. It is a useful clinical tool, since transfer of heat can be investigated with safe and minimally invasive methods in conscious persons. Investigations of the female genital organs (vagina, uterus, and urethra) are examples of this potential.

Vaginal flushing with saline (room temperature) or saline infusion into the balloon of a Foley catheter positioned close to the cervix induced cooling of the uterus through local transfer of (negative) heat between the vaginal-uterine veins and the uterine arteries. The temperature was measured every two seconds at 2, 4, or 8 points using ELLAB equipment (www.ELLAB.com). The temperature decreased in the corpus of the uterus, but not in the tubal corner of the uterus in menopausal women. The results indicate that the arterial supply to the tubal corner originates from the ovarian and not the uterine artery since the cooling was associated with the arterial supply (48, 49). Results obtained in younger, cycling women indicate that the border between the arterial supply moves some centimeters during the ovulatory cycle due to a local influence of the ovarian hormones (Cicinelli and Einer-Jensen, personal communication).

As a result of local transfer, vaginally applied progesterone will have a higher local effect on the endometrium than if the hormone were administered by intramuscular injection (50). Vaginal application of progesterone is now standard procedure to secure a secretory endometrium during *in vitro* fertilization procedures. Vaginal administration of small lipid-soluble cytostatic agents for treatment of uterine and possibly ovarian cancer should be considered prior to surgery, since local transfer would induce a relatively high local concentration in the arterial blood reaching the involved organ. The drugs would also penetrate to the local lymph vessels and provide local treatment of eventual metastases in the lymph glands.

Cooling of the vagina also induces local cooling of the urethra in menopausal women. The cooling was measured with a 4-point temperature probe with a diameter of 0.7 mm (51). This provides a rational basis for vaginal treatment with estrogens for menopausal urinary incontinence. A low estrogen dose will be sufficient and provide local impact on the urethra. The position of the hormone within the vagina seems important. Low vaginal application favors distribution to the urethra, while a high vaginal application favors distribution to the uterus (Cicinelli, personal communication).

Brain cooling

The brain, particularly after traumatic brain injury (TBI) or ischemia, is highly sensitive to increases in its temperature. During heat stress, including high fever, irreversible damage is induced in the brain before any other organ is endangered. Consequently, nature has over time developed a local brain cooling system to increase survival. Well-developed systems are found in many hunting and hunted mammalian species, where maximal muscular efforts otherwise might increase the brain temperature to dangerous levels (52).

The cooling system is very simple in principle. The respiratory air passing the nasal cavities cools the nasal surface, which cools the blood flowing through the surrounding tissues. The temperature of the nasal venous blood is therefore some degrees lower than the core temperature. Eventually, this cooler blood reaches the base of the brain via the infraorbital vein. The cold venous blood in the cavernous sinus is flowing in the opposite direction to the blood in the embedded carotid artery and is therefore able to cool the arterial blood to the brain. Many animal species, e.g., cats, pigs, and cows, have a special structure expanding the cooling surface of the carotid. It is called the rete mirabile, which consists of a large number of thin, short, parallel arteries within the cavernous sinus. In addition to the cavernous sinus, both animals and man have several other sinuses where transfer may take place (53).

In addition to brain cooling, the possible local transfer of substances from brain veins to brain arteries opens a huge number of possible local regulatory mechanisms of brain function. Transfer of substances has been documented in animals (54, 55), but not yet in man. Secretion of hormones from a brain center may reach other brain centers in a semi-selective manner, since only a minor fraction of the venous content is transferred. The principle may be most effective in the regulation of basic functions, such as mood. The therapeutic aspect is also promising since nasal application of a substance could provide a semi-selective port of administration (similar to the cooling effect described below).

Man does not have a rete mirabile and the presence of a brain cooling mechanism is controversial. In 1993, a heated discussion took place in two articles in the same journal between pro-cooling and no-cooling authors (56, 57). A major part of the "pro-evidence" was based on measurements of the tympanic temperature and the disputed assumption that tympanic temperature followed the brain temperature closely. Since then there have been several papers based on invasive brain measurements in neurosurgical patients; some indicate signs of brain cooling, others do not (58-60).

By tradition, many scientists and clinicians expect the brain temperature to be similar to the body core temperature. It may, however, be lower due to local cooling, but higher during conditions where the local blood flow is impaired. The brain set point may also be different from the body temperature set point due to local damage. The mistake may harm an unknown number of patients; since the brain may suffer from overheating while the body temperature is normal.

If one wants to know the brain temperature, it must be measured inside the brain, since no method at present can reliably measure the brain temperature from outside the head. Development of a non-invasive method to measure brain temperature would be a major step forward, especially if continuous measurement were possible. Neurosurgical patients often undergo craniotomy and insertion of a catheter to measure the intracranial pressure, since increased pressure is as destructive as increased temperature. Today, disposable combination brain catheters that measure both temperature and pressure are available. Such catheters could be used to validate the hypotheses below without any additional risk for the patient, but with a huge potential of benefit.

Autoregulation of brain temperature appears to be based on a special arrangement of the nasal venous outflow, though this is poorly understood. The blood may take two routes: a) a deep pathway through the infraorbital vein to the cavernous sinus providing cooling of the carotid blood, and b) a superficial pathway through the facial veins by-passing the cooling system (61). A muscular sphincter on the facial vein close to its origin is able to redirect the blood from the superficial to the deep pathway. The bottom line seems to be that cooling takes place on demand. A hypothermic brain may avoid cooling while a hyperthermic brain could have very active cooling. Some of the clinical investigations probably overlooked this basic physiological mechanism.

Brain cooling is based on the cooling effect of the respiratory air. Disruption of the airflow must obviously interfere with brain cooling. Tracheal intubation of anesthetized animals or humans provides a model of potential importance. An animal model was created that easily could be adapted to a clinical situation (62). Young pigs were anesthetized, intubated, and supported on artificial ventilation. Anesthesia was maintained with oxygen, nitrous oxide and isoflurane. A hollow catheter for ventricular pressure measurement was inserted into the third ventricle through a burr hole. A temperature probe was inserted inside the catheter with the tip positioned in the third ventricle. A rectal temperature probe was also inserted. The temperatures were measured every 2 sec and transferred to an ELLAB computer program (www.ellab.com). Two catheters were inserted deep into the nasal cavities and oxygen flow established for 15 min followed by a similar recovery period before each new session. Different flow rates (2 - >10 l/min) as well as oxygen temperatures of 5°C and 23°C were investigated. Saline was injected into the nasal cavities in some cases. The results showed a flow dependent temperature decrease in the brain (0.5 – 2°C) without affecting the rectal temperature with the physiological range of oxygen flow selected. We found no obvious difference between the effects of the saline compared to cold air. Finally, the pig was transitioned from the gas anesthesia to intravenous barbiturate. The tracheal tube was removed when spontaneous respiration was adequate. The transfer from the tube to nasal respiration decreased the brain temperature by 0.6°C. The experiments indicate a clear cooling effect of nasal airflow on the brain temperature (62).

A similar experiment was conducted on large, anesthetized rats (63). They were breathing spontaneously through a tracheal catheter and two needle temperature probes were inserted with a stereotactic instrument into brain tissue through burr holes. The rectal temperature was also measured. Nasal flushing with 100–1000 ml/min induced a decrease in the brain temperatures similar to that in the pigs (0.5 – 2°C) (57). The highest, more-than-physiologic oxygen flow also decreased the body temperature. The rat results are interesting since they show that the rete mirabile is not necessary for significant cooling. This is essential for the present discussion of brain cooling in man, since man does not have a rete mirabile.

Man and brain cooling

Scientists like to regard themselves as objective. However, they also tend to perform and evaluate experiments in a way that support their own hypotheses. The discussion for and against brain cooling is an example, as one finds believers and non-believers. This section will suggest that brain cooling in man is possible. It will concentrate on two hypotheses:

1. Intubation bypasses the normal brain cooling mechanism in man and may eventually induce brain damage in hyperthermic patients.
2. The brain damage caused by hyperthermia can be diminished by a nasal gas flow.

Many mammals have a brain cooling system. It is fair to assume that this is part of the general selection and development involved in evolution, and that it should be present in man also. Selective brain cooling is logical since the brain is the first organ to be damaged by an increased temperature, while other organ systems may actually benefit from a small increase in body temperature. Since primates are mammals, one would expect that a brain cooling system would be present. However, man has recently (from a developmental point) developed a unique method to diminish heat stress: a sparse hair coating supplemented with clothes and heating when needed. Thus a brain cooling mechanism may rarely be essential and active in man. An individual may simply adjust the environment to feel comfortable. In addition, investigations in normal man into whether or not a cooling mechanism exists may underestimate the potential of the mechanism, since it is normally dormant and/or the effect diminished through autoregulation of the route of the venous outflow. In addition, it is difficult and/or unethical to measure the brain temperature in man, since reliable non-invasive methods do not yet exist. Tympanic temperature measurements may represent brain temperature, but this is controversial, making any studies based on this method suspect. Brain and core temperature are frequently different, but measurements of core temperature (e.g., rectal or esophageal) are important for comparison.

Clinical studies should be performed on the "right" patients. One approach for investigations could be to study patients under heat stress (a hot environment or hard physical work) or patients with an endogenous increase in brain temperature (infections or brain trauma). The "right" methods should also be selected. Unfortunately, this involves invasive methods at present, since this is the only way to measure temperature in the brain.

The demands above cannot be met in healthy persons, where application of invasive methods would be unethical. A group of patients may, however, be studied without ethical concerns, e.g., patients being monitored for increased intracranial pressure (ICP). The recent development of disposable catheters for simultaneous measurement of intra-ventricular pressure and temperature allow brain temperature measurements without any additional risk.

Patients suspected of long term increased ICP may develop hydrocephalus. This may be treated by insertion of a valve regulating the outflow of ventricular fluid. The intracranial pressure is measured after the insertion for a prolonged period during which the patient is conscious. During this period it may be acceptable to also measure the brain and esophageal/rectal (core) temperature and even induce moderate heat stress to observe potential differences between the two temperatures. It may also be possible to ask the heat stressed patient to alternate in 15 min periods between breathing through the mouth and through the nose. This will deactivate and activate the brain cooling mechanism and possibly induce variations in the brain temperature and the brain-rectal temperature difference.

Tracheal intubation is commonly performed for anesthesia and intensive care. It is without any doubt a safe and frequently lifesaving procedure. However, special groups should be investigated for potential side effects induced by intubation: patients with hyperthermia and patients with TBI (64). After intubation, the nasal airflow is stopped, thus preventing selective brain cooling. An increased brain temperature may be present in both cases, perhaps more so because of the intubation. Measurement of intracranial pressure via a ventriculostomy is common in patients with severe TBI and risk of increased ICP. There would be no added risk to inserting a pressure-temperature catheter to follow intracranial pressure and temperature in addition to the core temperature. One could then investigate the effects of selective brain cooling established by gas flow through the nasal cavities. The gas used may be sterile oxygen, nitrogen or atmospheric air. It may be at room temperature and humidified. The flow should be applied for 15 min periods in stepwise increases, starting with normal tidal volume (5 l/min) increasing to maximal ventilation (30-40 l/min) or more. One may expect a "dose-response" cooling effect in man based on the pig and rat results, and the results from one trial in man (Einer-Jensen and De Thomassi, personal information) (Figure 14-2).

If the feasibility of selective brain cooling in man can be documented, large-scale preventive brain cooling through nasal flushing with air or oxygen could be initiated at an early stage in patients with acute insults to the brain, perhaps already in the ambulance. Indications could include global brain ischemia (cardiac arrest), stroke, TBI, asphyxiation, or heat stroke. The rationale is that even a limited decrease in brain temperature may benefit long-term neurologic function. The procedure is safe and cheap. Nasal oxygen is often administered therapeutically anyway; the whole change would be an increase in flow. Given the ease of use and low cost of implementation, a multi-center study looking at outcome could be performed once a physiologic effect in man is demonstrated.

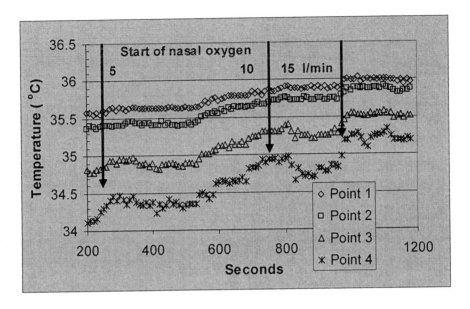

Figure 14-2. Brain temperature measured with a 4-point temperature probe inserted into a human brain before removal of a deep tumor. The patient was intubated during the procedure, thus stopping the natural airflow through the nasal cavities. The points were each separated by 7 mm; point 1 in the tip of the probe was inserted approximately 35 mm. The nasal cavities were flushed with 5, respectively 10 and 15 l/min oxygen. The tissue temperature at start was low and increasing; the nasal oxygen prevented the increase or actually decreased the brain temperature, indicating a brain cooling effect in man of nasal administration of oxygen (Einer-Jensen and De Thomassi, personal communication)

INTRAPERITONEAL COOLING

Skin surface cooling is slow and cumbersome. The peritoneal surface offers significant advantages including a much larger surface area and a contained space so that cold fluid could be instilled and drained in a controlled manner. Instillation of cold fluid into the peritoneal cavity has been utilized clinically for treatment of severe hyperpyrexia (65). For rapid cooling to mild hypothermia levels, peritoneal cooling was explored by Xiao, et al (66). Two liters of Ringer's solution at 10°C was instilled into the peritoneal cavity of dogs. The fluid was left for 5 min, then allowed to drain. Tympanic temperature decreased by 0.3°C/min, while pulmonary artery temperature decreased by 0.8°C/min. The target temperature of 34°C was achieved in 12 min for tympanic temperature and 5 min for pulmonary artery temperature. There were no specific complications secondary to placement of the peritoneal catheter. Use of peritoneal cooling plus surface cooling improved neurologic outcome compared to normothermia after prolonged cardiac arrest.

For more profound cooling needed for surgery with hypothermic circulatory arrest, Fujiki, et al (67), filled the abdominal cavity of beagles with crushed ice. Once esophageal temperature had reached 30°C, left heart bypass was initiated to complete the cooling process. Eleven of 18 animals had normal recoveries. The authors concluded that the abdominal cooling was useful for protecting the abdominal organs, but additional protection is needed for the heart and lungs.

OVERVIEW

Table 14-1 shows an overview of different cooling techniques and discusses the pros and cons. External cooling techniques like a cooling cap are easy to handle, however, their cooling capacity is low compared to methods using the arterial blood supply of the brain for cooling. Another disadvantage is the lack of homogeneity of the temperature in the brain. However, in some species the vertebral arteries could be occluded to create a more homogeneous temperature field in the brain, while using the carotid arteries for brain cooling, though this is not clinically relevant. Heat exchangers acting on the blood are invasive and often need major surgical interventions. This may often be unwelcomed. The nasopharyngeal cooling may work well as it generates a homogeneous temperature field in brains of animals with a complete, or only partially degenerated, carotid rete. However, in animals and humans without a rete, the cooling effect is very small and affects only the surface of the larger brain (37, 68, 69). Selective brain cooling in humans has been discussed in a very controversial manner (68, 70, 71), but some points are clear: the human brain is very large in comparison to animals and there is no rete system in humans. These facts decrease the probabilities of natural selective brain cooling, but selective cooling of the brain via the nasopharynx should be explored in man.

Peritoneal cooling deserves further study. This may be more invasive than some other techniques. Since diagnostic peritoneal lavage has been used for trauma victims to rule out hemoperitoneum for years, the feasibility has been established.

The use of natural blood circulation for body and/or brain cooling results in a high cooling efficiency and a homogeneous temperature field. Extracorporeal carotid heat exchangers acting on the arterial blood allow the independent control of brain and core temperatures at a predetermined level. Intravascular venous heat exchangers acting on the venous blood allow cooling and control of core temperature with minimal surgical interventions only. Intravascular catheters for maintenance of normothermia or mild cooling are already available.

All in all, there is no ideal cooling method. The aim (systemic vs. selective cooling) and the general clinical conditions determine which method of cooling is the proper one.

Table 14-1. Overview of cooling methods

Method	Cooling efficiency	Brain temperature	Core temperature	Practical use
External conduction: cooling cap	Low	Major temperature gradient	Minimally effective	Easy to use, Non-invasive
External conduction: nasopharyngeal cooling	Low	Variable homogeneity	Minimally effective	Easy to use, minimally invasive
Intravenous Cooling	Medium	Homogeneous	Effective control	Minimally invasive
Intravascular cooling acting on the venous blood	Medium to high	Homogeneous	Efficiency depends on flow rate and heat exchange area	Minimally invasive
Venovenous Cooling	High	Homogeneous	Effective control	Minimally invasive
Extracorporeal heat exchangers acting on arterial blood	High	Homogeneous	Effective control	Invasive Needs major surgical intervention

REFERENCES

1. Tooley JR, Satas S, Porter H, et al. Head cooling with mild systemic hypothermia in anesthetized piglets is neuroprotective. *Ann Neurol* 2003; 53:65-72.

2. Iwata O, Iwata S, Tamura M, et al. Brain temperature in newborn piglets under selective head cooling with minimal systemic hypothermia. *Pediatr Int* 2003; 45:163-168.

3. Thoresen M, Simmonds M, Satas S, et al. Effective selective head cooling during posthypoxic hypothermia in newborn piglets. *Pediatr Res* 2001; 49:594-599.

4. Gelman B, Schleien CL, Lohe A, Kuluz JW. Selective brain cooling in infant piglets after cardiac arrest and resuscitation. *Crit Care Med* 1996; 24:1009-1017.

5. Horn M, Schlote W, Henrich HA. Global cerebral ischemia and subsequent selective hypothermia. A neuropathological and morphometrical study on ischemic neuronal damage in cat. *Acta Neuropathol* 1991; 81:443-449.

6. Kuluz JW, Gregory GA, Yu AC, Chang Y. Selective brain cooling during and after prolonged global ischemia reduces cortical damage in rats. *Stroke* 1992; 23:1792-1796.

7. Dennis BH, Eberhart RC, Dulikravich GS, Radons SW. Finite-element simulation of cooling of realistic 3-D human head and neck. *J Biomech Eng* 2003; 125:832-40.

8. Diao C, Zhu L, Wang H. Cooling and rewarming for brain ischemia or injury: theoretical analysis. *Ann Biomed Eng* 2003; 31:346-53.

9. Ku YT, Montgomery LD, Webbon BW. Hemodynamic and thermal responses to head and neck cooling in men and women. *Am J Physic Med Rehab* 1996; 75:443-50.

10. Wang H, Olivero W, Lanzino G, et al. Rapid and selective cerebral hypothermia achieved using a cooling helmet. *J Neurosurg* 2004; 100:272-7.

11. Mellergard P. Changes in human intracerebral temperature in response to different methods of brain cooling. *Neurosurg* 1992; 31:671-7.

12. The Hypothermia after Cardiac Arrest Study Group. Mild therapeutic hypothermia to improve the neurologic outcome after cardiac arrest. *N Engl J Med* 2002; 346:549-556.

13. Bernard SA, Gray TW, Buist MD, et al. Treatment of comatose survivors of out-of-hospital cardiac arrest with induced hypothermia. *N Engl J Med* 2002; 346:557-563.

14. Bernard S, Buist M, Monteiro O, Smith K. Induced hypothermia using large volume, ice-cold intravenous fluid in comatose survivors of out-of-hospital cardiac arrest: a preliminary report. *Resuscitation* 2003; 56:9-13.

15. Schmutzhard E, Engelhardt K, Beer R, et al. Safety and efficacy of a novel intravascular cooling device to control body temperature in neurologic intensive care patients: A prospective pilot study. *Crit Care Med* 30: 2481-2488, 2002.

16. Doufas AG, Akca O, Barry A, et al. Initial experience with a novel heat-exchanger catheter in neurosurgical patients. *Anesth Analg* 2002; 95:1752-1756.

17. Jessen C. Independent clamps of peripheral and central temperatures and their effects on heat production in the goat. *J Physiol (Lond)* 1981; 311:11-22.

18. Jessen C, Mercer JB, Puschmann S. Intravascular heat exchanger for conscious goats. *Pfluegers Arch* 1977; 368:263-265.

19. Bergland H-P Mercer JB. The effect of rate of cooling, time of the day and light regime on the shivering response in rabbits. *Acta Physiol Scand* 1992; 145:413-421.

20. Behringer W, Safar P, Wu X, et al. Veno-venous extracorporeal blood shunt cooling to induce mild hypothermia in dog experiments and review of cooling methods. Resuscitation 2002; 54:89-98.

21. Nozari A, Safar P, Stezoski SW, et al. Mild hypothermia during prolonged cardiopulmonary cerebral resuscitation increases conscious survival in dogs. *Crit Care Med* 2004; 32:2110-2116.

22. Jessen C, Feistkorn G. Some characteristics of core temperature signals in conscious goats. *Am J Physiol* 1984; 247:R456-R464.
23. Jessen C, Felde D, Volk P, Kuhnen G. Effects of spinal cord temperature on the generation and transmission of temperature signals in the goat. *Pfluegers Arch* 1990; 416:428-433.
24. Kuhnen G, Jessen C. Thermal signals in control of selective brain cooling. *Am J Physiol* 1994;267:R355-R359.
25. Kuhnen G, Bauer R, Walter B. Controlled brain hypothermia by extracorporeal carotid blood cooling at normothermic trunk temperatures in pigs. *J Neurosci Methods* 1999; 89:167-174.
26. Walter B, Bauer R, Kuhnen G, et al. Coupling of cerebral blood flow and oxygen metabolism in infant pigs during selective brain hypothermia. *J Cereb Blood Flow Metab* 2000; 20:1215-1224.
27. Kuhnen G, Jessen C. Threshold and slope of selective brain cooling. *Pfluegers Arch* 1991; 418:176-183.
28. Schubert A. Side effects of mild hypothermia. *J Neurosurg Anesthesiol* 1995; 7:139-147.
29. Taylor CA. Surgical hypothermia, in Schönbaum E, Lomax P (eds): *Thermoregulation: Pathology, pharmacology, and therapy*. New York, Pergamon Press, 1991, pp 363-396.
30. Clifton GL, Allen S, Berry J, Koch SM. Systemic hypothermia in treatment of brain injury. *J Neurotrauma* 1992; 9:S487-S495.
31. Frank SM, Fleisher LA, Breslow MJ, et al. Perioperative maintenance of normothermia reduces the incidence of morbid cardiac events: A randomized clinical trial. *JAMA* 1997; 277:1127-1134.
32. Kurz A, Sessler DI, Lenhardt RA. Study of wound infections and temperature group: Perioperative normothermic to reduce the incidence of surgical-wound infection and shorten hospitalization. *N Engl J Med* 1996; 334:1209-1215.
33. Ohta T, Kuroiwa T, Sakaguchi I, et al. Selective hypothermic perfusion of canine brain. *Neurosurgery* 1996; 38:1211-1215.
34. Schwartz AE, Stone JG, Finck AD, et al. Isolated cerebral hypothermia by single carotid perfusion of extracorporeally cooled blood in baboons. *Neurosurgery* 1996; 39:577-581.
35. White RJ, Locke GE, Albin MS. Isolated profound cerebral cooling with a bi-carotid heat exchanger shunt in dogs. *Resuscitation* 1983; 10:193-195.
36. Kuhnen G, Jessen C. Effects of selective brain cooling on mechanisms of respiratory heat loss. *Pfluegers Arch* 1992; 421:204-208.
37. Langer T, Nielsen B, Jessen C. Non-thermometric means of assessing changes of brainstem temperature: The question of selective brain cooling in humans, in Milton AS (ed): *Temperature regulation. Recent physiological and pharmacogical advances*. Basel, Birkhaeuser Verlag, 1994, pp 145-149.
38. Schmidt-Nielsen K. Counter current systems in animals. *Sci Am* 1981; 244:118-128.
39. Waites GMH, Setchell BP. Physiology of the mammalian testis. In: Lamming GE, ed. *Marshall's Physiology of Reproduction*. Edinburgh, London & New York: Churchill Livingstone, 4th Edn, Vol. 2, Ch. 1, 1998:1-105.
40. Glad Sørensen H, Lambrechtsen J, Einer-Jensen N. Efficiency of the counter current transfer of heat and 133xenon between the pampiniform plexus and testicular artery of the bull under in vitro conditions. *Int J Androl* 1991; 14:232-40.
41. Einer-Jensen N, Waites GWH. Testicular blood flow and a study of the testicular venous to arterial transfer of radioactive krypton and testosterone in the rhesus monkey. *J Physiol* 1977; 267:1-15.
42. Grinsted J, Blendstrup K, Andreasen MP, Byskov AG. Temperature measurements of rabbit antral follicles. *J Reprod Fert* 1980; 60:149–155.

43. Hunter RHF, Bøgh IB, Einer-Jensen N, et al. Pre- ovulatory graafian follocles are cooler than neighbouring stroma. *Hum Reprod* 2000; 15:273-83.

44. Luck MR, Griffiths S, Gregson K, et al. Follicular fluid responds endothermically to aqueous dilution. *Hum Reprod* 2001; 16:2508-2514.

45. Gillet JY, Koritké JG, Muller P, Juliens C. Sur la microvascularisation de l'ovaire chez la lapine. *CR Soc Biol* 1968; 162:762-766.

46. Einer-Jensen N. Counter current exchange in the ovarian pedicle and its physiological implications. *Oxford Reviews of Reprod Biol* 1988; 10:348-381.

47. Einer-Jensen N, Hunter RHF. Physiological and pharmacological aspects of local transfer of substances in the ovarian adnexa in woman. *Hum Reprod Update* 2000; 6:132-138.

48. Einer-Jensen N, Cicinelli E, Galantino P, et al. Preferential vascular-based transfer from vagina to the corpus but not to the tubal part of uterus in postmenopausal women. *Hum Reprod* 2001; 16:1329-1333.

49. Einer-Jensen N, Cicinelli E, Galantino P, et al. Uterine first pass effect in postmenopausal women. *Hum Reprod* 2002 ; 17(12):3060-3064.

50. Cicinelli E, Cignarelli M, Sabatelli S, et al. Plasma concentrations of progesterone are higher in the uterine artery than in the radial artery after vaginal administration of micronized progesterone in an oil-based solution to postmenopausal women. *Fertil Steril* 1998; 69(3):471-473.

51. Cicinelli E, Einer-Jensen N, Galantino P, et al. Model of counter current transfer from vagina to urethra in postmenopausal women. *Hum Reprod* 2001; 16:2496-2500.

52. Jessen C. Brain Cooling: An economy mode of temperature regulation in Artiodactyls. *News Physiol Sc* 1998; 13:281-286.

53. Rhoton AL, Harris FS, Fujii K. Anatomy of the cavernous sinus. In: Kapp JP, Schmidek HH, ed. *The cerebral vascular system and its disorders*. Orlando, Fla: Grune and Stratton, 1984; (?):61-91.

54. Skipor J, Grzegorzewski W, Krzymowski T, Einer-Jensen N. Local transfer of testosterone from the nasal mucosa to the carotid blood and the brain in the pig. *Pol J Vet Sci* 2000; 3:19-22.

55. Einer-Jensen N, Larsen L. Transfer of tritiated water, tyrosine, and propanol from the nasal cavities to the brain arterial blood in rats. *Exp Brain Res* 2000b; 130:216-220.

56. Cabanac M. Selective brain cooling in humans: "fancy" or fact? *FASEB* 1993; J7:1143-1147.

57. Brengelmann GL. Specialized brain cooling in humans? *FASEB* 1993; J7:1148-1153.

58. Harris BA, Andrews PJD: The rational for human selective cooling. In: Vincent J, ed. *Yearbook of Intensive Care and Emergenc*. Berlin: Springer Verlag, 2002;1:738-747.

59. Mellergård P, Nordström C-H. Epidural temperature and possible intracerebral temperature gradients in man. *British J Neurosurg* 1990; 4:31-38.

60. Mariak Z, Bondyra Z, Piekarska M. The temperature within the circle of Willis versus tympanic temperature in resting normothermic humans. *Eur J Appl Physiol* 1993; 66:518-520.

61. Caputa M, Perrin G, Cabanac M. Reversal of human ophthalmic vein blood flow: selective cooling of the brain. *Acad Sci Hebd Seances Acad Sci D* 1978; 287:1011-1014.

62. Einer-Jensen N, Khorooshi MH, Petersen MB, Svendsen P. Rapid cooling in intubated pigs through nasal flushing with oxygen: Prevention of brain hypothermia. *Acta Vet Scand* 42:459-464, 2001. *Acta Veterinaria* 2001; 42:461-466

63. Einer-Jensen N, Khorooshi MH. Cooling of the brain through oxygen flushing of the nasal cavities in intubated rats: An alternative model for treatment of brain injury. *Exp Brain Res* 2000; 130:244-247.

64. Einer-Jensen N, Baptiste KE, Madsen F, Khoroshi MH. Can intubation harm the brain in critical care situations? (A new simple technique may provide a method for controlling brain temperature). *Medical Hypotheses* 2002; 58:229-231.

65. Horowitz BZ. The golden hour in heat stroke: Use of iced peritoneal lavage. *Am J Emerg Med* 1989; 7:616-619.

66. Xiao F, Safar P, Alexander H. Peritoneal cooling for mild cerebral hypothermia after cardiac arrest in dogs. *Resuscitation* 1995; 30:51-59.

67. Fujiki M, Misumi K, Sakamoto II, Kanemoto I. Circulatory arrest under hypothermic anesthesia using abdominal cavity cooling. *J Veterinary Med Sci* 1998; 60:1237-1242.

68. Jessen C, Kuhnen G. Selective brain cooling in mammals: general and regional modes of operation, in Kosaka M, Sugahara T, Schmidt KL, Simon E (eds): Thermotherapy for neoplasia, inflammation, and pain. Tokyo, Springer-Verlag, 2001, pp 207-214.

69. Jessen C, Kuhnen G. No evidence for brain stem cooling during face fanning in humans. *J Appl Physiol* 1992; 72:664-669.

70. Brengelmann GL. Specialized brain cooling in humans? *FASEB J* 7:1148-1152, 1993.

71. Cabanac M. Keeping a cool head. *NIPS* 1986; 1:41-44.

Chapter 15

DETRIMENTAL EFFECTS OF HYPOTHERMIA

Ram Nirula, MD, MPH[1], Larry M. Gentilello, MD[2]
[1]*Medical College of Wisconsin, Milwaukee, WI, USA*
[2]*University of Texas Southwestern Medical School, Dallas, TX, USA*

INTRODUCTION

Hypothermia in humans is defined as a core temperature below 35°C. Primary accidental hypothermia occurs as a result of overwhelming cold stress, such as cold water immersion or exposure. Secondary accidental hypothermia is a result of alterations in thermoregulation and heat production. Secondary hypothermia occurs more frequently, and injuries are the common etiologic factor. Mild hypothermia frequently occurs in the operating room. This chapter will review the organ-specific effects of hypothermia and potentially detrimental effects of hypothermia on trauma and postoperative patients.

DETRIMENTAL EFFECTS OF HYPOTHERMIA

Cardiovascular

Hypothermia leads to a progressive decrease in cardiac output and, subsequently, a decrease in blood pressure. Osborn ("J") waves and atrial flutter/fibrillation can be seen below 32°C. Below 30°C, bradycardia and ventricular dysrhythmias are common; asystole occurs at around 24-28°C.

In addition to the hemodynamic changes, hypothermia causes a leftward shift in the oxyhemoglobin dissociation curve, increasing the affinity of hemoglobin for oxygen. Despite initial conservation of the balance between oxygen supply and demand, the overall net result is cellular dysfunction due to depletion of adenosine triphosphate stores, and lactic acidosis (1).

Hypothermia can also elicit a significant catecholamine response. In human volunteers (2), a 0.7°C decrease in core temperature resulted in a 4-fold increase in circulating concentrations of norepinephrine; a 1.2°C decrease in temperature resulted in a 7-fold increase in norepinephrine. This adrenergic response was associated with systemic vasoconstriction and increased blood pressure.

Shivering may also contribute to hypothermia-induced cardiovascular complications because of increased metabolic demands. Frank, et al, found that shivering was associated with a significant increase in myocardial ischemia (36%), angina (18%), and a reduction in PaO_2 in elderly patients undergoing elective vascular surgery (3). They also demonstrated that shivering is associated with a 40% average increase in metabolic rate in elderly patients (4)

Renal , Gastrointestinal, and Metabolic

Renal tubular dysfunction may result in "cold diuresis" when core temperature approaches 30°C. Intense peripheral vasoconstriction may increase central venous pressure and increase urine output despite the presence of hypovolemia. Hypovolemia may be further aggravated by third-spacing of fluids. In addition, the release of anti-diuretic hormone (ADH) and ADH receptor responsivity are decreased by hypothermia. The resultant hypovolemia can contribute to "rewarming shock".

Hypothermia has been associated with gastric erosions, ileus, bowel wall edema, decreased hepatic drug detoxification, hyperamylasemia, and, rarely, hemorrhagic pancreatitis. These findings are generally attributed to splanchnic vasoconstriction, which, when combined with the peripheral vasoconstriction, often results in anaerobic metabolism and metabolic acidosis.

Hypothermia suppresses insulin release and blocks insulin receptor sites often producing hyperglycemia; exogenous insulin administration is unwarranted, as "rebound hypoglycemia" may occur during rewarming.

Acidosis is present in approximately one third of the patients due to respiratory depression, lactic acid generation, and/or hepatic metabolism depression. Shivering, as well as blood loss or under-resuscitation of the trauma victim, may greatly aggravate lactic acidosis.

Hematology and Coagulation

Exposure hypothermia often causes an increase in hematocrit due to plasma losses through leaky capillaries. A leukocytosis or leukopenia can also occur.

The control of hemorrhage in hypothermic patients with associated platelet and clotting factor depletion is often impossible (5, 6). The extent to which hypothermia intensifies coagulopathic bleeding is underestimated clinically because tests such as the prothrombin time (PT), partial thromboplastin time (PTT), and thrombin time (TT) are temperature standardized to 37°C by all hospital clinical laboratories.

To quantify the effect of hypothermia upon clotting, Reed, et al (7), used a fibrometer that was modified to conduct coagulation assays at 35°C, 33°C and 31°C using human plasma with normal clotting factor levels. They compared the results with those obtained from Factor IX depleted plasma assayed at 37°C. The PTT of the normal plasma was prolonged to the same extent as occurred when Factor IX levels were depleted to 39%, 16% and 2.5% of normal, respectively (7, 8). These results are further supported by a prospective examination of 112 patients with an Injury Severity Score (ISS) >9 that revealed a significant reduction in clotting enzyme activity at a temperature ≤34°C (9).

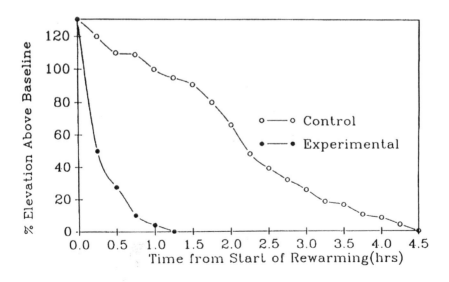

Figure 15-1. Effect of continuous arteriovenous rewarming (CAVR) (solid dots) vs. external rewarming on Ivy bleeding time. Bleeding time is reduced to baseline more than 3 h faster in the CAVR group.

Hypothermia also reduces platelet numbers and function. The amount of blood loss in patients with coagulopathic bleeding most closely correlates with the bleeding time (Duke or Ivy method), which is primarily a measure of platelet function (10, 11). Valeri induced systemic hypothermia to $32°C$ in baboons, but kept one forearm warm using heating lamps and a warm blanket (12). Simultaneous bleeding time measurements in the warm arm and cold arm were 2.4 and 5.8 minutes, respectively. Thus, cold-mediated platelet dysfunction may result in coagulopathic bleeding despite a normal platelet count.

In the trauma patient, a dilutional coagulopathy often coexists with hypothermia. Low concentrations of platelets and coagulation enzymes, plus the additional effect of hypothermia-mediated alterations in kinetic activity, may make attempts at achieving hemostasis futile. In such cases, platelet and clotting factor repletion without rewarming may not adequately restore clotting mechanisms (13). Restoration of normal clotting and bleeding times can be achieved with rapid rewarming methods (Figures 15-1 and 15-2).

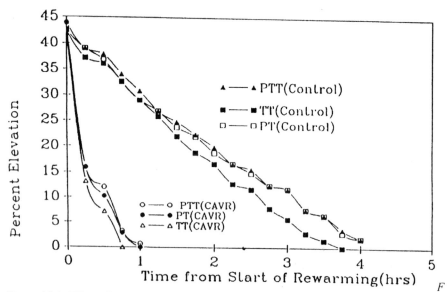

Figure 15-2. Effect of continuous arteriovenous rewarming (CAVR) vs. external rewarming on prothrombin time (PT), activated partial thromboplastin time (aPTT), and thrombin time (TT). All tests were performed at the core temperature of the subject. All coagulation tests normalized as much as 3 h faster with CAVR.

Infection

Hypothermia may lead to a decrease in white blood cell counts. More importantly, neutrophil and macrophage function may be inhibited. With prolonged hypothermia, the risk of infection increases dramatically (14).

HYPOTHERMIA IN TRAUMA PATIENTS

Some degree of hypothermia is reported to occur in nearly half of major trauma victims, with 10-15% of cases being severe (15-17). Gregory and colleagues reported that 57% of trauma patients became hypothermic at some time during their admission, with heat loss being most severe in the emergency department (16). In a report from Seattle, the average initial temperature for 94 intubated major trauma victims was 35°C, with 24% having a body temperature of 34°C or less (15). Another study noted that 42% of adult trauma victims with an ISS ≥25 developed a core temperature below 34°C; 23% were below 33°C and 13% were below 32°C (18). However, the incidence of hypothermia appears to be decreasing in recent years as a result of increased attention to heat conservation measures during resuscitation and, in particular, avoidance of the infusion of cold blood products and room temperature crystalloid solutions.

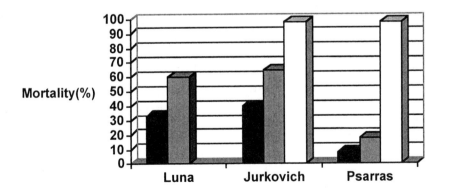

Figure 15-2. Three separate studies demonstrate a stepwise increase in mortality as body temperature decreases.

There is a difference in the risk of mortality associated with different types of hypothermia. In a multi-center study of 401 cases of primary hypothermia the mortality rate was only 21% when core temperature was below 32°C (19). Nearly every death was a result of underlying co-morbidity, not the hypothermia. In contrast, a core temperature reduction to only 35°C is associated with an increase in mortality in an injured patient, and a temperature of 32°C or less is almost always lethal. (Figure 15-3) (15, 18, 20).

Several theories as to the etiology of hypothermia in the injured patient have been proposed. One hypothesis is that shock causes hypothermia as a compensatory response (21-24). Shivering is inhibited by hypotension or hypoxemia (23, 25). This decrease in the shivering set-point is equivalent to a decrease in the temperature, which the body accepts as being normal during shock. In one study, shivering was noted to occur in only one of 82 severely injured hypothermic trauma patients (25). It may be that down-regulation of body temperature is a teleologic mechanism designed to gain a protective effect of hypothermia during shock (26, 27).

An alternative hypothesis is that the physiologic derangements that occur in the trauma patient contribute to the development of pathologic hypothermia. Shock is defined as a decrease in oxygen transport to tissues to the point where the normal rate of oxygen consumption (combustion) can no longer be maintained, and anaerobic metabolism occurs. Thus, by definition, shock always causes a pathologic decrease in oxygen consumption, and therefore, a decrease in heat production. The contribution of pathologic reductions in oxygen consumption to the presence of hypothermia may explain the strong correlation between body temperature and the magnitude of shock. This is also consistent with the frequent clinical observation that patients who are well resuscitated generally experience a relatively rapid return to normal core temperature. The frequent presence of lactic acid accumulation in cold, seriously injured patients supports the theory that hypothermia is a form of metabolic failure, rather than a compensatory survival mechanism.

Other factors that contribute to development of hypothermia in trauma patients include exposure, opening body cavities, and administration of sedatives, analgesics, and anesthetics, which decrease the patient's response to hypothermia. In addition, alcohol or drug ingestion by the patient prior to injury may play a role.

Effect on Trauma Outcomes

The degree of hypothermia in trauma patients is proportional to injury severity. Therefore, it has been difficult to determine if the increased mortality associated with hypothermia is a result of the severity of injury or the hypothermia itself. Hypothermia was associated with an adverse outcome in a review that focused on lowest recorded core temperature, stratified by ISS, blood and fluid requirements, and the presence or absence of shock (Table 1) (18). Patients who became hypothermic had significantly higher mortality rates than similarly injured patients who remained warm. Mortality was 100% if core body temperature dropped to 32°C, even in mildly injured patients.

Steinemann, et al (17), attempted to account for the confounding factors by stratifying patients using a combination of anatomic and physiologic factors (TRISS methodology). In this study, hypothermic patients did not have higher mortality rates when severity of injury was controlled. It may not be appropriate to stratify hypothermic patients with a physiologic index of injury severity because hypothermia itself adversely affects physiology, which would make patients with more minor injuries appear to be more severely injured. This would result in inappropriate comparisons between warm and cold groups. In this same study, when patients were stratified using the ISS, a strictly anatomic index of injury severity, hypothermic patients had significantly higher mortality rates than patients with the same ISS who remained warm. Overall, in this study, hypothermic patients had a mortality rate of 63%, while none of the euthermic patients died.

There are limitations to the use of retrospective data to form conclusions about the effects of hypothermia that occurs in trauma patients. A reduction in body temperature naturally occurs during the process of dying, and hypothermia may simply identify patients who are succumbing to their injuries. Only prospective studies using treatment of hypothermia as an independent variable can answer this question.

In one prospective study, a group of hypothermic trauma patients were treated with slow rewarming methods, and the mean duration of hypothermia was 3.2 hours (28, 29). In a second (non-randomized) group, an extracorporeal continuous arteriovenous rewarmer (CAVR) was used to treat hypothermia, which resolved within 39 minutes. The more aggressive therapy was associated with a significant decrease in fluid and blood product requirements, organ failures episodes, and length of ICU stay (Figure 15-4). Two additional prospective, but non-randomized studies have demonstrated the potential for improvements in outcome when protocols designed to minimize heat loss were utilized (30, 31).

The results of the first randomized, prospective trial to assess the effect of rapid rewarming from hypothermia on outcome from trauma were recently reported. Patients who were hypothermic on arrival to the intensive care unit after major injury were randomized to standard (slow) rewarming or to rapid rewarming using CAVR. Patients undergoing rapid rewarming required less fluid resuscitation to achieve the same resuscitation endpoints (32). At sixteen hours, 42% of the patients randomized to slow rewarming died, compared to 7% in the CAVR group. This trial was not designed to have sufficient statistical power to study overall mortality to hospital discharge, however, there was a six-fold increase in mortality during resuscitation in the group randomized to slow rewarming (p=0.05) .

The above body of literature suggests that the hypothermia in trauma victims is an independent predictor of mortality. The current Advanced Trauma Life Support recommendations for trauma management state that every effort should be made to prevent hypothermia from occurring in the trauma patient, and that aggressive efforts to restore normothermia should be undertaken. The detrimental effects of hypothermia extend to metabolic derangements and hypocoagulability that are associated with an increase in mortality in trauma patients. Evidence demonstrates that rapid temperature homeostasis leads to an improvement in these derangements, and decreases the risk of mortality during resuscitation.

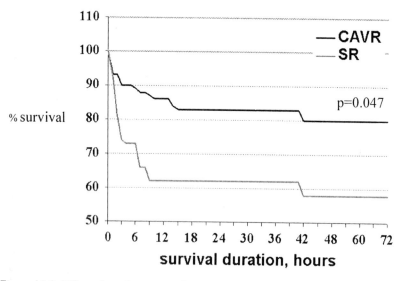

Figure 15-3. Effect of continuous arteriovenous rewarming (CAVR) vs. standard rewarming (SR) on mortality in a randomized trial of hypothermia trauma patients. CAVR decreased early mortality.

HYPOTHERMIA AND BRAIN INJURY

The effects of hypothermia upon cerebral metabolism have been extensively examined in animal models. Cerebral blood flow declines in parallel with cerebral oxygen and glucose metabolism, suggesting that the balance between oxygen supply and demand is maintained until hypothermia is severe ($< 26°C$) (33-36).

The use of hypothermia to reduce metabolic demands during periods of oxygen supply limitation and successful use of induced hypothermia in animal studies have prompted the use of induced hypothermia in clinical studies of brain injured patients. Despite initial enthusiasm, these studies have failed to show a consistent improvement in neurologic outcome, and have been associated with an increased risk of pneumonia and other septic complications (37-41).

The first of these efforts consisted of a randomized clinical trial of induced hypothermia in brain injured patients (40). Patients were excluded if they had a history of hypotension or significant hypoxia; thus, the sample primarily consisted of stable patients with isolated brain injuries. After ICU admission 82 patients were randomized to surface cooling to a core temperature of 33°C for 24 h, or to standard therapy. Post hoc analysis revealed that a subset of patients with a Glasgow Coma Score of 5 to 7 had improved neurologic outcomes at six but not twelve-month follow-up. However, neurologic outcomes of patients with a Glasgow Coma Score of 5-7 in the normothermia group in that study had worse outcomes than are typically reported, with 80% having died, or being severely disabled or in a vegetative state. The outcome of the induced hypothermia group was similar to what has been reported in other studies where no novel therapies were used (42).

This trial was followed by a National Institutes of Health-sponsored multi-center trial of patients with traumatic brain injury. The hypothermia patients were cooled to 33°C for 48 h. The trial was subsequently terminated early due to lack of efficacy. There were more complications in the hypothermia group, including prolonged hypotension with organ failure (p=0.01), prolonged bradycardia with hypotension (p=0.04) and more hospital days during which any complication was recorded (p=0.005) (38). There was also a trend towards worse outcomes with hypothermia in patients older than 45 years (p=0.08), and significantly more complications (p=0.002). Retrospective analysis of body temperature on admission showed that an admission temperature of 35.0°C or less had an adverse effect on outcome; however, temperatures above 35.0°C had no effect. This finding supports the relationship between hypothermia and mortality in critically injured patients.

One criticism of the multi-center study was that patients may have had such severe brain injury that any treatment modality would be doomed to failure (mean Glasgow Coma Score=5.6). However, a subsequent randomized trial of induced hypothermia in less severely injured patients also found no benefit (43). Furthermore, during the initial 2 weeks post-injury, the incidence of pneumonia, meningitis, leukocytopenia, thrombocytopenia, hypernatremia, hypokalemia, and hyperamylasemia were all significantly higher in the hypothermia group.

This same group sought to determine if core temperature reduction to 33°C was inadequate in the most severely injured patients. In patients with intracranial hypertension refractory to mild hypothermia (34°C), they induced moderate hypothermia 31°C) (44). There was no therapeutic benefit. As brain temperature was reduced from 34 to 31°C, the requirements for intravenous fluid and dopamine increased significantly. Despite these treatments, mean arterial blood pressure and heart rate decreased significantly, with a resultant increasing metabolic acidosis and a decrease in serum potassium concentration, white blood cell and platelet counts.

Attempts to detect a potential benefit of hypothermia in brain-injured patients continue to be disappointing. Additional studies are ongoing.

PERIOPERATIVE HYPOTHERMIA

Cardiac Morbidity

Hypothermia is common in the perioperative period due to open body cavities, cold room temperature, administration of cold or inadequately warmed fluids, and anesthetic induced impairment in thermoregulation. With standard management strategies, half of the patients undergoing major operative procedures develop hypothermia to a core temperature of <36°C; one third to <35°C (3). These levels of hypothermia can cause a sympathetic discharge and shivering, which can increase metabolic demands. The increased demands on a patient with coronary artery disease may lead to myocardial ischemia or infarction, particularly in the post-operative period, after the potentially protective effects of anesthetics have subsided.

Frank, et al (45), examined the effect of perioperative hypothermia on cardiac morbidity in a prospective, randomized trial of patients with known coronary disease or high risk of coronary disease undergoing major thoracic, abdominal, or vascular procedures. Patients were managed with standard rewarming techniques vs. supplemental warming with a forced air heating blanket during the operation and the early post-operative period. After the operation, core temperature was lower in the standard rewarming group (35.4±0.1°C) than in the supplemental warming group (36.7±0.1°C) (p<.001). The degree of vasocontriction, assessed by the forearm to fingertip skin-surface temperature gradient, was greater in the hypothermic patients. The incidence of perioperative cardiac events (cardiac arrest, myocardial infarction, or unstable angina/ischemia) was 1.4% in the normothermic group and 6.3% in the hypothermic group (p=.02). Hypothermia was an independent predictor of morbid cardiac events by multivariate analysis. Maintenance of normothermia resulted in a 55% reduction in risk. Postoperative ventricular tachycardia also occurred less frequently in the normothermic group than in the hypothermic group. The differences in events between groups were present in the post-operative, not intra-operative, period. This suggests either that anesthetics are protective or that intra-operative effects of hypothermia set the stage for subsequent cardiac events.

Infection

Hypothermia may cause intense vasoconstriction, which can decrease tissue oxygenation. This may be particularly detrimental in surgical wounds, in which the inflammatory response and collagen deposition are critical to normal healing without wound infections. Decreased tissue oxygen tension, can decrease neutrophil oxidative killing and decrease collagen deposition. In addition, hypothermia can directly impair immune function by decreasing neutrophil chemotaxis and phagocytosis, macrophage motility, and antibody production. Kurz, et al (46), explored the effect of hypothermia on wound infections in patients undergoing colorectal procedures. Patients were randomized to standard temperature management using a forced air blanket with ambient temperature (hypothermia) vs. more aggressive warming using a forced air blanket at 40°C (normothermia). Intraoperative temperature was 34.7±0.6°C in the hypothermia group and 36.6±0.5°C in the normothermia group (p<0.001). Surgical wound infections occurred in 18 of 96 patients in the hypothermia group and 6 of 104 in the normothermia group (p=0.009). In addition, in the hypothermia group, sutures were removed later and hospital length of stay was prolonged compared to the normothermia group.

SUMMARY

Hypothermia can cause multiple detrimental effects to individual organ systems and the organism as a whole. In patients with severe trauma, the presence of hypothermia is independently associated with worse outcomes. Similarly, in the perioperative period, hypothermia is associated with cardiac events and infections. The standard of care continues to include aggressive measures to prevent hypothermia and to reverse it if it occurs. As the use of therapeutic hypothermia is further explored in a variety of patient populations, the potential risks of hypothermia, particularly when prolonged, need to be considered.

REFERENCES

1. Hochachka PW. Defense strategies against hypoxia and hypothermia. *Science* 1986; 231(4735): 234-241.
2. Frank SM, Higgins MS, Fleisher LA, et al. Adrenergic, respiratory, and cardiovascular effects of core cooling in humans. *Am J Physiol* 1997; 272:R557-R562.
3. Frank SM, Beattie C, Christopherson R, et al. Unintentional hypothermia is associated with postoperative myocardial ischemia. *Anesthesiology* 1993; 78:468-476.
4. Frank SM, Fleisher LA, Olson KF, et al. Multivariate determinants of early postoperative oxygen consumption in elderly patients. Effects of shivering, body temperature, and gender. *Anesthesiology* 1995; 83:241-249.
5. Sharp KW, Locicero RJ. Abdominal packing for surgically uncontrollable hemorrhage. *Ann Surg* 1992; 215:467-474.
6. Burch JM, Ortiz VB, Richardson RJ, et al. Abbreviated laparotomy and planned reoperation for critically injured patients. *Ann Surg* 1992; 215:476-483.
7. Reed RL 2nd, Bracey AW Jr., Hudson JD, et al. Hypothermia and blood coagulation: dissociation between enzyme activity and clotting factor levels. *Circ Shock* 1990; 32:141-152.
8. Johnston TD, Chen Y, Reed RI. Relative sensitivity of the clotting cascade to hypothermia. *Surg Forum* 1989; 40:199.
9. Watts DD, Trask A, Soeken K, et al. Hypothermic coagulopathy in trauma: effect of varying levels of hypothermia on enzyme speed, platelet function, and fibrinolytic activity. *J Trauma* 1998; 44:846-854.
10. Harker LA, Malpass TW, Branson HE, et al. Mechanism of abnormal bleeding in patients undergoing cardiopulmonary bypass: acquired transient platelet dysfunction associated with selective alpha-granule release. *Blood* 1980; 56:824-834.
11. Czer LS, Bateman TM, Gray RJ, et al. Treatment of severe platelet dysfunction and hemorrhage after cardiopulmonary bypass: reduction in blood product usage with desmopressin. *J Am Coll Cardiol* 1987; 9:1139-1147.
12. Valeri CR, Feingold H, Cassidy G, et al. Hypothermia-induced reversible platelet dysfunction. *Ann Surg* 1987; 205:175-181.
13. Reed RL 2nd, Johnson TD, Hudson JD, Fischer RP. The disparity between hypothermic coagulopathy and clotting studies. *J Trauma* 1992; 33:465-470.
14. Dripps RD. *The physiology of induced hypothermia*. Washington, DC, National Academy of Sciences 1956;447.
15. Luna GK, Maier RV, Pavlin EG, et al. Incidence and effect of hypothermia in seriously injured patients. *J Trauma* 1987; 27:1014-1018.
16. Gregory JS, Flancbaum L, Townsend MD, et al. Incidence and timing of hypothermia in trauma patients undergoing operations. *J Trauma* 1991; 31:795-798.
17. Steinemann S, Shackford SR, Davis JW. Implications of admission hypothermia in trauma patients. *J Trauma* 1990; 30:200-202.
18. Jurkovich GJ, Greiser WB, Luterman A, Curreri PW. Hypothermia in trauma victims: an ominous predictor of survival. *J Trauma* 1987; 27:1019-1024.
19. Danzl DF, Pozos RS, Auerbach PS, et al.; Multicenter hypothermia survey. *Ann Emerg Med* 1987; 16:1042-1055.
20. Psarras P, Ivatury RR, Rohman M. Hypothermia in the trauma patient: Incidence and prognostic significance. Proceedings of the Eastern Association for the Surgery of Trauma 1988: Longboat Key, Fl.
21. Wood SC: Interactions between hypoxia and hypothermia. *Annu Rev Physiol* 1991: 53:71-85.

22. Little RA, Stoner HB. Body temperature after accidental injury. *Br J Surg* 1981; 68:221-224.

23. Stoner HB, Marshall HW. Studies on the mechanism of shock. Thermoregulation during limb ischaemia. *Br J Exp Pathol* 1971; 52:650-655.

24. Bastow MD, Rawlings J, Allison SP. Undernutrition, hypothermia, and injury in elderly women with fractured femur: an injury response to altered metabolism? *Lancet* 1983; 1(8317):143-146.

25. Stoner HB. Effect of injury on the responses to thermal stimulation of the hypothalamus. *J Appl Physiol* 1972; 33:665-671.

26. Best R, Syverud S, Nowak RM. Trauma and hypothermia. *Am J Emerg Med* 1985; 3:48-55.

27. Little RA: Heat production after injury. *Br Med Bull* 1985; 41:226-231.

28. Gentilello LM, Cortes V, Moujaes S, et al. Continuous arteriovenous rewarming: experimental results and thermodynamic model simulation of treatment for hypothermia. *J Trauma* 1990; 30:1436-1449.

29. Gentilello LM, Cobean RA, Offner PJ, et al. Continuous arteriovenous rewarming: rapid reversal of hypothermia in critically ill patients. *J Trauma* 1992; 32:316-325.

30. Satiani B, Fried SJ, Zeeb P, Falcone RE. Normothermic rapid volume replacement in vascular catastrophes using the Infuser 37. *Ann Vasc Surg* 1988; 2:37-42.

31. Satiani B, Fried SJ, Zeeb P, Falcone RE. Normothermic rapid volume replacement in traumatic hypovolemia. A prospective analysis using a new device. *Arch Surg* 1987; 122:1044-1047.

32. Gentilello LM, Jurkovich GJ, Stark MS, et al. Is hypothermia in the victim of major trauma protective or harmful? A randomized, prospective study. *Ann Surg* 1997; 226:439-447.

33. Watanabe T, Orita H, Kobayashi M, Washio M. Brain tissue pH, oxygen tension, and carbon dioxide tension in profoundly hypothermic cardiopulmonary bypass. Comparative study of circulatory arrest, nonpulsatile low-flow perfusion, and pulsatile low- flow perfusion. *J Thorac Cardiovasc Surg* 1989; 97:396-401.

34. Frietsch T, Krafft P, Piepgras A, et al. Relationship between local cerebral blood flow and metabolism during mild and moderate hypothermia in rats. *Anesthesiology* 2000; 92:754-763.

35. Krafft P, Frietsch T, Lenz C, et al. Mild and moderate hypothermia (alpha-stat) do not impair the coupling between local cerebral blood flow and metabolism in rats. *Stroke* 2000; 31:1393-1400.

36. Tanaka J, Shiki K, Asou T, et al. Cerebral autoregulation during deep hypothermic nonpulsatile cardiopulmonary bypass with selective cerebral perfusion in dogs. *J Thorac Cardiovasc Surg* 1988; 95:124-132.

37. Clifton GL, Allen S, Barrodale P, et al. A phase II study of moderate hypothermia in severe brain injury. *J Neurotrauma* 1993; 10:263-271.

38. Clifton GL, Miller ER, Choi SC, et al. Lack of effect of induction of hypothermia after acute brain injury. *N Engl J Med* 2001; 344:556-563.

39. Hayashi N, Hirayama T, Udagawa A, et al. Systemic management of cerebral edema based on a new concept in severe head injury patients. *Acta Neurochir Suppl* 1994; 60:541-543.

40. Marion DW, Penrod LE, Kelsey SF, et al. Treatment of traumatic brain injury with moderate hypothermia. *N Engl J Med* 1997; 336:540-546.

41. Jiang J, Zhu C. Mild to moderate hypothermia: the hope for improving outcome of severe head injured patients. *Chin J Traumatol* 2001; 4:6-7.

42. Rosner MJ, Rosner SD, Johnson AH. Cerebral perfusion pressure: management protocol and clinical results. *J Neurosurg* 1995; 83:949-962.

43. Shiozaki T, Hayakata T, Taneda M, et al. A multicenter prospective randomized controlled trial of the efficacy of mild hypothermia for severely head injured patients with low intracranial pressure. Mild Hypothermia Study Group in Japan. *J Neurosurg* 2001; 94:50-54.

44. Shiozaki T, Nakajima Y, Taneda M, et al. Efficacy of moderate hypothermia in patients with severe head injury and intracranial hypertension refractory to mild hypothermia. *J Neurosurg* 2003; 99:47-51.

45. Frank SM, Fleisher LA, Breslow MJ, et al. Perioperative maintenance of normothermia reduces the incidence of morbid cardiac events: a randomized clinical trial. *JAMA* 1997; 277:1127-1134.

46. Kurz A, Sessler DI, Lenhardt R. Perioperative normothermia to reduce the incidence of surgical-wound infection and shorten hospitalization. Study of Wound Infection and Temperature Group. *N Engl J Med* 1996; 334:1209-1215.

Chapter 16

FUTURE DIRECTIONS

Samuel A. Tisherman, MD[1], Fritz Sterz, MD[2], Wilhelm Behringer, MD[2], Patrick Kochanek, MD[1]

[1]Safar Center for Resuscitation Research, University of Pittsburgh, PA, USA
[2]Medical University of Vienna, Vienna, Austria

Hypothermia research has come a long way over the past 50 years. We have asked many questions about how hypothermia works and in which situations is it beneficial. From a mechanistic standpoint, our understanding of the effects of hypothermia, both beneficial and detrimental, are much more complex than just direct effects on oxygen metabolism, as was first thought.

Laboratory studies have demonstrated benefit of therapeutic hypothermia in cardiac arrest caused by ventricular fibrillation, asphyxiation, or exsanguination, as well as traumatic brain injury, stroke, hemorrhagic shock, myocardial infarction, hepatic failure, and even pulmonary failure with sepsis. Additional studies are needed to more clearly define the optimal timing of hypothermia in terms of induction and duration, and the optimal depth, which are likely to be different for each insult. As we move forward in translating these findings to clinical studies, there may be appropriate indications to perform studies, if not done already, in animals that are high on the phylogenetic scale to hopefully better predict what will happen in humans.

The pathophysiologic mechanisms behind the molecular, cellular, organ, and organism level changes that occur after the various disease states addressed in this book are quite complex. So far, however, there has been little research into multifaceted therapeutic interventions that include hypothermia. Better understanding of the biochemical and molecular mechanisms behind the effects of hypothermia should allow us to develop synergistic pharmacologic approaches that perhaps could complement or potentate the beneficial affects of hypothermia, as well as decrease the detrimental effects. It is naive to think, however, that therapies aimed at one pathway will have an overall beneficial affect with such complex disease processes in critically ill patients. It is not surprising that so many single drug clinical trials have failed to show benefit.

Hypothermia affects many pathways simultaneously, and thus may have more hope for benefit. The fact that two randomized controlled clinical trials demonstrated benefit of hypothermia in diverse groups of patients after cardiac arrest, even when induced relatively slowly, is encouraging, particularly since drug studies have been disappointing. This success should help the endeavors to proceed with clinical trials after other insults. By the same token, the overall negative results of the most recent trial of hypothermia after head injury should not discourage further studies in this area. We should learn lessons from this study regarding the potential for different outcomes with different subpopulations, the need for close attention to detail regarding protocolized patient care algorithms, and timing of hypothermia induction.

Even when positive studies are published, clinical research should not stop there. Additional studies are needed to improve the techniques for inducing hypothermia and to better define the optimal parameters, timing and depth. Ideally, we should develop key endpoints for resuscitation that help us decide when to cool, how deep, and when to rewarm. Patient selection should also be better defined.

Dissemination of research findings and development of clinical practice guidelines related to hypothermia become the next steps. It was impressive how quickly the American Heart Association and the International Liaison Committee on Resuscitation picked up on the studies showing benefit of hypothermia after cardiac arrest and published statements encouraging the use of hypothermia.

We've come a long way in laboratory and clinical research into the potential benefits of therapeutic hypothermia in a variety of situations. With this momentum, we should anticipate that hypothermia will be applied to even more disease states, perhaps ones that have not even been thought of yet. Rigorous research from the molecular level to the bedside needs to continue. Although hypothermia may not have the scientific appeal of the most recently described cytokine pathway, monoclonal antibody, or genetically engineered animal, funding agencies need to recognize the great potential for hypothermia to have impact upon complex disease states in acute care medicine. There is no doubt that hypothermia, when applied in the appropriate manner at the appropriate time, can help save lives.

INDEX